The Diabetes
Comfort Food Diet
C O O K B O O K

The Diabetes Comfort Food Diet COOKBOOK

200 **DELICIOUS DISHES**

TO HELP YOU LOSE WEIGHT AND BALANCE BLOOD SUGAR

LAURA CIPULLO, RD, CDE,
and the editors of **Prevention**

RODALE

Printed in the United States of America
Rodale Inc. makes every effort to use acid-free ∞, recycled paper ♻.

Photographs by Mitch Mandel/Rodale Images
Book design by Christina Gaugler

Library of Congress Cataloging-in-Publication Data is on file with the publisher.
ISBN 978–1–62336–141–9   direct hardcover
2   4   6   8   10   9   7   5   3   1   direct hardcover

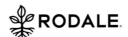

We inspire and enable people to improve their lives and the world around them.
For more of our products, visit rodalestore.com or call 800–848–4735.

To my family: Dennis, Gene, Richard, and Joan

CONTENTS

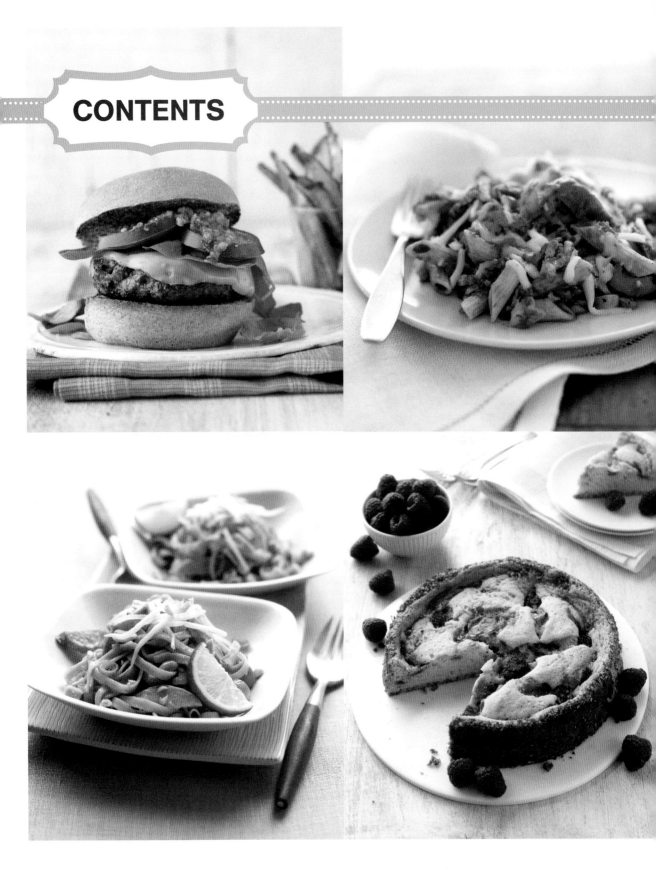

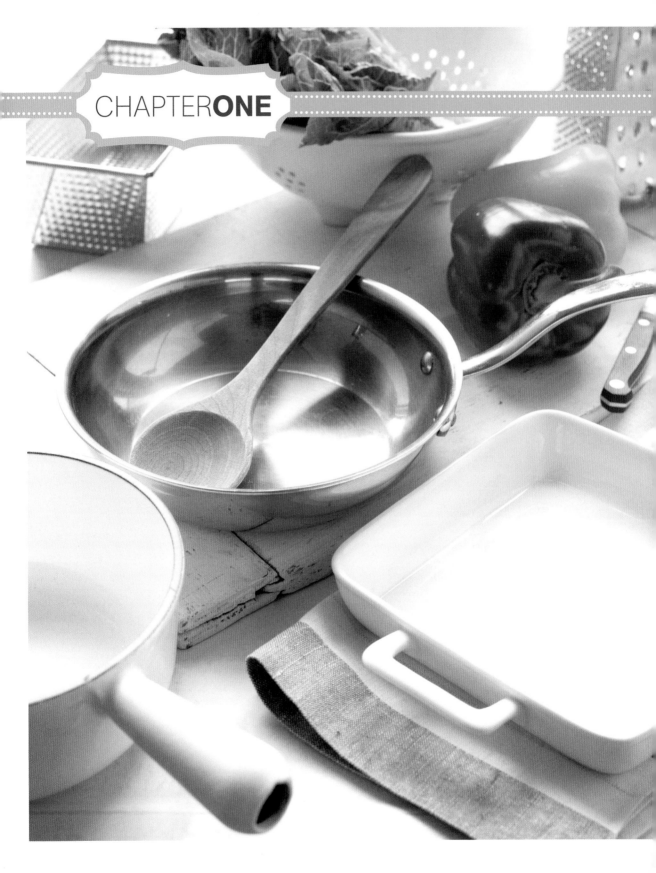

CHAPTER**ONE**

The Lowdown
on Diabetes

Like · many people, you might think your life is over if you receive a diagnosis of prediabetes or type 2 diabetes. Suddenly, meals and lifestyle choices that you didn't think twice about before must come under scrutiny, and needing to make changes can be scary. You can't help but panic. Your mind just shuts down. You close your ears to the doctor's advice and explanations about blood sugar and insulin. It all sounds like a pronouncement that life's pleasures for you are over . . . forever. "Now I must be on a diet for the rest of my life," you may find yourself thinking. "Restaurants, favorite foods, holiday feasts, and all social events will become tainted and nearly impossible to enjoy." Well, think again. This does not have to be your reality. There's no need to plan your own pity party!

Diabetes is definitely not a doomsday diagnosis. You can still eat—and yes, even some of your favorite foods, like hot, crusty bread or sweet, silky ice cream, can stay on the menu! Research clearly supports the fact that there really are no foods off-limits for individuals with prediabetes or diabetes. You *can* have it all—you just need to be smart about how you do it. That's where *The Diabetes Comfort Food Diet Cookbook* comes in. This cookbook is designed to give you the tools you need to manage or reverse insulin resistance while continuing to eat the foods you love. As a registered dietitian, I have directly witnessed this amazing nutrition plan in action with my clients. You'll read their stories over the next few chapters and be wowed by their results. Read on to learn how to transform your life, your diet, and your health. You can continue to love your food—and not fear what it will do to your blood sugar. Just implement the three simple steps to make over any meal so you can balance blood sugar, lose excess weight, and beat this disease. We'll talk about these three steps specifically in Chapter 2. First, though, let me help you understand a little more about diabetes and how to manage it.

Note: When discussing prediabetes or type 2 diabetes in this book, we will refer to the diagnosis simply as "diabetes." While the advice in this cookbook is aimed at those who have the ability to prevent or reverse insulin resistance, the recipes themselves can also benefit individuals with type 1 diabetes and even people who want to eat healthier to lose weight, improve their heart health, or just promote general good health and wellness.

THE EASY EATING SOLUTION THAT WORKS FOR LIFE

Please keep this important reality in mind: The main goal of diabetes management is to learn how to best and most effectively balance your blood sugar levels through food and physical activity. The Diabetes Comfort Food Diet is about living your life to the fullest by learning to eat in ways that are beneficial to your body—and especially understanding how different foods influence your blood sugar levels and endocrine system. And though this daily diet will likely result in weight loss, you must recognize that this is a lifetime methodology, not a fad plan.

You will see positive changes in just a few weeks, but you should not stop this diet when you feel you have reached your goals. Rather, it's a diet to learn thoroughly, implement totally, and follow diligently. You must make it your healthy nutrition habit for the rest of your life. The good news is that it is easy to learn and will help you look and feel great . . . and you'll still get to eat all the foods you enjoy! We'll show you how to make enjoyable foods work for you and ultimately help you beat diabetes.

Definition of *diet*:
1. Food and drink regularly provided or consumed, 2. Habitual nourishment[1]

Look up the definition of *diet* in Webster's Dictionary and you'll see the noun defined as "habitual nourishment." The Diabetes Comfort Food Diet focuses on this definition so that you, the reader, recognize this is a lifelong approach to nutrition and health. Stop thinking of a diet as restrictive and start thinking of it as providing the building blocks that nourish your body each day.

There's no reason to feel overwhelmed with despair when a doctor diagnoses you with prediabetes or diabetes! To immediately help dispel your fears, let's cover the basics of diabetes so that you better understand your body and why you need to fuel it in specific ways.

ALL ABOUT BLOOD SUGAR

When we talk about blood sugar, what we really mean is blood glucose. This is a measure of the sugar also known as glucose present in your blood at any given time. When you sit down to a meal, your body digests the food and breaks it down into three macronutrients known as carbohydrates, proteins, or fats. Carbohydrates, whether

THE LOWDOWN ON COMMON CARBOHYDRATES

Carbohydrates include many different sugars. Below are common carbs you may read about or see on a food label. Your body digests the simplest form of sugar, known as monosaccharides, the fastest and takes the longest to digest the more complex sugars known as polysaccharides. Be aware that the body may not digest or may only partially digest some carbs falling under the category of polysaccharides, including cellulose and inulin. Use caution when eating these carbs or increasing your consumption of them, as they are healthy but can cause gas!

Three Common Monosaccharides

Fructose: found in honey and fruits such as apples, peaches, and watermelon

Galactose: found in dairy products such as milk, yogurt, and ice cream

Glucose (also known as dextrose): found in a wide range of foods, such as fruits, sweet corn, and honey

Three Common Disaccharides

Sucrose (table sugar, from sugarcane) = glucose + fructose

Lactose (sugar found in milk) = glucose + galactose

Maltose (malt sugar found in germinating grains) = glucose + glucose

Three Common Polysaccharides

The indigestible: cellulose (found in broccoli, celery), pectin (apples, pears), and algal substances like seaweed. These polysaccharides are bulking agents that slow digestion.

The partially digestible: inulin (wheat, onions, and artichokes), raffinose (beans, cabbage, Brussels sprouts), and stachyose (beans and legumes). These polysaccharides are likely culprits of gas and bloating.

The digestible: starch and dextrin (grains and starchy vegetables) and glycogen (meat products and seafood—it's stored in muscle)

they are monosaccharides, disaccharides, or even some of the digestible polysaccharides, are further converted or broken down into the simple form of sugar known as glucose, which is then absorbed into your bloodstream. That glucose gets transported throughout your body for your muscles and organs to use as fuel. Most glucose is used immediately; however, excess glucose is converted to glycogen (which gets stored for use in your muscles and liver) or fatty acids (which are stored in your adipose tissue—a.k.a. your love handles and other visible body fat).

But how does the body know to use that glucose? The endocrine system is the body's active metabolic map that directs the "where, when, what, and how much" of hormones that help the body convert food into sugar and then energy. Insulin is one of the endocrine hormones produced by the pancreas. This organ releases insulin, which functions to open your cell doors and take up sugar from your blood. Sugar is mostly converted into energy when it enters the cells. This process helps you do everything from running a marathon to simply staying awake at your desk during that after-lunch slump. If this sugar gets locked out of your cells due to a malfunction with insulin, you are likely to feel shaky, sweaty, mentally foggy, and anxious. This means your blood sugar is likely very high. When this starts to happen, you probably have developed insulin resistance.

Insulin resistance is a condition in which the body does not use insulin properly. The muscle, fat, and liver cells do not respond appropriately to insulin; thus, the body thinks it needs more insulin to lower its blood sugar. The pancreas consequently goes into overdrive, pumping out more insulin. After years of being in overdrive, the pan-

SWEET**FACT**

Our brains use only the form of sugar known as glucose.

creas can eventually begin to burn out, resulting in prediabetes and diabetes. Insulin resistance is evident by both elevated blood sugar and elevated insulin levels.[2]

Prediabetes

As defined by the American Diabetes Association (ADA), prediabetes is diagnosed when a person's blood glucose levels are higher than normal (an A1C of 5.7 to 6.4 percent) but not high enough to qualify as type 2 diabetes (an A1C of 6.5 percent or higher). People who have prediabetes are more likely to develop type 2 diabetes in the future and may already have some problems stemming from the disease.

The good news is that you can take steps right now to reverse insulin resistance and prevent diabetes. Research shows that you can lower your risk of type 2 diabetes by 58 percent. The trick is to focus on one magic number: 7. By losing 7 percent of your current body weight, you can balance your blood sugars and get back to feeling great again. The Diabetes Comfort Food Diet can help—by eating healthy (we'll show you how!) and by exercising just 90 to 150 minutes per week. You will achieve these goals and consequently bring your blood sugar back to the normal range.[3] If you don't need to lose weight, well, don't worry. Our easy eating plan is flexible enough to decrease your blood sugar and help you live a healthier lifestyle.

KNOW YOUR BLOOD TESTS

Hemoglobin A1C (A1C): Hemoglobin A is another name for red blood cells. This test specifically measures how much glucose is attached to hemoglobin in your blood over the life of the cell—a 3- to-4-month period. This test is now used alone or in conjunction with a fasting plasma glucose test to diagnose prediabetes or diabetes. An A1C value of 5.7 to 6.4 percent is consistent with a diagnosis of prediabetes. If this value is 6.5 percent or greater, it is consistent with a diagnosis of diabetes.

Fasting Plasma Glucose (FPG): Commonly used to diagnose prediabetes, this blood test measures your blood sugar after you have fasted approximately 12 hours. If your blood sugar falls in the range of 100 to 125 mg/dl, you are considered to have an impaired fasting glucose and are diagnosed with prediabetes. If your FPG is 126 mg/dl or higher, your results indicate diabetes.

Oral Glucose Tolerance Test (OGTT): This test is also used to diagnose diabetes. You are given a beverage with 75 grams of a sugar solution to drink after fasting for 12 hours. Your blood glucose is then measured every hour, and a plasma glucose of 140 to 199 mg/dl on the second hour is considered an impaired glucose tolerance and diagnosed as prediabetes. If it is higher than 200 mg/dl at 2 hours postconsumption, you are diagnosed with diabetes.

Type 2 Diabetes

If your doctor diagnoses you with type 2 diabetes, this indicates that your body has difficulty with insulin. Either your pancreas is not able to produce enough insulin or, for some unknown reason, your body's cells are ignoring the hormone. If your body is unable to obtain sugar from your bloodstream and move it into your cells, your blood sugar levels rise and can cause complications such as heart disease, nerve damage, and kidney disease. As mentioned above, this diagnosis is made when your A1C is equal to or greater than 6.5 percent or your blood sugar measures greater than 126 mg/dl on a fasting plasma glucose test.

CALCULATE YOUR RISK

If you are worried about diabetes but haven't yet been tested for it, use the list above to determine your risk. The American Diabetes Association recommends you get tested for prediabetes and type 2 diabetes—even if you have no symptoms— if you are overweight or obese and have one or

SWEET**FACT**

Hyperglycemia, or high blood sugar, can be identified by excessive thirst, frequent urination, and unexplained weight loss.[4, 5]

more additional risk factors. For people without these risk factors, testing should begin at age 45 and be repeated a minimum of every 3 years if tests are normal.

Risk factors for prediabetes and diabetes—in addition to being overweight or obese or being age 45 or older—include the following:

- Being physically inactive
- Having a parent or sibling with diabetes
- Having a family background that is African American, Alaska Native, American Indian, Asian American, Hispanic/Latino, or Pacific Islander
- Giving birth to a baby weighing more than 9 pounds or being diagnosed with gestational diabetes (diabetes during pregnancy)
- Having high blood pressure—140/90 mmHg or above—or being treated for high blood pressure
- Having HDL ("good" cholesterol) below 35 mg/dl or a triglyceride level above 250 mg/dl
- Having polycystic ovary syndrome (PCOS)
- Having impaired fasting glucose (IFG) or impaired glucose tolerance (IGT) on previous testing
- Having other conditions associated with insulin resistance, such as severe obesity or a condition called acanthosis nigricans, which is characterized by a dark, velvety rash around the neck or armpits
- Having a personal history of cardiovascular disease[6]

SO YOU'VE BEEN DIAGNOSED . . . NOW WHAT?

When I first became a certified diabetes educator, I learned two profoundly valuable take-home messages that still lead the way for diabetes self-management and self–blood glucose monitoring. The first message: A carbohydrate is a carbohydrate is a carbohydrate. The second: Meet you, the client, where you are in terms of food and fitness—then empower you to make the lifestyle changes you need. The Diabetes Comfort Food Diet is an extension of these messages.

In October 2012, the most recent standards for professionals—the National Standards for Diabetes Self-Management Education and Support—were published in the journal *Diabetes Educator*. These standards are designed for both individuals with prediabetes and those with diabetes and are intended to help encourage daily healthy behavior changes, both physically and mentally. The Diabetes Comfort Food Diet will use these standards to

DIABETES: THE ASSOCIATED DISEASES

Elevated blood sugar can lead to a host of problems besides diabetes. By controlling your blood sugar, you help to minimize the prevalence or severity of damage from the following:

Heart disease	Nerve damage	Depression
Lipid abnormalities	Hypertension	Kidney disease

help you not only determine your starting point and progress through the next several weeks but also keep your eye on the prize—maintaining lifelong changes.[7]

Remember, this will be your diet routine for the rest of your life. As the educator, it is my job to help provide nutrition education and support so that you can successfully attain and sustain these self-care behaviors. Many dietitians, as do I, use a model called the Stages of Change to help clients identify where they are in terms of readiness to make nutrition changes. The Diabetes Comfort Food Diet has adapted these stages into a unique program, just for you! This plan is called START. First identify where you are using the chart below. Then begin moving through each stage at your own pace to ensure that this new way of eating will be most effective at helping you turn your health—and your life—around. Carefully read each stage's description and see which one you relate to most. For more information on START and specific advice for each stage of the program, flip to Chapter 3.

START

Read the descriptions of each stage to identify your current level of readiness.

SHOCK	You have just been diagnosed with prediabetes or diabetes. You may be in shock or denial. This is the time to raise your level of personal awareness. Perhaps you notice how awful you feel when you have high blood sugar. Think about your nutrition choices. Do you think you need to make any dietary changes? Identify education resources like this book as well as a support system to help you understand what prediabetes or diabetes means to you and your daily life. List pros and cons for making dietary and fitness changes.
TIPTOEING	You dabble with a few new choices but continue to have resistance and skepticism. You recognize the need to change your lifestyle for the purpose of preventing or beating diabetes. You read this book and are even willing to try new foods such as whole wheat bread and salmon or to take a walk for just 5 minutes to start decreasing your blood sugar. You focus on decreasing your list of cons from the previous phase by reducing these barriers. You are thinking about the need for lifestyle change. Temptations like eating out seem overwhelming and may prevent you from advancing to the next phase.
ACHIEVING	You are starting to do what you need to do. You reduce temptations and triggers such as eating out or ordering in by grocery shopping weekly, prepping meals in advance on weekends, or planning a healthy-themed dinner party. You get as much support as possible from family members, your personal dietitian, or this book. You are ready to start a fitness program and begin curbing your carbs. Notice how your sleep, mood, and energy level improve as you continue to make changes.
REPEATING	You are now a doer. You are implementing your new behaviors with the emphasis on the three tips to make over any meal (see Chapter 2). You are action oriented. This is one of the busiest stages as you incorporate the new behaviors encouraged in these chapters, such as food shopping, prepping, cooking, and the best part: eating! You are learning to curb carbs, increase fiber, and choose healthy fats. This is where you start to see results. The process doesn't seem like such a process anymore, because the pounds seem to be falling off you.
TIME	You have new, healthy self-care habits promoting balanced blood sugar. After 6 months, your nutrition changes are part of your daily routine, and you can foresee a bright, manageable future. Curbing carbs is a way of life, but so is going out to dinner every Friday night. Focus is on eating all foods in moderation so you can stick with these healthy behaviors. You know how to eat a piece of cake without risking a binge or high blood sugar. Life is literally sweet again.[8]

Not everyone will need to start at the Shock phase. It's okay to start this process at whichever stage represents your level of readiness. Your nutrition goals must be written specifically considering your present stage. We'll talk more about START and how to write nutrition goals in Chapter 3, but for now, just keep in mind that no matter where you start, you need to proceed in order through all remaining stages. For example, if you fit the description consistent with Tiptoeing, do not expect to skip to Repeating right away. Pace yourself! Reading this book may help you get from Tiptoeing to Achieving by realizing you can manage diabetes while still enjoying a serving of potatoes (truly—check out our recipe for Creamy Mashed Potatoes on page 283). The Achieving phase may consist of food shopping for one recipe from this book or reading nutrition labels for grams of carbohydrates. This is the time to plan for any possible triggers that may cause old behaviors (such as eating two large bowls of pasta). Repeating could be regularly preparing recipes from this cookbook and finally seeing results (such as pants fitting loosely around your smaller waist).

How Do We Know This Works?

By using the recipes and other tools in *The Diabetes Comfort Food Diet Cookbook,* you really will achieve better blood sugar control and lose weight. We have the evidence right here! Now that you know just where you fall on the START chart, start thinking about how to get to the next stage. Remember, you cannot skip a stage. Just know that you really can use this process—and the recipes and other tools in this cookbook—to achieve better blood glucose control and lose weight.

In 2002, the results of a major research study called the Diabetes Prevention Program (DPP) were published in the *New England Journal of Medicine.* The goal of this study was to determine if a small amount of weight loss through dietary changes and increased physical activity could prevent or delay the onset of type 2 diabetes. The research found that by eating properly, exercising regularly, and changing daily behaviors, study participants reduced their risk of developing diabetes by 58 percent. Even better, participants older than 60 reduced their risk by 71 percent. This reinforces the message that diet and physical activity together are the most effective ways to prevent uncontrolled blood sugar—and it's never too late to get started!

The DPP focused on decreasing calories, cutting saturated fat, and exercising 150 minutes a week (that's 30 minutes 5 days a week), along with learning new behaviors such as keeping a food log.[9] The Diabetes Comfort Food Diet takes these steps—particularly the nutrition guidelines—and goes further, so you don't have to sacrifice the comfort foods you love to get back on the path to health. You will learn how to make any meal healthier by addressing not only carbohydrates but also fiber and fat content.

FOOD BASICS: UNDERSTANDING YOUR CHOICES

You now know how diabetes works—and that prevention or reversal is absolutely possible. So let's talk about the food that will get you there. Prepare to learn everything you need to know about eating in ways that will either prevent or manage diabetes.

THE THREE MACRONUTRIENTS

- **Carbohydrates** (examples: fruits, vegetables, grains, low-fat dairy, beans, table sugar, and syrups)
- **Proteins** (examples: poultry, meats, fish, eggs, dairy, tofu, beans, nuts, and nut butters)
- **Fats** (examples: oils, butter, lard, margarine, nuts, nut butters, avocados, dairy, and seeds)

As shown above, there are three basic macronutrients—carbohydrates, proteins, and fats. When you digest these macronutrients, your body responds with hormones that help get the macronutrients where they need to be. Whenever you eat carbohydrates of any kind—whether table sugar, agave, an apple, or a slice of bread—insulin opens the cell doors that transport the sugar from the bloodstream into the cells.

When you eat any form of carbohydrate, your blood sugar rises to a certain degree. However, when you eat carbohydrates with protein or fat, this does not happen. That's because it takes the body longer to break down proteins and fats, which are much more complex. If you eat a modest amount of carbohydrate with either protein or fat—or both—your blood sugar levels will not rise as high, because the sugar enters the bloodstream more slowly so there is less sugar available at any one point.

Therefore, if you moderate how many carbohydrates you consume at each meal and spread your intake throughout the day, your pancreas will not be overwhelmed by overproducing insulin. This will prevent further aggravation of insulin resistance. At the same time, by limiting carbs, you decrease your overall caloric intake.

A Carb Is a Carb Is a Carb

Research in the *Journal of the American Dietetic Association* reports that the primary determinant affecting your after-meal blood sugar levels is the total amount of carbohydrates consumed at meals, regardless of whether the source is sucrose or starch.[10] In other words, the most important factor is your meal's total number of carbohydrates, whether they come from potato chips, a bowl of berries, or a muffin. Timing your intake is also important: You can't save all of your carbohydrates, no matter their source, for one meal during the day—and especially not the last meal of the day, as so many people do. This also tells you that sucrose, otherwise known as table sugar, can stay on your table. You can actually consume up to 35 percent of your total daily intake in the form of sucrose without adversely affecting your blood sugar control. That means if you follow a daily diet of 60 grams of carbohydrates per meal, you could potentially eat a piece of cake or a scone without triggering a negative glycemic response. However, I don't suggest you do that often—while the cake may not budge your blood sugar, it doesn't have as many nutrients as a starchy vegetable or another healthier source of carbs. I simply mention cake as an example to set your mind at ease that you can

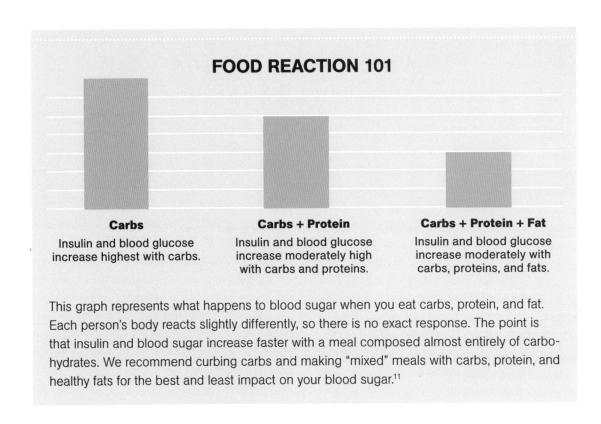

FOOD REACTION 101

Carbs	Carbs + Protein	Carbs + Protein + Fat
Insulin and blood glucose increase highest with carbs.	Insulin and blood glucose increase moderately high with carbs and proteins.	Insulin and blood glucose increase moderately with carbs, proteins, and fats.

This graph represents what happens to blood sugar when you eat carbs, protein, and fat. Each person's body reacts slightly differently, so there is no exact response. The point is that insulin and blood sugar increase faster with a meal composed almost entirely of carbohydrates. We recommend curbing carbs and making "mixed" meals with carbs, protein, and healthy fats for the best and least impact on your blood sugar.[11]

safely indulge your occasional cravings—or even enjoy a little sweet snack every day.

And don't think you'll be relegated to artificial sweeteners. In fact, it may be better to have the real stuff. Research has suggested that noncaloric sweeteners—Splenda, Sweet'N Low, Equal, and others—may affect appetite and energy intake, further disrupting your feelings of hunger and fullness. Plus, overly sweet foods make you crave more sweet foods. Furthermore, the Third National Health and Nutrition Examination Survey found that individuals who drank diet soda—soda with noncaloric sweeteners—had poorer glycemic control overall.

When all is said and done, you need to learn how to manage your sugar intake, and eating the real deal is less likely to cause brain and body confusion.[12]

This isn't permission to start adding sugar at every meal, however. The goal of the Diabetes Comfort Food Diet is to show you how you can enjoy all foods in moderation. Eating real, natural, wholesome meals as often as possible is ideal. This is a lifelong approach to beating diabetes, and there is a way to eat all foods—you just need to know when and how much.

Determining Just When to Eat—And How Much!

If you have prediabetes or diabetes, food is one of the best medicines you can give yourself. The trick is to determine what to eat the majority of the time and how to finesse your favorite foods into your meal plan. The ADA makes many recommendations on how to do this successfully, and the Diabetes Comfort Food Diet builds them into the plan that will help you lose weight and get your blood sugar back on track. If you have pre-diabetes or diabetes, our recommendations are as follows:

- Aim to lose 7 percent of your body weight if you are overweight or obese. Our plan will show you how!

- Follow an eating plan that is lower in carbohydrates, saturated fat, and calories and higher in healthy fats.

- Consume about 22 grams of dietary fiber per day (based on a 1,600-calorie diet) if you are at risk of diabetes.

- Limit intake of sugar-sweetened beverages if you are at risk of diabetes.

- Work up to getting 90 to 150 minutes of physical activity per week. (Read more about the importance of daily movement and daily diet on page 12.)

If you already have diabetes:

- Eat mixed meals—include carbohydrates, proteins, and fats at each meal.

- Monitor carbohydrate intake via carbohydrate counting or experienced-based estimation. (We'll talk more about this in Chapter 2.)

- Limit saturated fat and minimize trans fats while increasing intake of healthy fats such as omega-3 fatty acids.

- If you choose to drink alcohol, drink moderately—one serving per day for women and two or less per day for men—and with a meal.

- Follow individualized meal planning.

- Spread exercise over at least 3 days a week and do not skip more than 2 consecutive days.

- Perform strength training 2 days per week, if approved by your doctor.

- Self-monitor blood glucose in addition to making the fitness and nutrition changes above.

The Diabetes Comfort Food Diet Cookbook incorporates the above nutrition recommendations in all 200 recipes. The most important thing to remember is to curb carbs. "Curbing carbs" is basically a fun way of saying "consistent carbohydrate counting." This is the most effective way to control blood glucose, especially after meals. Every individual differs in nutrition and movement needs, degrees of medical risks, and, of course, willingness to change. Eating to beat diabetes is about addressing these needs while maintaining the pleasure and joy of eating.[13]

JUST IMAGINE . . . WEIGHT LOSS, TOO!

Your effort to curb carbs and calories isn't just about your blood sugar—it's also a means to lose weight. Many weight-loss programs use body mass index (BMI) as an across-the-board way to determine whether you need to lose weight. However, it is extremely important to recognize that BMI is not considered a perfect measure of your overall health. Having a BMI greater than 25, defined as overweight and/or obese, does not necessarily mean you need to lose weight. Consider this: Most gymnasts and other athletes would be considered overweight or obese according to their BMIs. Higher weight can be a result of muscle mass, not just fat mass.

The diabetes community recognizes this flaw

and encourages a different assessment. All you need is a tape measure. A waist circumference greater than 35 inches for women or greater than 40 inches for men is a more definitive measurement that takes into account excess abdominal fat. This excess fat, also referred to as adipose tissue, increases your risk of complications such as cardiovascular disease. Again, even this measurement is not "one size fits all."

If you do need to lose weight, your focus should be on changing your behaviors and letting weight loss happen secondarily to your new, consistent, daily habits. Diabetes can be prevented with just 7 percent weight loss, and you are more likely to fend it off for the long haul if you then maintain a 5 percent loss for 3 years. For example, if you weigh 180 today and lose about 12 pounds, and then keep off at least 9 of those pounds, you will be successful! As evidence proves, this is attainable. You can do this!

Losing weight is a great strategy for reversing insulin sensitivity, but it's no secret that it is also highly challenging. If dropping a lot of weight is important to you, be very realistic when setting your goals. We choose to think slow and steady,

because this is about a healthy lifestyle, not a fad diet. Start with the nutrition changes, as they will most dramatically affect your blood sugar, and add in exercise as soon as you are ready.

Don't let slow weight loss frustrate or discourage you. Instead, focus on making the positive behavior changes that we mention in Chapters 2 and 3, such as food shopping and meal planning. Simply making healthier food choices is effective at staving off diabetes. By incorporating a Mediterranean-style diet, you can decrease your risk of diabetes by 52 percent. Yes, diet—one that focuses on fruits, vegetables, whole grains, legumes, and healthy fats such as olives and nuts—is effective enough.[14] This is fantastic news, because we all know how extremely hard it is to lose weight once we have gained it, despite the fact that we may be eating less and even exercising more. That's why the Diabetes Comfort Food Diet gives you so many helpful tools, such as recipes that incorporate the beneficial Mediterranean fats, to make healthy changes easy, enjoyable, and livable.

Complementing Your Daily Diet with Movement

As mentioned previously, regular physical activity is a critical component for both weight loss and diabetes management. Reliable evidence suggests that to achieve significant weight loss, you must move for 60 minutes daily,[15] but if you aren't already that active, it's important to build up slowly. It's valuable to move daily because, in addition to burning calories, research shows that physical activity actually improves blood glucose control, regardless of weight loss! Physical activity also reduces cardiovascular risk and enhances overall well-being. If you have type 2 diabetes,

SWEET**FACT**
Exercise Benefits Extend Beyond Weight Loss

Aerobic exercise lowers LDL cholesterol by about 5 percent.
Blood glucose remains lower for 2 to 72 hours after mild and moderate-intensity exercise.
Both aerobic exercise and weight training are recommended to aid in blood sugar control.

The Lowdown on Diabetes

working up to meeting a weekly activity goal of 90 to 150 minutes is ideal. Whether you walk 30 minutes 5 days a week or take a Spinning class 2 days and do Zumba for 3, try to meet your movement goals. Most commonly, people choose walking for their physical activity, but your surest path to success is to find a form of movement you love. This will ensure you stick with it.

What exactly do we mean by "physical activity," "movement," and "exercise"? We're not just talking about running on a treadmill or lifting weights. There are all kinds of ways to get out of your seat and get moving. Many types of movement benefit blood sugar balance, heart health, and weight management.

The key to long-term blood sugar control is to make sure that no more than 2 days pass without physical activity. So if you exercise on Monday, be sure to get back to moving by Thursday. If reading all of the material presented here seems overwhelming, please don't fret. Just begin by assessing your level of readiness using START, and we'll help you put together an action plan in Chapter 3.

Meeting Your Minutes

Getting cleared for exercise by your doctor is the first step to meeting the recommended 90 to 150 minutes of movement per week. Then simply begin to walk or move. If you feel ready to take action, consider walking for 5 minutes a day 2 days a week, and continue building on this. If you can take a 5-minute walk every evening after dinner, that's even better. Then you can work your way to increasing your walk to 20 and then 30 minutes to obtain the most benefits. Not only does walking or light exercise help lower your blood glucose and, consequently, your insulin levels, but physical activity also makes your body more sensi-

SWEET**FACT**
More Reasons to Move

Hyperinsulinemia (high levels of insulin in the blood) is also associated with high blood pressure, heart disease and heart failure, obesity (particularly abdominal obesity), osteoporosis (thinning bones), and certain types of cancer, such as colon, breast, and prostate. In contrast, having low circulating insulin levels is associated with greater longevity; most centenarians without diabetes have low circulating insulin levels.[16]

tive to insulin. So if your body was not responding to insulin before, the addition of physical activity means less insulin is needed to open up your cells to receive sugar. Physical activity without weight loss is also associated with improved cholesterol—specifically, as waist circumference decreases, so does total cholesterol.[17]

Again, this is just more evidence that making nutrition and exercise changes can only improve your health and overall lifestyle. There will always be benefits from making these changes.

There you have it. A sweet life *is* possible when preventing diabetes or managing the disease. Eating real food (including real sugar) and losing just a small amount of weight is your new diet-and-lifestyle prescription. Let it sink in. Restaurant meals, holiday feasts, and even birthday celebrations will be a part of your future to enjoy—not just observe. The magic starts with curbing carbs, increasing fiber, and focusing on healthy fats. Check out Chapter 2 to learn how these three steps will help you make change that is realistic and delicious!

My Diabetes Success Story

Rebecca Weiss found her way to my New York City private nutrition practice in January of 2012. At age 40, this communications and marketing director at a New York City auction house and mother of two felt physically awful. She was fatigued, sluggish, and had difficulty sleeping. She felt depressed and soothed herself with emotional eating. To top it off, Rebecca was often sick and had terrible gastric reflux. She was living on Maalox. Every morning she had swollen ankles, diarrhea, and a puffy body.

"I'd wake up each morning feeling like I had a hangover—with nausea, a headache, and a stomachache from eating sweets before bedtime," Rebecca says. This smart and savvy woman was losing herself to food and was on the path to diabetes.

One major risk factor working against Rebecca was that she had been diagnosed with gestational diabetes during both of her pregnancies. After delivering her second child, she was told she had a 50/50 chance of developing diabetes. Her weight had climbed to 235 pounds and rather than help her come up with a plan to avert diabetes, her doctors shamed her, telling her she was too fat and that she needed to lose 50 to 100 pounds—but not how to achieve this goal.

When her A1C hit 5.6, on the border of prediabetes, Rebecca decided to get support from a registered dietitian so that she could get her health on track and be a positive role model for her young children. When she learned how to count carbohydrates—with the manageable goal of losing 7 percent of her weight—she felt capa-

ble and ready. "I felt empowered, realizing I could eat all foods, but that I had to make choices about when and how much. I would have done this long ago, if someone had just told me to look at my behaviors and start small."

Together we looked at her lifestyle and how food was woven through it. The easiest change for Rebecca was to stop eating at the most problematic part of her day: She was consuming one-third of her entire day's calories at night, between 9 and 11 p.m. Rebecca began journaling and realized she needed to take that time for herself in a new way. She was binge eating for 2 hours to numb her painful emotions rather than learning to face those emotions. For food to be comforting, she realized it should make her feel good—not sick. Soon, her self-care routine changed from soothing with food to de-stressing each night by riding her recumbent bike and reading fun, non-mommy magazines like *US Weekly* and *People*. Rebecca is shocked by her new love of physical activity. She feared sweating and was always told no one liked to exercise. "No one could be more surprised than me! I love that bike," she says.

Rebecca easily gave up fake sugar and diet foods like diet drinks (except one diet soda a day), diet ice creams, and sugar-free pudding. Through journaling and using the IRS hunger/fullness scale (see page 39), Rebecca gained a new level of awareness. This mindfulness helped her to realize she actually preferred savory foods to the sweets she had been eating. And she didn't feel restricted by her new carbohydrate guidelines—she learned how to eat enough of the right foods during meals and snacks throughout the day to prevent blood sugar spikes and combat cravings and nighttime eating. Buying lunch at the local salad cafés became one of Rebecca's favorite discoveries. She loves trying the different dressings and varying her high-fiber salad toppings, such as sun-dried tomatoes and chickpeas. When it comes to high-carb sources like pasta, she can't discern a difference in taste between whole wheat pasta and white pasta, but she knows which makes her body feel better—the whole wheat! Rebecca also knows she cannot just eat half of a bagel for breakfast (one half bagel has 30 grams of carbs versus a whole bagel with 60 grams of carbs), so instead she opts for bagel chips, which are just 15 grams, with a side of hummus at snack time to keep her carbs curbed and her appetite for bagels satiated. Rebecca feels empowered knowing she is her own nutrition gatekeeper.

Her new outlook on food and diabetes prevention has paid off! When Rebecca first came to my office, she weighed 222 pounds. In 6 months she lost 10 percent of her original body weight (that's 22 pounds) and dropped from a size 16 to a size 14. Rebecca can cross her legs again and shop at any store for clothes, no longer relegated to the plus-size section. Her husband constantly reminds her how great she looks. Rebecca's blood pressure remains high, but she no longer needs additional medication to manage it. She has prevented prediabetes, and her doctor said her liver and gallbladder readings have normalized.

She no longer takes antacids, nor does she even buy them. The nausea, the stomach pain, the diarrhea, and the nighttime eating have been replaced with exercise, energy, and renewed self-esteem. Rebecca has become protective of her bike, and her husband now knows it is neither his laundry basket nor his closet. It is Rebecca's bike: providing 35 minutes of freedom, sweat, and self-fulfillment almost daily.

Now she spends 2 hours a day on herself, doing the things she loves. "A fog has lifted. I'm awake and ready for the day. I now love my walk to and from Penn Station. I used to resent that walk, and now this mile and a half round-trip is my favorite part of the day." She's more productive at work and has started a regular date night with her husband—and they enjoy a renewed sex life, too.

"Basically when I was told to focus on behaviors, small changes, and small weight loss, I learned I actually loved foods that were lower in carbs, like hummus and vegetables. These foods work with my body rather than against me."

Another plus: When Rebecca stopped eating dessert, so did her children. They typically don't even ask for it anymore, she says. If they do, Rebecca is happy to give it to them. She is ecstatic that everyone in her family has benefited from her nutrition changes. Now she looks forward to getting weighed at her doctor's office. It will be the first time in 10 years she weighs less than 200 pounds. And now she can finally sleep through the night, free from the fear of diabetes.

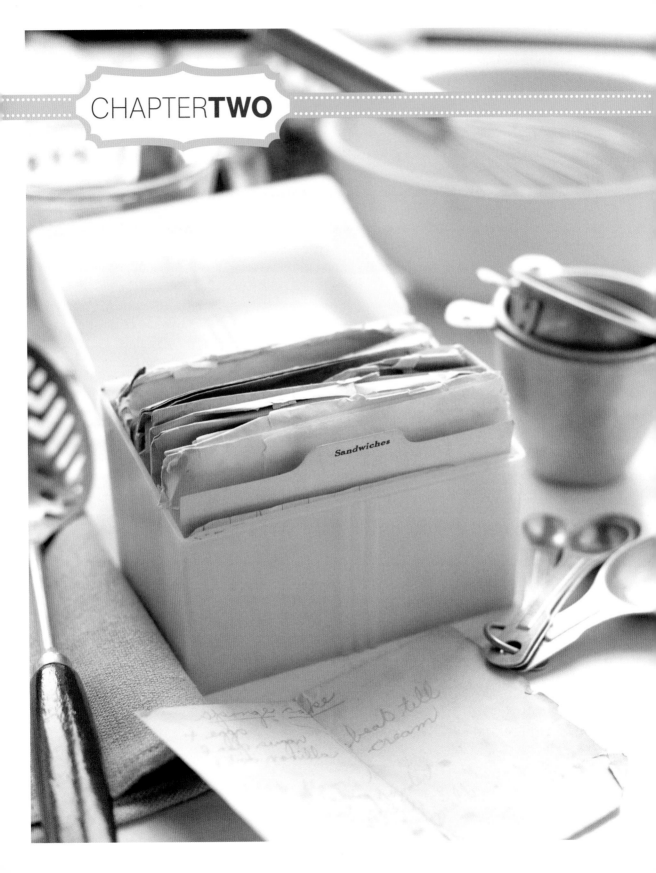

CHAPTER**TWO**

Change Your Recipes,
Not Your Life

Why call it "comfort food" when it actually makes you feel uncomfortable? These rich, traditionally carb-laden dishes make a person with insulin resistance feel lethargic, shaky, emotional, and perhaps even guilty. Well, forget that! It's time to learn how to make comfort food what it should be: energizing, balancing, and stabilizing. You can take almost any meal you love—mac 'n' cheese, mashed potatoes, or fried chicken—and transform it into a recipe that works *with* your body, not *against* it. Ideally, your meals should fuel your body without raising your blood sugar to a harmful level. This new, harmonious way of eating will allow you to reverse insulin resistance, lose weight, and lower your risk for disease. All you need to remember are these three steps to make any dish defeat diabetes. They are:

Step 1: Curb carbs. The average woman should consume 45 grams of carbs at every meal, while the average man should consume about 60 grams of carbs. The trick to managing diabetes is to hit that magic number consistently during each meal throughout the day. This is one of the easiest ways to improve blood sugar, lose weight, and be free from deprivation.

Step 2: Fill up on fiber. For every 6 grams of fiber you add to a meal, you can cut 6 grams of carbs off your total! That means opting for whole grains, leafy greens, and other fibrous foods that are a cinch to incorporate into classic dishes.

Step 3: Favor fats. When it comes to fats, you want to make sure you're getting the right kind. You want to decrease your intake of harmful saturated fats and increase the diabetes-friendly fats—monounsaturated fatty acids (MUFAs) and omega-3 fatty acids.

STEP 1: CURB CARBS

Your recipe for success lies in "curbing your carbs." This means women should consume up to 45 grams of carbohydrates at breakfast, lunch, and dinner, or no more than 135 grams at all three meals. In addition, each woman has the option of adding one to three snacks throughout the day, at an average of 15 to 30 grams of carbohydrates per snack. Men should consume up to 60 grams of carbs at breakfast, lunch, and dinner (no more than 180 grams at mealtimes), plus one to three 30-gram snacks.

Curbing carbs is a solution that can work for anyone, in part because it's easy to customize. By including snacks, you can tailor your daily diet to meet your individual needs. If three meals a day sounds limiting to you, don't worry. Just start by consuming three meals and three snacks. On the other hand, if three meals and three snacks sounds like too much food (especially for someone who has been inactive or is older than 60 years of age), you can start with three meals and slowly add in snacks as your metabolism increases with the addition of physical activity. Most importantly, be sure to meet at least 45 grams of carbohydrates per meal (or a minimum of 130 grams of digestible

Nutrition Facts

Serving Size
Servings Per Container

Amount Per Serving

Calories 0	Calories from Fat 0

	% Daily Value*
Total Fat 0g	0%
Saturated Fat 0g	0%
Trans Fat 0g	
Cholesterol 0mg	0%
Sodium 0mg	0%
Total Carbohydrate 0g	0%
Dietary Fiber 0g	0%
Soluble Fiber 0g	0%
Insoluble Fiber 0g	0%
Sugars 0g	
Protein 0g	

Vitamin A 0%	•	Vitamin C 0%
Calcium 0%	•	Iron 0%
Phosphorus 0%	•	Magnesium 0%

* Percent Daily Values are based on a 2,000 calorie diet. Your daily values may be higher or lower depending on your calorie needs:

		Calories:	2,000	2,500
Total Fat	Less than		0g	0g
Sat Fat	Less than		0g	0g
Cholesterol	Less than		0mg	0mg
Sodium	Less than		0mg	0mg
Potassium			0mg	0mg
Total Carbohydrate			0g	0g
Dietary Fiber			0g	0g

Calories per gram:

carbs per day) to ensure your body is properly fueled.[1]

All the recipes in this book have been uniquely designed to help prevent you from exceeding the 45-to-60-gram carbohydrate allotment. As long as you are not taking medication for diabetes, don't fret if your carb intake falls below the 45 or 60 grams for some of your meals. If this is the case, just be sure you achieve the minimum of 130 grams of total carbs per day. When making over a dish or a meal, be sure you know what carbohydrates are and where to find them on a food label. Did you know vegetables are carbohydrates? Yes, broccoli and lettuce are carbs—and so are beans! Some foods are even considered both carbs and proteins. But don't worry about the nitty-gritty details; we'll take care of that for you. Let's just get familiar with the foods in the carbohydrate category: grains, beans, low-fat dairy, fruits, vegetables, and of course, sugar. When we talk about any carbohydrate, the ideal form is the least processed and most wholesome.

The Go-To Grains

When it comes to grains, aim for whole grain options whenever possible. When making muffins and other baked goods, substitute oat bran or whole wheat flour for refined white flour. If you are cooking pasta, always choose the whole wheat or sprouted grain varieties. Did you know whole wheat pasta is better for you than brown rice pasta? That's right; whole wheat pasta contains more natural fiber per serving. When shopping, aim for the least processed foods. You can find them by reading the ingredients. Choose products that have short ingredient lists and that include sugar as the third ingredient or beyond. Then compare nutrition fact labels and choose the food higher in total natural fiber.

What is natural fiber? There is no legal definition, but we consider it to be foods that have not been stripped of the bran and the germ or are in the least-modified state, so they are less processed and much healthier. Breads, cereals, cookies, and other foods with "added fiber" such as the partially digestible polysaccharide inulin or foods marketed as low-carbohydrate products are typically not high in fiber until fiber is added through food processing. We do not encourage you to focus on eating these foods in large quantities. Rather, seek out products like sprouted wheat bread or cereal with millet and flax that have not been refined or altered to meet fiber recommendations for marketing purposes. In fact, a 2003 study of thousands of men and women showed that including more fiber-rich whole grains in your diet can prevent diabetes.[2] At the beginning of the study, the participants were ages 40 to 69, and none had been diagnosed with diabetes. After

(continued on page 22)

CLUES FOR CURBING CARBS AND INCREASING FIBER

Cereal: Opt for 30 grams of carbs or fewer and 5 grams of fiber or more per serving.

Bread: Opt for 15 to 20 grams of carbs or fewer and about 3 grams of fiber per slice.

Pasta: Opt for 45 grams of carbs or fewer and about 5 grams of fiber per 2-ounce serving.[3]

BREAKDOWN ON BREADS

Beware of breads that are too high in fiber (we recommend no more than 5 grams) or too low in carbs (we recommend no less than 15 grams). Below are different breads to choose from while curbing your carbs and filling up on fiber. **Minimize or avoid the breads with harder-to-digest added fiber like inulin and cellulose.**

BREAD	SERVING SIZE	INGREDIENTS	FIBER (G)	CARBS (G)
Arnold, 100% Whole Wheat **NO ADDED FIBER**	1 slice (43 g)	Whole wheat flour, water, sugar, wheat gluten, yeast, raisin juice concentrate, wheat bran, molasses, soybean oil, salt, monoglycerides, calcium propionate (preservative), calcium sulfate, DATEM, grain vinegar, citric acid, soy lecithin, whey, nonfat milk	3	20
Arnold, Double Fiber **ADDED FIBER**	1 slice (43 g)	Whole wheat flour, water, sugar, inulin (chicory root fiber), wheat gluten, wheat fiber, yeast, soybean oil, cellulose fiber, polydextrose, wheat bran, molasses, salt, DATEM, calcium propionate (preservative), monoglycerides, grain vinegar, calcium sulfate, citric acid, soy lecithin, calcium carbonate, whey, nonfat milk	6	21
Ezekiel 4:9, Sprouted Whole Grain Bread **NO ADDED FIBER**	1 slice (34 g)	Organic sprouted wheat, organic sprouted barley, organic sprouted millet, organic malted barley, organic sprouted lentils, organic sprouted soybeans, organic sprouted spelt, filtered water, fresh yeast, organic wheat gluten, sea salt	3	15
Stroehmann, Dutch Country Double Fiber Bread **ADDED FIBER**	1 slice (38 g)	Whole wheat flour, water, sugar, inulin (chicory root fiber), wheat gluten, wheat fiber, yeast, cellulose fiber, polydextrose, soybean and/or canola oil, salt, wheat bran, molasses, enrichment (calcium sulfate, vitamin E acetate, vitamin A palmitate, vitamin D_3), mono- and diglycerides, calcium propionate (preservative), DATEM, soy lecithin, citric acid, grain vinegar, sodium stearoyl lactylate, ethoxylated mono- and diglycerides, azodicarbonamide	5	19
Rudi's, 7 Grain with Flax **NO ADDED FIBER**	1 slice (40 g)	Water, organic whole wheat flour, organic evaporated cane juice, organic wheat gluten, organic quinoa flour, organic oat fiber, organic sesame seeds, organic millet, organic kamut flour, organic whole spelt flour, yeast, organic sunflower seeds, sea salt, organic high oleic sunflower/safflower oil, organic potato flour, organic flaxseed, organic rolled oats, organic oat bran, organic vinegar, organic molasses, organic wheat starch, ascorbic acid, natural enzymes	3	15

Change Your Recipes, Not Your Life

BREAD	SERVING SIZE	INGREDIENTS	FIBER (G)	CARBS (G)
Rudi's, 100% Whole Wheat **NO ADDED FIBER**	1 slice (43 g)	Organic whole wheat flour, water, organic cracked wheat, organic brown sugar, organic wheat gluten, organic wheat bran, yeast, organic high oleic sunflower and/or safflower oil, sea salt, organic vinegar, organic oat flour, organic molasses, cultured organic wheat starch, organic barley malt, ascorbic acid, natural enzymes	3	18
Vermont Bread Company, Organic Soft Multigrain **NO ADDED FIBER**	1 slice (40 g)	Organic wheat flour, water, organic whole wheat flour, organic grain and seed blend (organic cracked rye, organic cracked yellow corn, organic cracked wheat, organic cracked barley, organic steel-cut oats, organic flaxseed, organic hulled millet), organic cane sugar, contains less than 2 percent of each of the following: organic soybean oil, organic wheat gluten, yeast, organic molasses, salt, organic oat flour, organic potato flour, enzymes, organic cultured wheat starch, citric acid, organic reduced-fat soy flour, ascorbic acid, organic soy lecithin	3	21
Weight Watchers, 100% Whole Wheat **ADDED FIBER**	2 slices (41 g)	Whole wheat flour, water, wheat gluten, cellulose fiber, polydextrose, sugar, contains 2 percent or less of the following: yeast, oat fiber, molasses, salt, calcium, sulfate, vinegar, soybean and/or canola oil, soy protein isolate, dough conditioners (one or more of the following: DATEM, mono- and diglycerides, ethoxylated mono- and diglycerides, ammonium sulfate, sodium stearoyl lactylate, potassium iodate), calcium propionate (preservative), wheat flour,* guar gum, ferrous fumarate, folic acid, citric acid *trivial amount of wheat flour	6	16

10 years of follow-up, the researchers found that those who ate the most fiber-rich whole grains had a 35 percent lower risk of developing diabetes than those who ate the least. And even more shocking: Participants who ate the most fiber from cereals had an amazing 61 percent lower risk of developing diabetes. That's a greater reduction of risk than was seen in a study (page 8) that involved diet, exercise, and significant weight loss.

Ironically, many diets tell you to avoid cereal products like wheat, rye, corn, and rice, the only sources of cereal fiber! These wholesome foods, enjoyed in whole grain form, are abundant in our diet, making them the best way of all to stay healthy. Just make sure to stick with unprocessed foods. Be cautious: Those who consume processed foods such as Arnold's Double Fiber bread with added fiber (see highlighted ingredients in "Breakdown on Breads" on page 20) often report bloating and gas.

Besides wheat products, there is an entire world of other delicious whole grains to choose from: amaranth, barley, buckwheat, bulgur, millet, oat bran, and quinoa are all great choices. Barley is delicious as a side instead of rice. Quinoa can be used when stuffing peppers or even for a hot morning cereal. The options are endless. Check out Good Morning "Grits" (page 71) or Vegetable Sauté with Quinoa (page 256) to try this grain. From this point forward, trade white flour for whole wheat flour, oat bran flour, spelt flour, or sprouted wheat flour—or any naturally high-fiber grain. Not only can these whole grains help you manage your blood sugar, but they really taste great.

Balance with Beans

Beans are a superfood. These little powerhouses have both carbohydrates and protein. They are packed with vitamins, high in soluble fiber, and noted for their ability to lower cholesterol. Basically, you are getting two for one when eating beans. You are getting a nutritious carb that is not only diabetes friendly but also heart healthy! When choosing beans, it's okay to purchase dry and soak overnight, or buy the canned version, which can be much more convenient. Remember, the goal is to make over your meals, not have the ingredients sit in your cabinets. When you purchase any canned item, whether it is beans, vegetables, or soup, make sure the label says "no added salt" and read the ingredient list to make sure there are no added sugars or fats.

WATCH WORDS

Beware of fake sugars, added sugars, and added fats in the ingredient list.

Fake Foes—Avoid the Artificial

- Acesulfame K
- Equal, NutraSweet (aspartame)
- Nectresse
- Sweet'N Low, SugarTwin (saccharin)
- Splenda (sucralose)
- Truvia and PureVia (stevia and erythritol)

Sugar Fraud—Steer Clear

- High fructose corn syrup

Fat Foes—Beware of These Heartbreakers

- Cocoa butter
- Crisco
- Lard
- Olestra—fake fat replacer
- Monoglycerides and diglycerides—fat-based fat replacer
- Partially hydrogenated oil
- Palm kernel oil
- Shortening
- Vegetable shortening

Did You Know? Low-Fat and Fat-Free Dairy Are Carbs

Low-fat and even fat-free dairy options such as fat-free milk contain carbohydrates as well as proteins and must be counted when curbing your carbs. Typically, low-fat versions of milk, yogurt, and/or even low-fat frozen yogurts contain 12 grams of carbohydrates per cup or more. Only a few low-fat or fat-free dairy options are low enough in carbs, less than 10 grams per cup, that they can be counted as proteins. The low-fat dairy options that are considered proteins only are low-fat or fat-free Greek yogurt, unsweetened soy milk, unsweetened almond milk, and low-fat cottage cheese. In addition to these lower-carb, higher-protein dairy options, we recommend choosing low-fat dairy options rather than fat free or full fat. This means choose 1% milk (not fat free), low-fat yogurt, low-fat ice cream, or possibly the real thing—good old full-fat ice cream. The low-fat dairy options will have a small amount of fat to help satiate you, regulate your blood sugar, and keep the product wholesome. Minimizing the amount of saturated fat is heart protective; therefore, lower-fat options are typically the better choice for dairy. When it comes to cheese or a sweet food like ice cream that contains protein, vitamins, and minerals, opt for full fat but keep the quantity small. While curbing carbs is our

CARBS CLIMB WITH FAT-FREE FOODS

Taking the fat out of a food leaves two macronutrients, carbohydrates and proteins. Typically one of these nutrients increases in quantity, and more often it is the carbohydrates. Think about fat-free dressing or fat-free cookies. They may be sans fat, but they have plenty of sugars. Read this as a blood sugar bomb and stay away from these products. As you will read later in this chapter, fats like olive oil for dressing and avocado for sandwiches offer heart-protective benefits. You can't say that about artificial ingredients. Your new motto is "Low fat, not no fat."

Your one exception to this rule is dairy such as fat-free Greek yogurt. Instead of being mostly carbohydrate based like other yogurts, this fat-free option contains 14 to 21 grams of protein and between 7 and 22 grams of carbohydrates, depending on whether it is fruit flavored. Across the board, low-fat and fat-free Greek yogurts are winners and go-to options for beating diabetes.

SWEET**FACT**

Ripe fruit is more likely to raise your blood sugar; opt for the harder, less-ripe pieces.

....

focus, portion control automatically and advantageously curbs your calories, as well.

Although most grocery aisles are a maze, you will soon have them mapped out for your own success! So when turning down the milk aisle, for example, choose from these options to make sure your blood sugar stays balanced.

"MOO"RE ON MILKS

- Choose 1% milk only—if using cow's milk.
- Soy, almond, and sunflower milks need to be unsweetened and fortified with calcium and vitamin D.
- If using regular almond milk, ensure it is enriched with protein (typically 5 grams of protein or more per serving).
- Hemp milk is a great omega source that needs to be fortified with calcium and vitamin D.

Flavor with Fruit

Nothing in life is free, and this includes fruit. Fruits fall into the carbohydrate category. Many times, clients have told me about all of the nutrition changes they are making, yet they can't seem to get their blood sugar under control. That's when we review their food log to read about breakfast with a glass of orange juice to take their medications or vitamin, an extra-large fruit smoothie before hitting the treadmill, and lunch meals of only fruit. And let's not forget the entire bunch of grapes while watching TV at night. Bingo. Fruit is absolutely good for

us—but like anything, it must be eaten in moderation and preferably as part of a mixed meal, with a protein or a fat like cottage cheese or almonds. Go for two servings of fruit daily.

One piece of fruit like a big apple can be equal to 30 grams of carbohydrates. Therefore, small pieces of less-ripe fruit are best to work into your daily intake. These less-mature fruits remain in their complex forms, taking longer to break down. As the fruit ripens, the complex sugars known as starch are broken down into simple forms and can raise your blood sugar more quickly. If you love juice, you can find a way to work it into your intake. Just recognize that the juice should be 100% juice and it will count toward your carbohydrate allotment for that particular meal.

FIVE COMMON FRUITS FOR 15 GRAMS OF CARBS

- 1 small apple (4 ounces)
- 1 small banana (4 ounces)
- ¾ cup blueberries
- 17 small grapes (3 ounces)
- 1 small orange (6.5 ounces)[5]

Very Veggie

As astonishing as it may seem, veggies are considered carbohydrates. There are two categories of vegetables: starchy and nonstarchy. Starchy vegetables are typically the root of the plant and include beets, potatoes, sweet potatoes, turnips, jicama, and radishes. Other starchy vegetables include pumpkin, butternut squash, peas, corn, and zucchini. The nonstarchy vegetables include, but are not limited to, the cruciferous veggies such as broccoli and cauliflower as well as dark leafy greens like kale, spinach, collards, and Swiss chard.

These roots, leaves, and stems afford you the luxury of quantity! You need to consume many vegetables daily to affect your blood sugar. Three cups of raw, nonstarchy veggies (or 1½ cups of cooked, nonstarchy vegetables) equals 15 grams of carbohydrates. So as you can see, including many veggies at meals gives you the opportunity to get quantity and variety.

When making over your meals, double or even triple your vegetable quantity to help fill you up, plus meet your daily needs of veggies, while keeping the carb level curbed. Most Americans do not eat enough veggies, and many recipes fall short in the quantity of veggies they use. Eat at least three servings of veggies per day. Go ahead and make your meal colorful!

HAVING YOUR CAKE AND EATING IT TOO

Vegetables let us have our cake and eat it too. If you eat 1½ cups of cooked vegetables as your only carb source for a dinner meal, you will have 30 to 45 grams of carbohydrates left over to enjoy another form of carbohydrate at that same meal. The other form of carbohydrate is your choice, whether it is a fresh bowl of fruit, or a refined carb such as a cookie, or even a piece of cake. That's right, dessert. This is how you can easily manage eating a sweet dessert at a dinner party or a res-taurant. Eat protein, such as a piece of grilled chicken or salmon, paired with nonstarchy vegetables so that your carbohydrate allotment is not used up for that meal. Then when the waiter offers dessert, you can look on the menu for an option that will serve up less than 45 grams of carbohydrates. If you are at home, you can easily use one of the recipes in this cookbook to find a sweet dinner complement. If you are reading the menu and feel stumped, a safe bet would be to eat half of a smaller dessert. You *can* enjoy any food, when you do it smartly.

Opt for Organic

Grocery stores, fruit stands, and farmers' markets now offer organic and conventional options. Organic farms adhere to earth-friendly practices that rely on biological controls rather than chemical interventions and use methods that build soil fertility, such as crop diversity and crop rotation, to minimize pests and maximize produce output. Conventional produce, on the other hand, may come from a farm that uses synthetic pesticides. Organic fruits and vegetables aren't necessarily more nutritious than nonorganic produce, but it is recommended that individuals (especially pregnant women, children under the age of 5, and immune-compromised individuals) minimize their exposure to pesticides.[7] Though more research in this area is needed, studies have found links between exposure to certain pesticides and impaired liver function, blood sugar control, and obesity. Eating organic produce is the surest way to reduce your pesticide exposure. However, the best way to protect your health—and your wallet—is to focus on limiting the foods that are most likely to come into contact with these chemicals.

CINNAMON CONTROL

Did you know meals containing 3 to 6 grams of cinnamon can lower glycemic response? Go ahead and add 1 teaspoon of cinnamon to your meals to help defeat sugar spikes.[6] This versatile spice tastes fabulous in both sweet and savory dishes!

THE DIRTY DOZEN AND THE CLEAN 15

Every year, the nonprofit organization called the Environmental Working Group compiles two lists to help consumers identify produce containing higher levels of pesticides versus lower levels. Use this list to help you save time and money when deciding which organic produce items are worth the extra dollars. To lessen your exposure to pesticides, stay up-to-date and educate yourself on the most recent lists each year at ewg.org/foodnews/summary.php.

The Dirty Dozen: This produce is most likely to come into contact with pesticides. Choose organic and sustainable vendors whenever possible.

1. Apples
2. Celery
3. Bell peppers
4. Peaches
5. Strawberries
6. Nectarines (imported)
7. Grapes
8. Spinach
9. Lettuce
10. Cucumbers
11. Blueberries (domestic)
12. Potatoes

The Clean 15: It's okay to buy these fruits and veggies from a conventional farm.

1. Onions
2. Sweet corn
3. Pineapples
4. Avocados
5. Cabbage
6. Sweet peas
7. Asparagus
8. Mangoes
9. Eggplant
10. Kiwi
11. Cantaloupe (domestic)
12. Sweet potatoes
13. Grapefruit
14. Watermelon
15. Mushrooms

The Real Scoop on Real Sugar

There are sticky forms of sugar such as honey, agave, and maple syrup. There are the powdered varieties of raw sugar, brown sugar, and white sugar. Last but not least there is the controversial high fructose corn syrup. When it comes to using these sweeteners, the trick is to choose the form that is the least processed and most sweet—this way you can use less of it to satisfy your sweet tooth. Use the sweetness meter below to help you decide which sugars to favor. Though agave has been touted as a lower-glycemic sugar, there is no conclusive beneficial evidence.[8] The research also has mixed reviews on high fructose corn syrup, but because it is highly processed, it's best to avoid it.[9] The Diabetes Comfort Food Diet recommends you use as little added sugar as possible in a form that is the least modified and that minimally affects your blood sugar.

AVOID ARTIFICIAL SWEETENERS

Unfortunately, sugar has gained a bad reputation over the years, and many people try to avoid real

....

SWEET**FACT**
Sweetness Meter

Less is more when it comes to these common sweeteners—that is, the sweeter the source, the less of it you need to use for a satisfyingly sweet flavor. **Consider these serving sizes equivalent to 1 cup of white sugar:**

- 1 teaspoon pure stevia
- ⅔ cup agave nectar
- ¾ cup honey
- ¾ cup maple syrup
- 1 cup brown sugar

Change Your Recipes, Not Your Life

sugar at all costs. Thinking they can cut calories and "cheat" the effects of real sugar, many turn to artificial sweeteners, also known as nonnutritive sweeteners: aspartame (Equal, NutraSweet), saccharin (Sweet'N Low, SugarTwin), acesulfame K, neotame, and sucralose (Splenda). When substituting artificial sweeteners for the real deal, it's important to consider the pros and cons. While these little packs of white sweetness seem harmless, no matter how they may taste or look, artificial sweeteners are chemicals. Although they have no effect on glycemic response, one study found that people who drank one or more diet sodas (sweetened with aspartame) had a higher A1C than people who drank none.[10] Also, it is possible that eating these sweeteners makes you crave more sweet foods high in real or added sugars—and lots of calories.

Finally, consuming these "fake friends" can actually lead to long-term weight gain.[11] Remember that sugar free doesn't mean calorie free when it comes to food. The little packets may be without calories, but the foods they are used in certainly contain calories. With artificial sweeteners, we may trick ourselves into thinking we consumed less—when we actually end up consuming more. Artificial sweeteners often distort our perception of calories by satisfying our current cravings but causing our bodies to crave those sweet calories

later in the day.[12] With these factors in mind, we think eating real sugar is worth the calories and carbs when defeating diabetes.

What About Wine?

We can't forget about wine and other beverages. You should know that the easiest way to curb your carbs when talking drinks is to switch from diet drinks and caloric beverages like juice and soda to water or seltzer. Water and seltzer are refreshing, hydrating, filling, and don't add any extra calories, carbs—or other nutrition. You can slice oranges, lemons, or limes and toss them in for some zesty flavoring. Plus, increasing your water consumption will improve your digestion as you increase your fiber intake. Hydrating will help to prevent the fiber from binding to cause constipation.

But what about wine, beer, and liquor? Well, like everything else on the Diabetes Comfort Food Diet, you can have them, but in moderation. This means one serving of alcohol per day for women and two for men[13]—but you must drink alcoholic beverages with meals from now on. There are two reasons: firstly because alcohol is dehydrating, and secondly because it can cause hypoglycemia, low

---

SWEET**FACT**

Stevia is a form of natural sugar found in the leaves of the stevia plant. This natural sugar is about 200 times sweeter than regular table sugar and does not affect blood sugar. Pure stevia is a real sugar alternative. Read the labels of packaged stevia to ensure it is 100 percent pure. Beware—some brands may add the sugar alcohol erythritol.

ALCOHOL: COUNTING CARBS

12-ounce beer = 13 grams (regular)
or 5 grams (light beer)

4-ounce glass of red wine = 3 grams

4-ounce glass of white wine = 1 gram

1.5-ounce shot of liquor = 0 grams
in gin, rum, or vodka[14]

---

blood sugar. Even though it lowers blood sugar, you must still count that beer toward your total carb count at that meal. Decide if it's worth it and don't start drinking now if you don't already drink.

STEP 2: FILL UP ON FIBER
MAGIC CARBS

As you curb carbs, we have a little more magic for your toolbox. It's fiber. A carbohydrate contains fiber, and there are two types: soluble and insoluble. It doesn't matter which form of fiber you eat, but if your meal boasts greater than 6 grams of fiber per serving, part of your carbohydrate intake "disappears"! For instance, if your entrée tallies up to 56 grams of carbohydrates but has 12 grams of fiber, you can subtract the 12 grams of fiber from the total carbohydrates. This means 56 grams of carbs, minus 12 grams of fiber = 44 total carbohydrate grams. These magic carbs help prevent you from exceeding 45 or 60 grams of carbohydrates per meal.

This concept also allows you to choose cereal or other foods with higher total grams of carbohydrates. For instance, if you choose a cereal like Kashi Good Friends, you'll see from the nutrition facts label that it has 42 grams of total carbohydrates. You may think, "Not only is this cereal too high in carbohydrates, but I don't have enough carbs for my milk choice!" Well, think again. If you look below this number, you will see that the cereal also has 12 grams of dietary fiber per cup. This means your cereal choice is really equivalent to 30 grams of carbs. Thus this cereal is a great high-fiber, moderate-carbohydrate breakfast choice.

1 cup Kashi Good Friends cereal:
> 42 grams of carbs
> − 12 grams dietary fiber
> = 30 grams of carbs

½ cup 1% milk:
> + 6 grams carbs
> = 36 grams of carbs for breakfast

NOT NET CARBS

Don't confuse the popular concept of net carbs with our magic carbs. Most people subtract total fiber from total carbs and call this net carbs. For the best results, you must go a step further than net carbs. Subtract fiber from your carb count only if the fiber quantity is greater than 6 grams per serving.

WHY FIBER?

Numerous research studies support the benefits of fiber specifically in relation to blood sugar management.[15] Dietary fiber, especially soluble fiber, decreases insulin resistance and prevents prediabetes and diabetes.[16] Furthermore the American Diabetes Association recommends that *all individuals* consume on average at least 22 grams of fiber per 1,600 calories per day, and studies show that a diet with 44 to 50 grams of fiber daily improves blood sugar management.[17] In fact, in a study published in the *New England Journal of Medicine*, researchers reported that when patients with type 2 diabetes ate more fiber, they experienced dramatic health results.[18] Their blood sugar levels went down an average of 13 points, and their blood fats (cholesterol and triglycerides) also went down steeply. The fiber used in this study came from ordinary, natural foods, not supplements. This is the same source of fiber you'll find in this book.

So what else can fiber do for your diabetes? Research shows that fiber can actually reduce the need for medication in those with diabetes. In a study of men with diabetes who were running high blood sugar levels, adding fiber to their diets produced truly stunning results: The men who were

CURB CARBS WITH CEREAL

When curbing carbs and filling up on fiber, find cereals with nutrition facts similar to our favorites in the left column. First read the nutrition facts and then check ingredients to make sure the grains are wholesome options like stone-ground whole wheat, and look for the "watch words." Choose the better option and enjoy.

	Kashi GOLEAN	Kashi GOLEAN Crunch!
Serving size	1 cup	1 cup
Calories	140	190
Total fat	1 g	3 g
Saturated fat	0 g	0 g
Total carbs	30 g	39 g
Total fiber	10 g	8 g
Protein	13 g	9 g

	Kellogg's All-Bran Complete Wheat Flakes	Kellogg's Raisin Bran
Serving size	1 cup	1 cup
Calories	113	190
Total fat	0.6 g	1 g
Saturated fat	0 g	0 g
Total carbs	31 g	46 g
Total fiber	6 g	7 g
Protein	4 g	5 g

	Bob's Red Mill Granola, Natural	Bear Naked Granola Heavenly Chocolate
Serving size	½ cup	½ cup
Calories	170	260
Total fat	2 g	7 g
Saturated fat	0 g	2 g
Total carbs	33 g	42 g
Total fiber	3 g	4 g
Protein	5 g	6 g

WHOLE FOODS = HIGHER FIBER

Compare the fiber content of foods in the whole form versus a processed form.

WHOLE FOOD	FIBER (G)	PROCESSED FOOD	FIBER (G)
1 small apple	3.0	½ cup applesauce	1.8
1 cup bran flakes	5.0	1 cup frosted flakes	1.0
1 cup steamed kale	4.0	1 cup boiled kale	3.0
Natural granola bar	5.0	Chewy granola bar	1.0
¼ fresh mango (40 g)	4.0	7 pieces dried mango (40 g)	2.0
1 slice sprouted whole grain bread	3.0	1 slice white bread	1.0

taking oral diabetes medications all had their medication discontinued! And those taking insulin in doses of less than 30 units a day were able to discontinue their injections.[19] The message is clear: The more fiber you consume, the less likely it is that the carbs you eat will negatively affect your blood sugar.

Filling up on fiber is easy when you use the recipes in this book. Whole grains, beans, fruits, and vegetables are all naturally high in fiber, as discussed above. Be sure to use these foods in whole form. For example, the fiber in a whole apple with the skin on is greater than you'll find in a mini cup of applesauce.

STEP 3: FAVOR FATS

Now you know to spread your fiber-filled carbohydrates evenly throughout the day. What goes on the rest of your plate? For starters, lean proteins like beans, eggs, tofu, chicken, and fish should accompany your grains, veggies, and fruits. Most important is the word *lean*—meaning low in saturated fat. When curbing carbs, filling up with fiber, and decreasing saturated fat in your proteins, you automatically cut calories, which can help you lose weight. It's also important to eat plenty of healthy unsaturated fats. That's why step 3 of the Diabetes Comfort Food Diet is to favor fats! This essential step to making over your meals will keep you full, enhance your whole-body health, and further protect against diabetes.

Eat More MUFAs

In Chapter 1, we mentioned previously the benefits of a Mediterranean-style diet, which is high in monounsaturated fats, or MUFAs (found in olive oil, olives, and avocados), and omega-3 fatty acids (especially found in fish). Coupled with a healthy lifestyle (daily physical activity and no smoking, as discussed in Chapter 1), a Mediterranean-style diet is significantly associated with less weight gain and a smaller waistline.[20] Obtaining—and maintaining—a small waistline is crucial when preventing and/or managing blood sugar. A larger waistline for women and men is associated with diabetes and metabolic syndrome, so we must keep this in mind for prevention and treatment. Furthermore, this dietary pattern characterized by a higher consumption of plant foods, a higher intake of olive oil as the main source of fat, and a moderate intake of fish correlates with preventing the cognitive decline associated with diabetes. The diet is also beneficial for reducing complications of diabetes such as a fatty liver.[21] MUFAs are known to be heart protective and do not cause inflammation the way other dietary components do.[22] The evidence supports a diet rich in MUFAs as your primary source of fats. Simply put, eat more MUFAs.

Oh, Oh, Omega-3 Fatty Acids

The other fat to favor is the polyunsaturated fat called the omega-3 fatty acid. There are two

GO FISH

When it comes to selecting the most healthful sources of fish, go *wild*. Wild fish have higher levels of omega-3 fatty acids as well as lower levels of undesirable fats. Wild fish are more environmentally friendly and have not been exposed to growth hormones, antibiotics, or dyes—common practices when it comes to imported farmed fish. Some grocery chains, like Whole Foods, are making finding wild fish (also known as "sustainably farmed" fish) easy. All of their fish are labeled to indicate where the fish was sourced from. Fish raised in a sustainable farm have lived in a natural body of water free of chemicals unless warranted for therapeutic use.

There are now certifications and seals of approval to help make finding sustainable fish and/or wild fish simple no matter where you shop. Look for the labels such as the Marine Stewardship Council's "Fish Forever" and the label Friend of the Sea. To educate yourself refer to FriendoftheSea.org, FishWatch.gov, seafoodsource.com, and nmfs.noaa.gov/aquaculture.

If you do buy regular farmed fish, try to make sure it comes from the United States. Aim to get fish from a variety of different water sources, just in case one water source is contaminated with mercury or environmental toxins. But remember, in the end, it's still better for you to eat farmed fish twice a week than no fish at all!

forms of polyunsaturated fatty acids, the omega-3s and the omega-6s. The American diet is already high in omega-6 fatty acids, so you need to make a specific effort to increase the omega-3 fatty acids in your daily diet. This essential fatty acid is an anti-inflammatory agent, protects your heart, and helps to prevent diabetes. The latest research reveals diets high in total omega-3 fatty acids are directly related to a lower risk of developing diabetes.[23, 24]

Omega-3 fatty acids come in three forms: Docosahexaenoic acid (DHA) and eicosapentaenoic acid (EPA) are both found in fish, while alpha-linolenic acid (ALA) is found in plants. The vegetarian sources of ALA should be eaten daily. Get your daily dose from canola oil, walnuts, Brazil nuts, hemp seeds, sesame seeds, pumpkin seeds, chia seeds, and ground flaxseeds.

DHA surrounds your nerves and helps with nerve transmission, brain development, and even depression. Our bodies cannot make this essential fatty acid, so in order to get enough EPA and DHA, you must eat direct sources found in marine life. Aim to include these foods two or more times a week: salmon, trout, bass, bluefish, sardines, tuna, catfish, cod, and/or halibut. If choosing canned tuna, check the label and buy only "chunk light in water, no added salt." Chunk light tuna is lower in mercury than canned albacore tuna. To alleviate worries about chemicals such as polychlorinated biphenyls (PCBs) and mercury in your fish, eat different types of wild fish from different sources of water each week. To stay current on fish advisories, refer to the Environmental Protection Agency.[25]

Steer Away from Saturated Fats

Consuming foods high in saturated fats—such as sausage, buttery biscuits, or highly processed foods—can increase your level of bad cholesterol known as low-density lipoproteins (LDL). LDL cholesterol deposits into tissues, causing fatty streaks, plaque buildup, and damage to your blood vessels. Higher levels of LDL are associated with increased inflammation and risk of cardiovascular disease.[26] In fact, lowering your dietary intake of saturated fat can be more beneficial in lowering LDL levels than just decreasing dietary cholesterol. Decreasing dietary cholesterol to less than 200 milligrams per day lowers your cholesterol about 3 to 5 percent, whereas getting less than 7 percent of your daily calories from saturated fat has been shown to lower cholesterol by 8 to 10 percent.[27] Therefore, focus on eating foods lower in saturated fat and higher in monounsaturated fats, like almonds.

There is one exception: cheese. Though high in calories and saturated fat, cheese is a great source of protein and calcium, and thus can help to manage blood sugar levels and provide a hard-to-get mineral for bone density. Continue to include fruits, vegetables, low-fat dairy products, and whole grains and limit added sugars to help decrease your cholesterol and risk for cardiovascular disease associated with diabetes.

Combat Diabetes with Calcium

You've probably heard it time and time again: "Calcium helps build strong bones and teeth!" And it's true! Calcium is an essential mineral, and vitamin D helps the body absorb more of it. Consuming enough calcium and vitamin D is crucial, especially if you have prediabetes or diabetes, since high levels of insulin are associated with weakening of the bones, known as osteopenia, and loss of bone known as osteoporosis. Your goal should be to consume adequate calcium and vitamin D to prevent these bone diseases. Aside from

Change Your Recipes, Not Your Life

low-fat dairy products, good sources of calcium include green leafy vegetables, the stems of broccoli, and fortified milk alternatives like almond milk. Opt for four servings of low-fat dairy per day. Weight-bearing exercise can also help build bone mass—add it to your list of pros for building up your exercise routine!

Give Salt the Shake

One thing we haven't talked about yet is salt. Dietary salt intake is known to raise blood pressure. Be sure to check all nutrition labels for sodium content. The general recommendation for Americans is to limit salt intake to 2,300 milligrams of sodium daily—or, if you already have diabetes and therefore are at risk for high blood pressure, no more than 1,500 milligrams of sodium per day. That may look

SODIUM SLEUTH

Sodium chloride is what you call table salt. It is 40 percent sodium and 60 percent chloride. Sodium is a natural mineral also known as an electrolyte and is necessary for fluid balance in your body.

like a lot, but it's surprising how much hidden sodium lurks in the foods you eat every day. To help you keep your sodium under control, our rule of thumb is that entrées should have no more than 600 milligrams of sodium. Snacks and small meals should have no more than 400 milligrams. If you are eating three meals and three snacks, you need to reduce this even more, to about 400 milligrams per meal and snack. If you are eating three meals and

SATISFY YOUR SALT BUDS

Season with 'Shrooms

A good way to skip the saltshaker is to cook with mushrooms. Button mushrooms contain glutamic acid, which is an almost-sodium-free version of MSG (monosodium glutamate—the flavor enhancer found in many processed foods). In exchange for salting your food, season with 'shrooms for a dose of potassium, added texture, and of course, the salty flavor.

Substitute Spice

Another option to sidestep salt is to give your meal a kick of flavor. Chop up a variety of peppers to add hot spice and extra nutrition—the antioxidants vitamins A and C.[28]

Learn to Love Bitter Greens

Swiss chard and other dark bitter greens like beet greens naturally contain sodium, with as much as 300 milligrams per cup. Of course these flavorful leaves are nutritious, containing exceedingly high levels of vitamin A and even calcium. Bitter greens are not likely the culprit for your high blood pressure. Be sure to keep greens in your diet and instead focus on eating fewer processed and fast foods.[29]

THE LEAN PROTEIN AND FAVORED FAT CHEAT SHEET

Use the Lean Protein and Favored Fat Cheat Sheet as your new guide for grocery shopping, recipe modifications, and meal planning. This guide will make following the Diabetes Comfort Food Diet simple! It is ideal for recipes to contain sources of both or at least one favored fat: MUFAs and omega-3 fatty acids.

LEAN PROTEINS

Fish (shrimp, monkfish, tilapia)
White meat (skinless chicken, turkey)
Lean grass-fed beef (sirloin, round, and filet mignon)

Vegetable protein (tofu, lentils, and dried beans like lima beans, black beans, pinto beans, or split peas)

HEALTHY FATS—OMEGA-3 FATTY ACIDS AND MUFAS

OMEGA-3 FATTY ACIDS

Alpha-linolenic acid (ALA)—Eat daily

Canola oil	**Pumpkin seeds**
Chia seeds	**Flaxseeds**
Hemp seeds	**Walnuts**

Eicosapentaenoic acid (EPA) and docosahexaenoic acid (DHA)—Eat twice weekly

Salmon	**Cod**
Trout	**Bass**
Sardines	**Mackerel**
Tuna, chunk light canned in water, no added salt	**Bluefish**

MUFAS (MONOUNSATURATED FATTY ACIDS)—EAT DAILY

Olives

Avocados

Nuts (such as peanuts, almonds, cashews, and pecans)

Hummus (when possible, choose hummus without tahini)

Oils

- Olive oil is best used when cooking with low-to-medium heat.
- Canola oil is best used when cooking with medium-to-high heat.
- Coconut oil is not yet proven to be protective; limit use, if any.
- Peanut oil, specifically gourmet peanut oil, is okay, especially if cooking with high heat.
- Cold-pressed canola, peanut, and olive oils are great options.
- No vegetable oil or blends, as they are not specific to type or ratio of oils.

SATURATED FAT

Limit or eliminate.

Choose foods with labels showing 2 grams or less of saturated fat per serving.

If butter is used, there should be no added salt; preferably choose olive oil instead.

Avoid trans fat (partially hydrogenated oils).

Remove all visible fat.

Choose lean proteins that are low in saturated fat.

Limit whole and reduced-fat milk.

Choose low-fat dairy and yogurt with the exception of cheese.

Choose harder cheeses and use small quantities.

Change Your Recipes, Not Your Life

three snacks and already have diabetes, be sure to use 250 milligrams as your rule of thumb. Most importantly, do not use a saltshaker, and if you are eating processed foods, check the nutrition label. First, identify how many servings are in the package. Many times, processed foods such as a can of soup have 800 milligrams of sodium per serving but pack two servings per can. This means that if you ate all of the soup in the can, you would be taking in 1,600 milligrams of salt! That is an entire day's worth of sodium for someone with diabetes. See "Satisfy Your Salt Buds" (page 33) for three strategies to get a salty flavor without damaging your health.

MIX UP YOUR MEALS

Your plate needs to have a balance of carbohydrates (especially foods high in fiber), lean proteins, and healthy fats such as canola oil, nut butters, salmon, walnuts, and flaxseeds. You want to eat these foods together. Because fat and protein slow the absorption of sugar into the bloodstream, eating mixed meals containing carbohydrates, proteins, and fats is the ideal way to manage blood sugar, insulin resistance, and diabetes.

PLANNING, PREPPING, AND PLATING

The recipes in this cookbook are all designed to satisfy you as only your favorite comfort foods can—and to be absolutely healthy. But for real success, planning ahead for a week's worth of meals and snacks is highly recommended. This means choosing one day a week to write up a meal plan and grocery shop. When planning, think about how much time it will take to prep a recipe. Perhaps cutting the veggies the night before or buying precut vegetables will make your new lifestyle easier and your

goals attainable. Think about the little things as they add up to big change, such as weight loss.

Planning

Stock your pantry with healthy essentials like olive oil, canola oil, low-fat and low-salt chicken broth, olives canned in water, chunk light tuna with no added sodium, canned beans with no added salt, and whole grains like whole wheat pasta. Keep spray cans of canola oil and olive oil on hand at all times. White wine and lemon juice are other great staples for cooking and eating healthy with flavor. Olive oil, canola oil, chicken broth, wine, and lemon can all be great mediums for sautéing and stir-frying. Check out the chart on page 41 for a complete list of staples to keep in your pantry, fridge, and freezer.

FRESH IN THE FRIDGE

Always keep one dozen fresh eggs on hand. Use real eggs rather than egg substitutes with food colorings and other artificial ingredients. You can use egg whites, but recognize that your blood sugar will increase more than if you had just kept the fat, specifically the yolk. The yolk does contain saturated fat, but it is also a great source of nutrition, especially vitamin A, and helps to keep your blood sugar at bay, making it worthy of eating some of the

(continued on page 38)

....

CANOLA: THE HIGH-HEAT OIL

Use canola oil when stir-frying or sautéing over high heat. It has a higher smoke point and will not smoke as quickly as olive oil. Plus this means it will not become carcinogenic, since it is not burning.[30]

The Diabetes Comfort Food Diet

Make your life easy with this weekly meal planner. Use this chart as a guide to plan out your meals for the week. You can put x's in the box when you are planning to dine out.

		Sunday	Monday	Tuesday	Wednesday
Meals (include 45–60 g Carbs, Lean Protein, and Healthy Fat)	Breakfast		Yogurt 16c (90c) ½ egg 2 bac (sm)		
	Lunch		Plain turkey w/ hummus		
	Dinner				
Snacks (include 15–30 g Carbs, Lean Protein, and/or Healthy Fat)	Snack #1 (optional)		3 Almonds Grapes		
	Snack #2 (optional)				
	Snack #3 (optional)				
DAILY TOTALS: Tally your servings of these four food groups for each day	Fish Servings (2x/week)	○	○	○	○
	Low-Fat Dairy Servings (4x/day)	○ ○ ○ ○	○ ○ ○	○ ○ ○	○ ○ ○ ○
	Vegetable Servings (3x/day)	○ ○ ○	○ ○ ○	○ ○ ○	○ ○ ○
	Fruit Servings (2x/day)	○ ○	○ ○	○ ○	○ ○

Vitamins X

36

Change Your Recipes, Not Your Life

Thursday	Friday	Saturday
◯	◯	◯
◯ ◯ ◯ ◯	◯ ◯ ◯ ◯	◯ ◯ ◯ ◯
◯ ◯ ◯	◯ ◯ ◯	◯ ◯ ◯
◯ ◯	◯ ◯	◯ ◯

New Recipes to Try This Week (Pick 1 or 2)

Pantry Refills

Refrigerator Refills

Freezer Refills

time. If you choose to use the egg whites, incorporate a healthy fat such as avocado in that meal to attain a mixed meal. Keep grated Parmesan and other hard cheeses in the refrigerator. Harder cheeses are naturally lower in saturated fat and great for flavor with the added benefits of calcium. When reading the nutrition labels, you will notice that provolone is usually lower in saturated fat and calories in comparison to other cheeses, especially the soft cheeses. Always read nutrition labels, even if you think you know the product. Ingredients and nutrition facts are constantly changing and are different for every brand.

Prepping

Now that you have chosen your recipes and stocked your pantry, think about cooking methods. As mentioned previously, olive oil and canola oil are the healthy oils to cook with. Use canola oil when cooking over high heat and olive oil when making dressings or using low heat. Canola oil is best for baking, as olive oil's strong flavors may overwhelm a quick bread or cookie.

The best methods for cooking vegetables are steaming or sautéing in a broth with a little bit of olive or canola oil and lots of garlic. If you sauté in broth (or white wine or lemon juice), incorporate that broth into the dish to get the full dose of vitamins. Many foods contain water-soluble vitamins that are lost in the liquid cooking method. So use this nutritious broth. You can drizzle it over the meal, serve the vegetables in it, or moisten grains with it.

If you are cooking lean proteins, baking is the best option. You can also roast, broil, and barbecue. If roasting, use a roasting rack. Also, drain off fat. Remove poultry skin and even visible fats before roasting or cooking. The skin and fat add flavor but are very high in saturated fat. When broiling or barbecuing, be sure to use a lower heat/flame with some form of moisture, such as a broth, lemon juice, or marinade to prevent burning (also known as charring). The black char you see on a steak or grilled piece of chicken is carcinogenic, meaning it has cancer-causing properties. You will be able to avoid charring with the use of moisture and a lower heat.[31]

Plating

Did you know something as simple as the color of your plate or the size of your glass can affect how much you consume? Dr. Brian Wansink of the Cornell Food Lab studies food psychology. The research suggests creating color contrast on your plate helps you decrease the amount of food you eat.[32]

This means you should use a white plate for brightly colored foods like steak with mashed sweet potatoes and green bean casserole. These foods will contrast with the white plate, and you will likely serve yourself less food and feel just as full. Using a colored plate for starchy and neutral-colored foods like pasta and white potatoes will create a stark contrast, helping you to decrease your intake these of hard-to-portion foods. The reverse is true for veggies. If you want to increase your intake of vegetables, serve a salad in a green bowl so there is less contrast and you will be more likely to eat more of those leafy greens.

Dr. Wansink's research also finds that tall, thin glasses can decrease your fluid intake. For caloric beverages like wine, juice, and smoothies, this is the way to go! Conversely, use a short, wide glass for water. Most people don't get enough water, so drinking water from a short, wide glass can be a great way to help you drink more.

Plate size is also an easy way to keep portions and calories under control. Dr. Wansink's study found that eating off a 10-inch plate helped participants eat less than those who dined off a standard 12-inch dinner plate. Plus, even though they ate less overall, the small-plate group didn't feel deprived.

Your Own IRS—Internal Regulation System

Another helpful hint for managing meal portions without feeling overly restricted is to use a hunger/fullness scale. This scale weighs the internal thoughts and feelings guiding your portion choices. The Diabetes Comfort Food Diet automatically curbs the grams of carbohydrates per meal. However, the lean protein and the healthy fat quantities are less specific. You can individualize your grams of protein and fat based on your personal physical needs (whether you are male or female, how active you are, and how much weight you want to lose all play a role), allowing this to be a long-term nutrition plan. Using your hunger level to identify the physical need for food versus emotional and behavioral eating gives you options. Eating for physical reasons, paying attention to your hunger and fullness cues, and using smart diabetes-friendly recipes from this book will leave you feeling balanced, empowered, and free. This is your path to weight loss. If you realize you are eating for emotional reasons, such as stress or even happiness, or for behavioral reasons, such as social eating or mindless eating while watching TV, you can address the "why" and choose whether to continue eating or stop until your body is physically hungry for more food. Use your IRS to prevent the deprivation and binge cycle associated with diet-

ing and food restriction. Take this opportunity to free yourself from externally focused diets and learn to eat for fuel, and some pleasure, without causing harm to your blood sugar.

THE HUNGER/FULLNESS SCALE

Truly understanding your unique levels of hunger and fullness is a very important element in developing a balanced and intuitive eating lifestyle. A person who is accustomed to eating mindfully understands the body's cues that indicate hunger and fullness or the levels in between. When adults are allowed to make choices regarding their food portions without overt restriction and guilt, they can access their internal hunger/fullness feelings for the purpose of portion control. This is called internal self-regulation. Use this scale in conjunction with the Diabetes Comfort Food Diet as a tool to empower choice and mindfulness.

The zero-to-10 scale noted on the next page (zero is "Starving, Sweating, and Shaking" and 10 is "Sugar Shock" or "Stuffed Like a Turkey") provides a useful guide for learning your own body's signals. Though you shouldn't wait longer than 3 to 4 hours between meals, and about 2 to 3 hours for snacks, a rating of 3 or 4 on this scale will tell you for certain that it's time to eat. Stop before you feel too full, however—somewhere between 6 and 7.

Use this scale to help determine when to eat and how food makes you feel at each meal. If you find yourself starting to eat at a 5 or 6, assess whether you may be eating for boredom or emotional reasons. If you are always starting at a 1, notice if you finish at a 9. Use this tool to gain mindfulness and identify what foods keep you full for about 3 hours on average. This will be easier to implement when used in conjunction with the three steps for a meal makeover to beat diabetes.

INTERNAL REGULATION SYSTEM

This scale is subjective and may vary for each individual.

0. You're probably feeling unsteady and woozy and possibly faint. You are starving, sweating, and shaking. You may have skipped one or even two meals, or waited longer than 7 hours in between meals. You are now hypoglycemic, which means your blood sugar is too low.

1. You're past hungry—not to mention irritable, shaky, and light-headed.

2. You're very hungry—just short of actually feeling "starved." You needed to eat an hour ago.

3. You really want to eat. Your brain and stomach are telling you it is time to eat. Your last meal was 3 to 4 hours ago.

4. You're a little bit hungry, and your body is trying to tell you it's time for a meal. You feel your blood sugar start to drop.

5. You feel content. You are satisfied, physically fueled. You are not hungry but also not feeling full. You will probably need to eat in the next 1½ hours. Your blood sugar is hopefully back in normal range or about there.

6. You feel almost full. One or two more bites would equal fullness. Wait 10 minutes to check in and see if you need a few more bites.

7. You're feeling energized and sated. Now is a good time to push your plate away or stand up from the table and recognize your body has fueled itself. You probably won't need to eat for another 3 to 4 hours.

8. You've passed a comfortable fullness. You took one or two more bites. You feel a little pressure in your belly/abdomen area.

9. You feel uncomfortable. You're overfull and on the verge of being stuffed.

10. You're superuncomfortable with belly pain and belly pressure, and it feels like your stomach is stretching—think of how you usually feel after Thanksgiving dinner. You need to rest in order to digest. Your blood sugar has gone through the roof. Your vision may be blurry, you feel agitated from hyperglycemia (high blood sugar), and you are sweating.

Ideally your color-contrasted 10-inch plate will have 45 to 60 grams of fiber, filling carbohydrates, some lean proteins, and favored fats. Your hunger fullness scale is a new tool to help you eat mindfully while eliminating emotional and behavioral eating. Now that you have your lunch box filled with tools and food, you can start your nutritious journey to prevent or reverse diabetes in Chapter 3.

STOCK UP: SMART CHOICES FOR YOUR PANTRY, FRIDGE, AND FREEZER

These regular items are great to keep in your kitchen at all times so you can whip up diabetes-reversing dishes at a moment's notice.

PANTRY POWERHOUSES

Grains
- Quinoa
- Spelt
- Whole wheat flour
- Whole wheat pancake mix
- Stone-ground oats
- Wheat berries
- Buckwheat
- Bulgur wheat
- Cereals that have 30 grams of carbs per serving or fewer and 5 grams of fiber per serving or more (Kashi GOLEAN, Kashi Warm Cinnamon Oat Heart to Heart, and Old Wessex Ltd. All-Natural 100% Whole Grain Irish-Style Oatmeal)

Beans—Dry or canned with no added salt
- Black beans
- Kidney beans
- Lentils
- Chickpeas

Canned goods— With no added salt or sugar
- Chopped tomatoes
- Hearts of palm in water
- Artichokes in water
- Olives in water
- Mandarin oranges
- Tuna, chunk light, low sodium, in water
- Salmon, low sodium

Nuts and seeds— Roasted or raw, unsalted
- Almonds
- Peanuts
- Pecans
- Walnuts
- Natural nut butters such as peanut or almond butter
- Ground flaxseeds
- Chia seeds
- Wheat germ

Spices—No added salt
- Basil
- Black pepper
- Chile powder
- Cinnamon
- Cumin
- Dill weed
- Garlic powder
- Onion powder
- Oregano
- Paprika
- Rosemary
- Sage
- Tarragon

Condiments
- Balsamic vinegar
- Low-salt, low-fat chicken or vegetable broth
- Mustard
- Natural olive oil spray
- Natural canola oil spray
- Cold-pressed olive oil
- Cold-pressed canola oil

REFRIGERATOR REGULARS

Fruits
- Apples
- Avocados
- Lemons
- Limes
- Oranges

Vegetables
- Broccoli

- Carrot sticks or baby carrots
- Cauliflower
- Garlic
- Spaghetti squash
- Onion

Dairy
- Low-fat or fat-free Greek yogurt

- 1% milk
- Hard cheeses such as Parmesan, Romano, and Pecorino

Protein
- Fresh eggs
- Tofu (optional)

Other
- Seltzer

My Diabetes Success Story

Kori Smith, 36, could never lose weight and keep it off, no matter what she tried—whether it was Body for Life, Weight Watchers, or the South Beach Diet. "I wasn't able to transfer those ways of eating into real life," Kori says. But by curbing her carbs, increasing her fiber, and favoring healthy fats, she discovered a realistic lifestyle diet that was easy to maintain.

Kori, an assistant principal at a public elementary school, was frustrated and confused when she received her diagnosis of insulin resistance. She thought her mostly vegetarian food choices were healthy: pastas, beans, tofu, and low-fat dairy. She always chose fat-free dressings for her salads, while eating lots of beans and rice for adequate vegetarian protein.

Not only was Kori following a lower-fat diet, but she had exercised consistently since high school, through college, and now as a career woman. She cheered competitively, danced, and ran one marathon, one half-marathon, and multiple 10-Ks. She continues to work out at the local gym three or four times a week, varying between Spinning and Zumba class. "I knew I worked really hard, but my body wasn't a physical representation of that. It was all in my stomach. I always looked bloated. I was so frustrated."

Kori's diagnosis of insulin resistance came last year, quite by surprise. She and her husband had decided to start a family, and because she was over 35 years of age, her pregnancy would be considered high risk. Her doctor, therefore, ran a battery of tests. Before she was even able to try to conceive, Kori was diagnosed with insulin resistance. Subsequently, her doctor stressed the risks of gestational diabetes as well as type 2 diabetes. Kori quickly cut her carbs, but she was scared and felt deprived. She thought diabetes was a sure thing for her. "Once I was told I needed to change my diet, I was more scared than anything. I really did not know what the new rules were."

After consulting with me and trying the Diabetes Comfort Food Diet recommendations, Kori turned an important corner. She learned this was not a diet of deprivation, but rather one of choices. She learned she could still go out to dinner with her husband. What really hit home for Kori was the fact that she was losing weight for the first time in her life! "After those sessions, I felt I had a road map and tools in my belt. It was more empowering than anything. Seeing the weight come off was exciting, and realizing the impact certain foods had on how I felt was eye opening." For example, many foods that Kori had thought were healthy were actually driving her carbohydrate intake way up.

"I took for granted that my favorite foods were high in carbs, such as fat-free dressings and even fruit!" Kori had grown up eating tortillas, rice, and beans. Her grandfather was Mexican, and these carbohydrates were part of the family's culture. Even though she had given up red meat long ago, she had replaced it with low-fiber pastas and breads. Now Kori incorporates carbs that are naturally high in fiber, such as spouted whole grain breads, whole wheat pasta, barley, and quinoa. "I just make different choices. Like when we eat out at a Mexican restaurant, I don't eat the chips on the table and I skip the rice. I still have beans, and some sort of grilled chicken or tofu. I love guacamole! At other restaurants, I choose bread or wine, and I order fish or poultry and a vegetable."

Kori was finally able to connect the dots and recognize that her body was not able to handle such large loads of carbohydrates at each meal. Now, equipped with reliable nutrition knowledge and a positive outlook, she is making active steps toward preventing diabetes and losing weight. And she feels so much better. "I didn't know that changing my food would have such a dramatic effect on how I felt overall, especially my energy. There was no more after-meal bloating or stomach pain."

Not only did Kori feel suddenly energized, but she also dropped 22 pounds between May and July. Her clothing size shrank from a 12 to an 8. The belly bloating and belly fat were gone.

And most surprising for Kori, she could breathe easier—she had never even realized she had difficulty breathing until then. When she returned to her elementary school position in August, her fellow educators were as surprised as she had been. Her colleagues had not seen her during summer recess, and the changes in Kori's appearance and energy levels were quite obvious.

Using the three steps to make over any meal allowed Kori to tackle her insulin resistance easily. But the best part was yet to come—Kori became pregnant! Regulating her weight and hormones helped her to start a family and has helped prevent her from getting gestational diabetes. As of her 17-week appointment, her doctor had found no indicators of diabetes.

She is grateful for her supportive family and friends who refrain from making any comments about her opting to skip the pre-meal bread in exchange for a grain with dinner. Because she knows she must choose between the bread basket and dessert, Kori makes her meal choices before she even walks into a restaurant. She knows her decision to reverse her insulin resistance and prevent diabetes and gestational diabetes is a very worthy choice—one that has helped her to feel better than ever, to be in the best shape of her adult life, and to finally start her family.

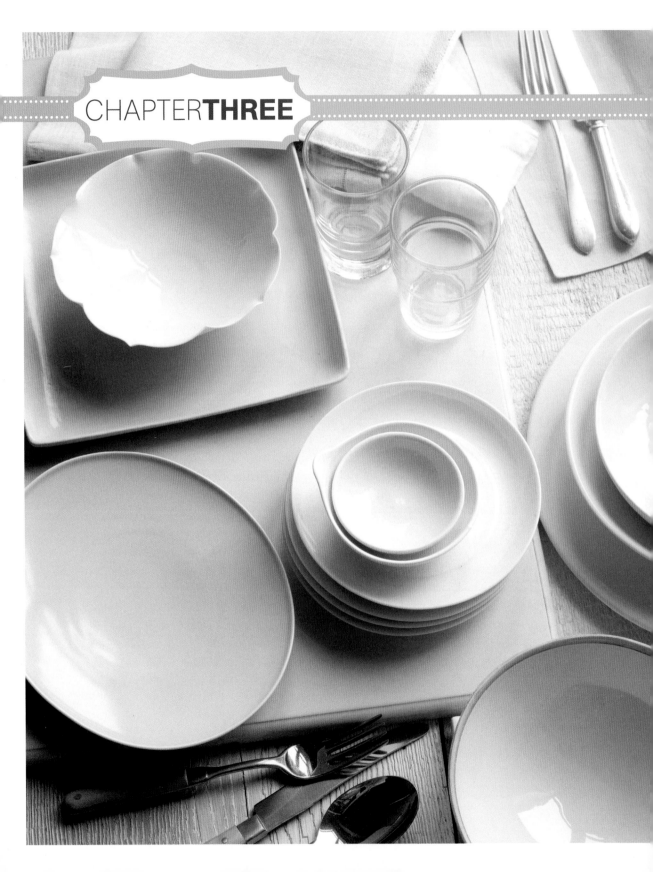

CHAPTER**THREE**

The Plan
to Defeat
Diabetes

Now you understand how blood sugar control works and you know the three essential steps to make over any meal—as well as the secrets to prepping, planning, and plating. Let's approach the action plan together so that you may implement your tools for dietary change to manage blood sugar, lose weight, and achieve long-term health. In Chapter 1, we introduced START. This five-stage plan is designed to help you make the lifestyle changes needed to avert diabetes and the risks associated with long-term insulin resistance.

Flip back to page 8, reread the descriptions, and figure out where you are on your journey, whether it is Shock, Tiptoeing, Achieving, Repeating, or Time. Remember that your nutrition goals will be tailored to your present stage. To make this system as easy to follow as possible, we have designed a five-step plan that is uniquely formulated to help you balance your blood sugar wherever you are. Recognize that some steps will naturally take longer than others; you may be beyond Shock, and perhaps at the Tiptoeing stage, which may take just a few days. But if moving from one stage to the next takes 6 months, that's normal too. Just focus on the action plans and move to the next step when you are ready. If you try to skip a stage, or start the next step before you have completed the previous stage, you run the risk of a "relapse"—returning to old thought patterns and behaviors that stand in the way of creating your very own diabetes success story.

Many readers will find they are ready to follow steps 2, 3, or even 4. The easiest way to figure out where you should start your action plan is to begin at "Step 1: Shock" and begin checking off every item on the action plan that you have accomplished. If you are missing three or more items, you must complete those exercises before moving on to the next step. Since everyone moves at his or her own rate, keep in mind that a step may take you 2 weeks or longer as you become accustomed to new routines and dietary changes. Remember: Don't rush to the next stage until you are ready. Moving too fast or skipping steps will backfire on you and make change seem harder than it really is! The goal is to be a success through consistent behaviors that ultimately become habits.

STEP 1: SHOCK

You are likely to identify with this stage if you have just learned you are at risk for prediabetes or have prediabetes or type 2 diabetes. Before you can start reversing your symptoms, you need time to absorb your new reality and truly consider the pros and cons of making lifestyle changes. You may find yourself looking for solutions that sound easier, like turning to medication, or wonder if you can get away with taking no actions at all. Give yourself permission to feel the anger, fear, and worry that you might be trying to push to the back of your mind. Don't turn to food now. Instead, grab a journal or write your answers below to release your emotions on paper. Here are some questions to ask yourself:

1. What were my first thoughts when the doctor told me I had prediabetes or diabetes? How did I feel and how do I feel now (possibly angry, mad, sad, or scared)? Why do I feel this? How can I cope with these feelings?

_____

_____

_____

_____

2. Did I exhibit signs of high blood sugar? (Check off the signs you felt.)

☐ Very thirsty   ☐ Sleepless   ☐ Other

☐ Sweaty after meals   ☐ Irritable

☐ Blurry vision   ☐ Lethargic

Do I understand why I wasn't feeling well?

☐ Yes   ☐ No

If Yes, write why.

If No, refer to www.diabetes.org

_____

_____

_____

3. What was I eating before that made me feel the symptoms above?

☐ Large portions (eating appetizers, entrées, and desserts when dining out)

☐ Sugary drinks (soda, smoothies)

☐ Fast food (hamburgers, fries)

☐ Restricting meals (during the day) and bingeing (during the evening)

☐ Skipping meals (brunch on weekends with no breakfast or lunch)

☐ High-carb meals without protein or fat

☐ Other

4. Am I ready to accept this diagnosis and make changes within the next week to the next 6 months? If yes, what changes seem possible?

_____

_____

_____

_____

5. Who will help me through this? (Identify who your support team may be. We will refer to this person as your "diabetes support person." Is it your spouse, partner, parent, sibling, or friend?)

☐ Spouse   ☐ Parent   ☐ Friend

☐ Partner   ☐ Sibling   ☐ Other

(continued)

6. What am I at risk for? See "Calculate Your Risk" on page 6.

_____

_____

_____

7. Identify education sources like the American Diabetes Association and magazines and books about diabetes.

_____

_____

_____

_____

8. What are three things I can easily change to be proactive without much effort? Scheduling my next doctor appointment? Reading this book from cover to cover? Can I ask my partner for help with the nutrition changes?

_____

_____

_____

_____

This is the time to talk and think. There is no expectation to make behavioral change this week. Your action plan is focused on getting in touch with your feelings, gathering education materials, starting to educate yourself, and getting inspired to make a change.

Your Action Plan This Week

- Identify what you are feeling and journal about these feelings to help address them. Is it denial, shock, anger, or sadness? Are you scared? See the sample journal on page 48.

- In your journal, make a list of pros and cons about making nutrition and exercise changes. To get started, look at the sample list on the opposite page.

- Find a support group at a local hospital or house of worship for individuals with diabe-

tes. Consider whether a mental health counselor may be useful in your acceptance of your new diagnosis of prediabetes or diabetes. Use this as an opportunity to understand and even embrace a diagnosis that you can prevent and reverse. Self-efficacy will favorably enable you to meet your soon-to-be lifestyle goals (nutrition and physical activity behaviors).

- Identify your support system and share with at least one person that you have diabetes.

- Observe how different foods make you feel (shaky, sweaty, energetic, tired, moody, content).

- Start to educate yourself about diabetes and the long list of complications that can arise, such as losing the ability to feel in your hands or feet. Visit www.diabetes.org for more information.

- Talk with your spouse and/or family about your diagnosis. Ask one person to attend doctor visits and diabetes education with you.

- Read Chapters 1 through 3 of this cookbook thoroughly, if you have yet to do so.

- Flip through the recipes in this cookbook. Make a mental note of a few you might like to try. Check out the sidebars to see how simple tweaking these foods for health can be!

- Think about what type of physical activity may be fun and not intimidating. Do you prefer to exercise alone or with others? Do you want to try a class at the local gym or do you prefer to be outside and move at your own pace?

- Read the stories of Rebecca (page 14), Kori (page 44), and Michael (page 60), who have successfully prevented diabetes and even lost weight. You can join them!

Pros vs. Cons: Preventing and Managing Diabetes through Nutrition and Exercise

Use this sample list to start generating your own pros and cons for committing to lifestyle changes that will prevent or reverse your diabetes.

Pros

- Manage blood sugar
- Prevent loss of vision, nerve, and kidney function
- Live longer
- Improve quality of life
- See the grandkids graduate
- Improve sex life
- Increase energy and endurance
- Positively affect cardiovascular health
- Reduce waist size
- Buy clothes more easily
- Be free from acid reflux
- Eat all food: Recipes in this book look comforting and delicious

Cons

- Planning meals in advance
- Drinking alcohol only with meals
- Finding time to move
- Reading nutrition labels
- Eating out sounds like a disaster
- Telling friends
- Feeling overwhelmed
- Needing medicine

STEP 2: **TIPTOEING**

After making your list of pros and cons, you have come to the conclusion that you must make changes for the better. *I need to change if I want to see my children or grandchildren graduate*, you may be thinking. Or perhaps learning you may lose sensations in your extremities was convincing enough. No matter your driving motivation, you have accepted that you will need to make dietary changes. You are feeling ready to start now but not necessarily 100 percent committed to the process. You aren't even 100 percent sure of what your process will look like.

You are willing to try the new high-fiber cereal your spouse purchased for you. You try it with an open mind. It tastes good, and you observe yourself feeling better after eating it. No lethargy, and you stay full until lunchtime. However, the next day the pancakes at the diner call louder than the high-fiber cereal. Or maybe you consider going to the gym for the second time since becoming a member 6 months ago. Your sore muscles prevented you from going back last time. This time, you plan to walk for 5 minutes on the treadmill and then hit the steam room for another 10 minutes. By planning for a gradual start to your nutrition and fitness routine, you understand you'll be more likely to achieve your goals and continue with them.

You are realizing that small, consistent change is better than no change or one big change that is so unrealistic you cannot commit.

Your Action Plan This Week

- Look back at your list of cons from last week. Create a mini action plan that will help you

turn those negatives into positives! Look at page 54 for some examples.

- Attend a support group if you are feeling overwhelmed or alone. If a support group doesn't feel sufficient, you may want to consider counseling. Reread individuals' success stories for beating diabetes. Think about how realistic this is for you.

- Decide which activity you will pursue and plan for one lifestyle modification such as taking the stairs or parking your car farther from the mall. Choose a physical activity that is realistic to pursue and decide when you can start this. We suggest starting with small movement goals and working up to regular activity. (Example: Walk for 5 minutes after dinner three nights this week, and move up to 10 minutes next week.) Decide if you prefer to be active alone or would rather identify exercise buddies.

- Draw up a food log in your journal or create one on your computer. Use it twice this week. If you have a glucometer (a device to measure your blood sugar from your doctor), you can add a section to log your blood sugar in mg/dl before and after meals. See page 54 for a sample food log you can copy.

- Reread Chapter 2 of this book. Highlight the things you can easily do. You do not need to do all of them now, but use this as a time to recognize what changes you can easily make. Choose two or three small goals for this week—perhaps to eat whole wheat pasta and use only olive oil–based salad dressing. The three main changes you can get ready to make are based on our three meal makeover guide-lines. If you feel able, choose one of these three to start pursuing.

1. **Curb carbs** at 45 grams per meal (if you are a woman) or 60 grams per meal (if you are a man) and determine whether you need zero, one, two, or three snacks a day (equal to 15 or 30 grams of carbs per snack depending on if you are a woman or a man). Reading food labels and identifying total grams of carbohydrates per serving in the foods you usually eat can help you to easily achieve this. Don't forget to make sure you identify how many servings you are really consuming. Food labels always provide information for one serving—but many foods have multiple servings per package.

2. **Fill up on fiber** and aim for 22 to 40 grams of total dietary fiber per day. You can achieve this goal the same way you count carbs—by reading food labels. But instead of looking at the carbohydrates, add up the dietary fiber. Remember: If your meal contains 6 or more grams of dietary fiber, you can subtract this amount of fiber from the total carbs of that meal.

3. **Favor healthy fats** such as the MUFAs and omega-3 fatty acids. You can find MUFAs in olive oil, canola oil, avocados, natural peanut butter, and many varieties of nuts and seeds. Vegetarian sources of omega-3 fatty acids include chia seeds, pumpkin seeds, and walnuts. Marine sources include salmon, trout, canned chunk light tuna, and bluefish.

- Begin developing mindfulness. Become aware of why you eat, whether due to physical hunger, emotional hunger, or behavioral hunger. Discerning why you eat will help you curb your overall intake of calories and help you learn to eat only when you are truly hungry. You can make notes about your motivation for eating on your food log as well.

- Check your pantry to see what foods you have and identify which items you should remove or begin to replace. Following are simple ways to start.

- Replace white bread with whole grains.

- Replace vegetable oil with olive and canola oils.

- Note how many grams of carbohydrates and fiber are in your cereals. Aim for brands with fewer than 30 grams of carbs but 5 or more grams of dietary fiber.

- Go food shopping with your spouse or diabetes support person. Stroll the aisles to see if there are new-to-you naturally high-fiber products like stone-ground wheat bread or cocoa-powdered almonds that you may want to try. Buy two or three new products to try.

- If you don't already have them at home, buy new dinner plates and glassware. Six 10-inch white plates and six 10-inch colored plates will be enough, plus a set of tall, thin glasses (for caloric beverages) and short, wide glasses (for water).

- Identify foods that might raise your blood sugar. Are you willing to modify certain ingredients, cooking techniques, or portion sizes to lessen the impact?

- Identify whether you need kitchen utensils or cooking tools to help you make new dietary changes.

  Chef knife

  Cutting board

  Can opener

  Garlic press

  Nonstick sauté pan

  Spatula

  Vegetable peeler

  Vegetable scrubber

  Whisk

Convert Your Cons into Pros

Con #1: Planning Meals in Advance → Pro:

- This is an excuse to try new recipes.
- You get to enjoy comfort food without the guilt—or the blood sugar spikes.
- You always know what you're eating.

Take Action: Spend 1 hour on Sunday planning meals with your diabetes support person; choose two recipes from this book to try.

Con #2: Drinking Alcohol Only with Meals → Pro:

- You can still enjoy a glass of beer or wine.
- When socializing, you don't have to feel like a stick-in-the-mud.

Take Action: Schedule "Sunday football beers" after a 10-minute walk at lunchtime; perhaps walk to the local bar in town, eat lunch, and enjoy a beer while watching football with friends.

Con #3: Finding Time to Move → Pro:

- You will start to feel energized.
- You may increase your muscle mass and will likely whittle your waistline.
- You get built-in time for yourself.
- You'll help your heart.
- You'll become a positive role model for your family.

Take Action: Start with 5-minute walks twice a week wearing your day clothes. Take the stairs at work. Research the cost of a gym membership or a personal trainer. Buy walking sneakers and consider a heart rate monitor.

Con #4: Reading Nutrition Labels → Pro:

- You'll become nutrition savvy.
- Soon you'll know what products are not only healthy but taste good. You can use the cheat sheets from this book!
- Even if you buy the wrong product, with the help of this book you know all foods fit, so you can still work them into your diet.

Take Action: Start by comparing the labels of pasta at the grocery store and choose the pasta with the most fiber. Make a note to compare carbs, fiber, and saturated fat on labels in the future.

Con #5: Eating Out Sounds like a Disaster → Pro:

- You can still dine out—many restaurants have diabetes-friendly options or can tailor menu items to your order.
- You can still have dessert and alcohol and enjoy your favorite foods in moderation.

Take Action: Go online to read the nutrition facts of your favorite meals at local restaurants (most chains make this available). Figure out how to make this meal fall into the range of 45 to 60 grams of carbohydrates.

Con #6: Telling Friends → Pro:

- You can tell others in your own time. Since you can still eat all foods, you won't automatically "out" yourself when dining with friends.

- You don't need to tell everyone, but we encourage you to confide in at least one person.

- If you decide to share with more people, you may find others who are also managing diabetes and you may have a greater support network.

Take Action: Expand your support network by sharing your diagnosis with your good friends with whom you dine out. Decrease triggers by requesting that bread not be served at the table so you can save your carbs for later, or order wine by the glass rather than the bottle.

Con #7: Feeling Overwhelmed → Pro:

- Using START and the many tools in this cookbook will make managing blood sugar easy—one step at a time.

- You will feel and look better.

- You can reverse prediabetes and prevent insulin resistance from progressing.

Take Action: Photocopy "The Lean Protein and Favored Fat Cheat Sheet" (page 34) and take it to the grocery store with you. Spend time talking with your support person.

STEP 3: **ACHIEVING**

You are committing yourself to change. You accept your diagnosis of prediabetes or type 2 diabetes. You feel empowered and know the new foods and recipes you've tried were not only edible, but also delicious. You realize that walking two times a week for 5 minutes is not only doable, but you want to move even more. You are taking advantage of your support system and you are ready to start curbing carbs when dining out. You are getting used to drinking water and seltzer (calorie free, sugar free) and natural beverage options. It's easier to replace the saltshaker with your own herbal mix to flavor your food (consider mixing oregano, basil, garlic, and lemon peel). Health, longevity, and a higher quality of life now seem attainable.

Your Action Plan This Week

- Talk to your doctor and consider getting a glucometer to see how food and exercise affect your blood sugar. This can be a turning point for some people. The glucometer measures your blood sugar in mg/dl. When you are ready, take your blood sugar immediately before eating and 2 hours after. Notice how each food and the combination of foods, especially mixed meals, affect your blood sugar and your mood.

- Curb carbs at 45 or 60 grams per meal. If you require one or more snacks per day, prepare some snacks with either 15 or 30 grams of carbs and carry them with you. See page 57 for "20 Grab-and-Go Snacks."

- Fill up on fiber and aim for 22 to 40 grams of total dietary fiber per day. Remember: If your meal contains 6 or more grams of dietary fiber, you can subtract this amount of fiber from the total carbs of that meal. Increase your fiber consumption slowly, as too much fiber too quickly can cause constipation and gas. Increase your water consumption when increasing fiber to prevent constipation. Add one glass more per day than usual.

The Diabetes Comfort Food Diet

Use this sample as a guide in logging your food and exercise. You can customize it with the number of snacks you eat and columns to track your blood glucose numbers if you have a glucometer. Be sure to note the time and location of your meals, how hungry you felt before and after eating, and your motivation for eating (was it physical hunger [P], emotional eating [E], or a behavioral response [B]?). There are also columns to note what you ate, how many grams of carbs and fiber those meals included, and whether there were healthy fats such as MUFAs and omega-3 fatty acids in your meals. At the bottom, there is

Today's Date		Time and Location	Hunger Scale Rating (0–10) (page 54)		Why Are You Eating? (P, E, B)	Foods/Calories Eaten
			Before	After		
	Breakfast					
	Snack #1 (optional)					
	Lunch					
	Snack #2 (optional)					
	Dinner					
	Snack #3 (optional)					
DAILY TOTALS		Calories _____ Carbs _____ g Fiber _____ g				
DAILY EXERCISE:						

The Plan to Defeat Diabetes

a place to tally up your daily total calories, carbs, fiber, protein, fat, and sodium intake. For blood sugar control, you'll absolutely want to track calories, carbs, and fiber—but the rest is optional and may be helpful if you are also tracking a weight-loss goal. Finally, at the bottom, you'll see a place to note your daily movement. Whether it is a 5-minute walk or a Pilates class, be sure to note the time and location, since you may see a correlation between your activity and your blood glucose numbers. We have left room for three separate entries over the course of 1 day.

Carbs (G)	Fiber (G)	Did You Include Healthy Fats (G)?	Pre-Meal Blood Glucose (Optional)	2-Hour Post-Meal Blood Glucose (Optional)

Protein _____ g   Fat _____ g   Sodium _____ mg

- Favor healthy fats such as the MUFAs and omega-3 fatty acids. Cut down on your saturated fat intake by eating lean protein and low-fat dairy and limiting fried foods. Use your IRS (internal regulation system) to aid in portion control of proteins and fats. Include fish two times a week.

- Replace soda, energy drinks, and other high-calorie beverages with seltzer and water.

- Rehab your pantry and refrigerator. Toss out or donate the rest of the tempting carb- and sugar-laden foods like cookies, crackers, and chips that are hard to portion. Stock eggs, hard cheeses, and fat-free Greek yogurt (plain or fruit flavored). Fill your cupboard and fridge with the suggestions on page 41.

- Plan a full week's worth of meals and snacks at the beginning of the week (see our sample meal plan in Appendix A on page 328). Follow it up with food shopping and any other prepping that will make cooking during the week quicker and easier. Refill any needed pantry essentials such as cinnamon, canola oil spray, and canned tuna.

- Plan to eat breakfast at home. You can dine out for lunch one or two times a week and pack your lunch the rest of the week. Prepare dinners 5 days a week and dine out a maximum of two times a week.

- Keep a food log for 3 to 7 days this week. Include your food, feelings, hunger/fullness ratings before and after meals, and your blood sugar, if you have a glucometer.

- Walk or move for 10 minutes per day, three times per week. Increase by 5 minutes per workout every week until you achieve 30 minutes of walking or physical activity per day. Each week, add 1 additional day of movement until you have achieved 90 to 150 minutes of movement a day.

- Schedule a doctor's visit 3 months from the day you started making nutrition changes to check your A1C.

- Plan a healthy potluck party and invite your guests.

- If you decide to weigh yourself, weigh one time a week or less and monitor for a trend. The goal is 7 percent weight loss. Be sure to weigh yourself at the same time every time: in the morning, after going to the bathroom, and before breakfast. We recommend weighing every Wednesday.

- If mindless munching is a problem you struggle with, carry an action plan in your wallet to prevent yourself from eating for nonphysical reasons. See the sample on page 60.

- Use your new dishes and glasses regularly. Eat colorful foods on the white plates and eat white and beige foods on the colorful plates. Drink water from short, wide glasses and drink caloric beverages from tall, narrow glasses.

Combat Mindless Eating

During this week, you should focus on becoming more aware of the habits that undermine your dieting success. Through journaling the past 2 weeks, you are becoming more mindful of your old, counterproductive habits and able to recognize when you eat for emotional and behavioral reasons instead of physical hunger. Design an action plan to

20 GRAB-AND-GO SNACKS

These snacks are great to pack if you're going to be away from home. Make a copy of this list and keep it close by for a quick and easy reference.

FOR WOMEN (~15 GRAMS OF CARBOHYDRATES)

- 6 ounces Greek yogurt, fat free, fruit flavored
- 6 ounces Greek yogurt, fat free, plain, topped with one small cookie
- 1 mini cheese round and 1 cup berries
- 1 part-skim cheese stick and a 4-ounce apple
- Higher-fiber, lower-carb, higher-protein bar (~5 grams fiber, 15 grams carbs, 7 to 14 grams protein); e.g., Almond Blueberry Zing bar and Gnu bar, all varieties
- 10 to 23 almonds and ½ large orange
- 2 teaspoons natural nut butter and 1 small banana
- 4 ounces low-sodium, low-fat cottage cheese and ¾ cup fresh pineapple
- 10 to 15 olives and five 1-ounce high-fiber crackers (size of a Wheat Thin)
- 2 tablespoons guacamole and ½ toasted whole wheat pita

FOR MEN (~30 GRAMS OF CARBOHYDRATES)

- 6 ounces Greek yogurt, fat free, fruit flavored, mixed with ½ cup berries and 1 tablespoon wheat germ
- 6 ounces Greek yogurt, fat free, plain, with 1 small apple and ½ cup berries
- 1 to 2 ounces (slices) hard cheese, 15 grapes, and 1 slice sprouted wheat toast
- 8 ounces unsweetened soy or sunflower milk with a 1.5-ounce mini cupcake (sometimes)
- 15 to 25 almonds with 1 large orange
- 2 teaspoons natural nut butter and 1 banana
- ¼ cup hummus, 1 cup carrots, and ¾ whole wheat/spelt pita, toasted and cut into triangles
- ¼ cup hummus and 20 to 25 (1.5 ounces) whole grain pretzels
- 1 granola bar (6 grams fiber, 25 to 28 grams carbs, 10 to 14 grams protein or healthy fats); e.g., Kind bars, Lärabars, and/or Zing bars
- ¼ cup guacamole with ~10 to 15 (1.5 ounces) low-sodium baked tortilla chips and 1 cup carrot sticks for dipping

My Diabetes Success Story

At age 59, Michael Sears* was shocked to learn he had prediabetes. In fact, with a fasting glucose of 124 mg/dl and an A1C of 6.4, he was bordering on a clinical diagnosis of diabetes.

"I knew I had a genetic predisposition to diabetes, but I did not think I would be facing diabetes or even prediabetes in my late fifties," he says. "My father has type 2 diabetes, but he is 89 years old."

When Michael first visited my office in May of 2012, I too was quite shocked by his diagnosis. He was a rather tall and thin man, though he did hold extra weight in his midsection, well disguised by his dress shirt, and had very little muscle, as he had started exercising only recently.

Michael's troubles started about 7 years ago, when he was diagnosed with high cholesterol. As an engineer, he would often work long hours under consistently high levels of stress. Finding time for exercise was hard enough, but eating regularly was even harder. He was skipping breakfast and eating lunch at his desk—if he was even lucky enough to find the time to eat lunch. When he wasn't traveling for work, Michael would eat dinner with his wife and teenage daughters, but dinner was usually late, around 8 p.m., and consisted of starchy dishes like pasta with sauce or chicken with white rice and vegetables.

Once he received his cholesterol diagnosis, Michael made diet changes, including decreasing red meat and butter. He was also put on cholesterol medication. While being treated for high cholesterol, he was also diagnosed with

high blood pressure. In addition to putting him on blood pressure medication, Michael's doctor advised him to lose weight and to exercise. In "type A" fashion, Michael did as his doctor recommended. He joined a gym next to his office and hired a personal trainer for two weekly sessions of weight training. He was seeing his doctor every 4 months to keep an eye on his blood pressure, when the doctor gave him more bad news—a diagnosis of prediabetes.

Michael was surprised and saddened, having thought he was doing everything right. He had been exercising twice a week for the past year and had even lost 11 pounds. However, he realized he still didn't feel "normal"—having mental fogginess, sleeping poorly, and making frequent trips to the bathroom at night. Plus, he experienced daily fatigue.

It was at this point that Michael came to see me. During his first nutrition session, he realized he was doing all the wrong things with his carbs. Rather than curbing carbs, he had mistakenly been increasing them by drinking fat-free smoothies and bingeing on fruit for nighttime snacks. With the tenets of the Diabetes Comfort Food Diet in hand, Michael left the nutrition session feeling ready to reverse prediabetes—and he has been quite successful! Over the course of about 6 months, he lost 5 more pounds and his blood sugar has really improved. His A1C gradually dropped from 6.4 in May 2012 to 6.0 in December of 2012. He is finally sleeping through the night, feels more energized during the day, and eats breakfast every morning.

The Plan to Defeat Diabetes

The easiest part of his new lifestyle was learning to incorporate three meals and three snacks daily. He has maintained this routine since his first day of dietary changes. He says this is especially easy at the office, where he keeps granola bars in his desk drawer for daily snacks. A typical day's meals may include a fat-free Greek yogurt with a piece of fruit for breakfast, a granola bar for a morning snack, a turkey sandwich on whole wheat bread and another piece of fruit for lunch, nuts or another bar for the afternoon snack, and then wild rice, veggies, and a lean protein such as fish or chicken for dinner. And he still enjoys a cookie every day as part of his carbohydrate intake.

Michael's greatest challenge has been curbing carbs on evenings and weekends, which often involve dining at restaurants and socializing with family and friends. The lack of structure throws his meal pattern off. Plus, since he and his family get home late, Michael is hungry and usually eats his dinner carbohydrates before dinner is even served. Many nights he just eats pasta for dinner, as it is easy and fast. Another challenge is adding in more exercise. He already does weight training twice a week and has added in one weekly run. Though this already meets the 150-minute exercise recommendation, he needs to increase his cardio routine—especially if he wants to lose more weight.

During Michael's most recent nutrition appointment, he set new goals to overcome some of his daily challenges.

1. **Vary afternoon snacks and incorporate a protein and a fat.** For example: ¼ cup hummus with 5 Ak-Mak crackers (1 ounce) and 1 cup carrots or 1 to 2 tablespoons natural, salt-free peanut butter on 2 pieces of Ezekiel bread.
2. **Eat mixed meals, especially at dinner.** Make grilled chicken breasts ahead of time on Sunday to add to dinners later in the week that are typically just carbs, such as pasta.
3. **Increase fiber.** Include carrots in the afternoon snack and change to whole wheat pasta or sprouted wheat pasta.
4. **Increase cardio to twice a week.** Change gym memberships to allow exercise near home on the weekends and add one Spinning class per weekend in addition to one weekly run.
5. **Skip the entrée carbohydrate when dining at restaurants on weekends.** By avoiding the baked potato with his steak, he'll leave the 60 grams of carbohydrate for a dessert choice after his meal.

Michael has made many changes and continues to make many more. He is happy to share that not only has his overall blood sugar improved, but his clothes fit better and he has dropped a pants size from 38 to 36. His wife notices his more muscular physique, and his whole family says that he just looks better.

"I am feeling better," he says. "I have a better mood, greater stamina, and I am less tired."

*A pseudonym has been used at the request of the client.

TAKE ACTION TO COMBAT MINDLESS EATING

1. Journal your feelings.
2. Get out of the house and walk to decrease anxiety.
3. Distract yourself by engaging in a hobby, such as playing games, listening to music, or going for a run.
4. Call a friend.
5. Tap into a creative outlet such as painting, drawing, knitting, or woodworking.

combat mindless eating or even binge eating. This list of alternatives will protect you from sabotaging your healthy efforts and can even help to improve social bonds or channel your energy to be productive. Above is a sample action plan to guide you in creating your own.

STEP 4: **REPEATING**

You are now a "doer." You are implementing your new behaviors. You are action oriented. This is one of the busiest stages, when you are incorporating the new behaviors encouraged in these chapters, such as food shopping, prepping, cooking, and eating. You are curbing carbs, increasing fiber, and choosing healthy fats. This is where you start to see results. The process starts to feel effortless and automatic.

By now, you are probably feeling pretty good! You likely have more energy, have even moods throughout the day, and are opening up your palate to a world of exciting new foods. You have learned that eating out is manageable—and that there's room for dessert! The Diabetes Comfort Food Diet is now a lifestyle. This is your present and your future. You may or may not have lost weight. Even if you have not lost weight, your after-meal blood sugars are decreasing! There are no ups and downs or constant highs when you test your blood sugar. If you don't test, don't worry. You can feel the difference in your blood sugar as evidenced by better moods, sleeping through the night, increased energy and productivity at work, and lessening of other symptoms that bothered you before you got your blood sugar under control. By your next blood test, don't be surprised if your A1C has decreased to less than 5.7—meaning you no longer have prediabetes. If you already have diabetes, I'll bet your A1C has decreased since your last appointment and you are managing your blood sugar typically to less than 140 to 160 mg/dl 2 hours after meals or even better.

Curbing carbs, filling up on fiber, and favoring fats is your prescription for inner and outer well-being. The foods you eat, the portions you choose, and your new body awareness are all habits now. These habits are relatively new and still need to be reinforced by continuing to reduce temptations and triggers.

Your Action Plan This Week

- Plan a full week's worth of meals and snacks at the beginning of the week (if you need inspiration, see our sample meal plan on page 328). Follow it up with food shopping and any other prepping that will make cooking during the week quicker and easier. Refill any needed pantry essentials such as cinnamon, canola oil spray, and canned tuna.

- Keep a food log for 3 to 5 days this week. Include your food, feelings, hunger/fullness ratings before and after meals, and your blood sugar, if you have a glucometer.

- If you are keeping track of your weight, weigh in weekly. Remember to weigh yourself at the same time every day, in the morning, after going to the bathroom, and before breakfast.

- If mindless munching is a problem you struggle with, carry an action plan in your wallet to prevent yourself from eating for nonphysical reasons.

- Prepare some snacks designed to have either 15 or 30 grams of carbs and carry them along with you.

- Use your IRS (internal regulation system) to aid in portion control of proteins and fats.

- Gather friends and host healthy potluck parties. Host the first one this Saturday night to set the tone. Impress your guests with the recipes from this book.

20 Ways to Reinforce the Diabetes Comfort Food Diet

1. Meet friends for exercise, not food.
2. Host a healthy dinner party weekly or monthly.
3. Make your carbohydrate choice *before* going to restaurants.
4. Eat 45 to 60 grams of carbohydrates at each meal, three times a day.
5. Continue to use the magic carb solution. If your meal totals more than 6 grams of fiber, subtract the total grams of fiber from total grams of carbohydrates to get your magic number at each meal.
6. Do not skip meals.
7. Recognize if you need snacks and plan accordingly.
8. Food shop at markets that offer wholesome foods, such as a farmers' market or local health food store.
9. Include healthy fats (such as avocado and olive oil) daily.
10. Eat fish two or more times a week. Select a different type of fish each week to minimize exposure to mercury and PCBs.
11. Purchase food items with less than 2 grams of saturated fat and 0 grams of trans fat per serving.
12. Use coping skills rather than emotional eating. (You can review those skills on page 54.)
13. Plan ahead when you want to include sweets or refined carbohydrates. There is no cheating on the Diabetes Comfort Food Diet—all you have to do is make trade-offs and be careful about your timing.

14. If you have been tracking your blood sugar with a glucometer, continue using it to gauge response to various foods and activities as needed.

15. Remember: Small changes are better than no changes, and small steps are better than no steps. If you can't get to the food store or the gym, look at this as an opportunity rather than a failure. You can choose a take-out food that meets your grams of carbohydrates, and you can break your 30 minutes of physical activity into three 10-minute increments—or just exercise on a different day.

16. Try at least one new recipe from *The Diabetes Comfort Food Diet Cookbook* per week for variety and adequate nutrition.

17. Continue eating all breakfasts at home, and dine out one or two times a week each for lunch and dinner.

18. Continue moving for 90 to 150 minutes a week, doing activities you love.

19. Continue to use "The Lean Protein and Favored Fat Cheat Sheet" (page 34) when grocery shopping.

20. Stay in touch with how you are feeling. If you've been maintaining a food log and feel that your new behaviors are now habits, you can choose to log less often.

STEP 5: TIME

This is your maintenance phase. You have made your lifestyle changes, and they are now healthy habits.

You can declare maintenance after you have implemented your new behaviors for greater than 6 months or up to 1 year. Following the Diabetes Comfort Food Diet has become your way of life. You love the foods you choose and feel proud knowing you have defeated diabetes by curbing carbs, filling up on fiber, and favoring the right fats to ultimately manage your blood sugar. Money is spent on food and fitness (and maybe new clothes in smaller sizes!) rather than over-the-counter gastrointestinal medicines, prescriptions, and junk food.

The 20 Ways to Reinforce the Diabetes Comfort Food Diet (page 61) have become second nature. Choosing to eat 45 grams of cake for dessert and forgoing a carbohydrate with the main meal is easy and enjoyable for you. You realize this diet is about making choices, not about deprivation. You feel empowered, successful, and beautiful. Diabetes no longer scares you. Going forward, you have this book for support and a constant reminder of what you can do rather than what you can't do.

Seven Guidelines for Maintaining the Diabetes Comfort Food Diet

1. Curb carbs at 45 grams per meal three times a day for women or 60 grams for men. Enjoy up to three snacks of 15 grams of carbs per day for women or 30 grams for men.

2. Fill up on fiber by choosing whole grains, legumes, vegetables, fruits, and even whole nuts and seeds.

3. Favor healthy fats found in nuts, seeds, oils, deep-sea fish, and other sources.

4. Continue to increase physical activity until you are moving for 30 minutes per day, 5 days per week.

5. If you have met a goal of losing 7 percent of your weight, your new goal is to keep off 5 percent. (If you haven't lost weight, don't worry as long as your blood glucose is normalized.)

6. Continue to use your IRS (internal regulation system) to aid in portion control of proteins and fats.

7. Continue regular doctor visits to monitor your A1C, fasting plasma glucose, and other markers for diabetes.

CHAPTER**FOUR**

Breakfast

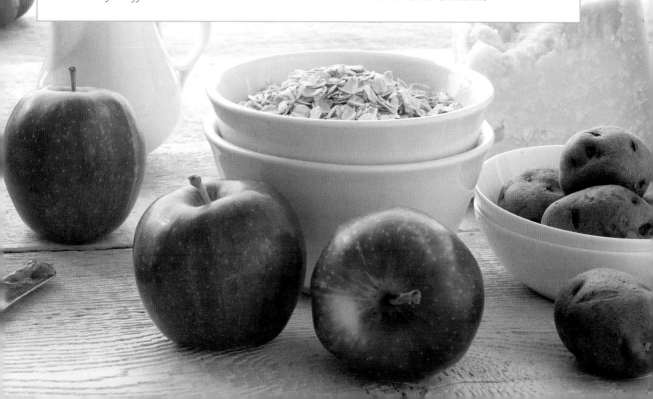

Makeover Magic

BEFORE		AFTER
318	CALORIES	226
20 g	FAT	16 g
7 g	SAT FAT	3 g
3 g	CARBS	5 g
1 g	FIBER	2 g
31 g	PROTEIN	17 g
596 mg	SODIUM	232 mg

Curb carbs: This dish is naturally low in carbs, so be sure to add some black beans and rice or a whole grain tortilla with 20 to 25 grams of carbs.

Fill up on fiber: The fiber in this recipe must come from your black beans or your whole grain wrap. You can get fiber only from carbohydrates, so put aside guilt and meet your 45 to 60 grams of carbs per meal.

Favor fats: Canola oil is a great source of both healthy fats, omega-3s, and MUFAs. You can add 2 tablespoons of avocado to this dish for even more MUFA power.

GRILLED STEAK AND EGGS

PREP TIME: **5 MINUTES** ■ TOTAL TIME: **25 MINUTES**

Makes 4 servings

2 tablespoons Worcestershire sauce

½ teaspoon paprika

¼ teaspoon salt-free onion powder

¼ teaspoon ground black pepper

8 ounces sirloin steak

2 teaspoons + 2 tablespoons canola oil

16 cups fresh spinach

4 eggs

1. In a small bowl, combine the Worcestershire sauce, paprika, onion powder, and pepper. Rub the mixture onto the steak.

2. In a grill pan, heat 1 teaspoon of the oil over medium-high heat. Grill the steak for 6 minutes, turning once, or until a thermometer inserted in the center registers 145°F for medium-rare. Let the steak rest for 10 minutes before slicing.

3. In a large skillet, heat 2 tablespoons of the oil over low heat. Cook the spinach for 1 minute or until it begins to wilt. Divide the spinach among 4 plates.

4. Heat the remaining 1 teaspoon oil in the skillet over medium-low heat. Crack the eggs into the skillet. Cook for 3 minutes, or until the egg whites are set. Serve with soft yolks, or cover and cook for 2 minutes or until the yolks are cooked through.

5. Place the egg on top of the spinach and serve with the sliced steak.

Breakfast

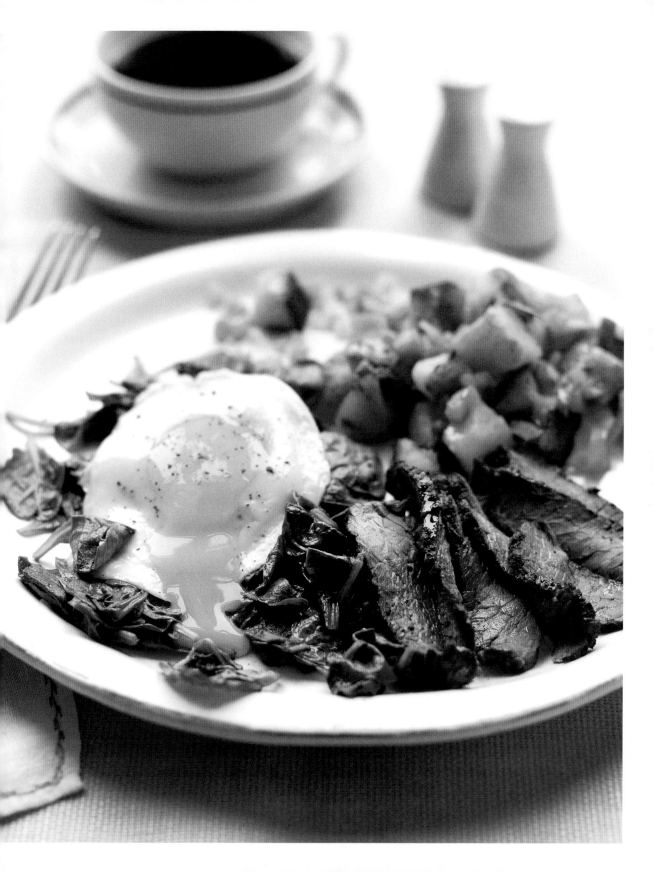

Makeover Magic

BEFORE		AFTER
840	CALORIES	322
39 g	FAT	12 g
13 g	SAT FAT	4 g
63 g	CARBS	29 g
5 g	FIBER	4 g
59 g	PROTEIN	24 g
1,205 mg	SODIUM	574 mg

Curb carbs: Choosing whole wheat 8" tortillas instead of a standard 10" white flour equivalent helps to curb carbs and balance your blood sugar.

Fill up on fiber: The whole wheat tortilla and spinach add fiber to keep you full.

Favor fats: Salmon is one of the best sources of DHA, the marine form of omega-3 fatty acids.

SALMON BREAKFAST BURRITO

PREP TIME: **5 MINUTES** ■ TOTAL TIME: **10 MINUTES**

Makes 4 servings

4 eggs

⅓ cup low-fat milk

1 cup spinach leaves, chopped

4 scallions, sliced

4 fat-free whole wheat tortillas (8" diameter)

8 ounces wild salmon, cooked and flaked into pieces

4 tablespoons crumbled feta cheese

1 teaspoon chopped fresh dill or ⅓ teaspoon dried

1. In a large bowl, whisk together the eggs, milk, spinach, and scallions.

2. Coat a nonstick skillet with cooking spray and heat over medium heat. Cook the egg mixture, stirring, for 2 minutes, or until scrambled and set.

3. Fill the tortillas with the eggs and salmon. Sprinkle with the cheese and dill. Fold the outer edges in and roll up.

SAYCHEESE

Cheese is a great source of protein, calcium, and vitamin D. The fat in cheese also helps to slow the breakdown of your breakfast meal and therefore aids in blood sugar balance.

CHEESY SCRAMBLED EGGS AND HAM

PREP TIME: **5 MINUTES** ■ TOTAL TIME: **10 MINUTES**

Makes 4 servings

4   whole eggs

8   egg whites

1   teaspoon canola oil

4   slices (4 ounces) low-sodium, nitrate-free, deli-style ham, cubed

1   green bell pepper, finely chopped

½   cup cherry tomatoes, chopped

4   tablespoons shredded Cheddar cheese

½   teaspoon ground black pepper (optional)

1. In a large bowl, whisk together the eggs and egg whites.

2. In a large nonstick skillet heat the oil over medium heat. Cook the ham, bell pepper, and tomatoes, stirring, for 2 minutes, or until the pepper pieces soften.

3. Add the eggs. Cook, stirring, for 2 minutes, or until the eggs are almost set. Stir in the cheese and black pepper, if using, and heat until set.

Makeover Magic

BEFORE		AFTER
383	CALORIES	178
33 g	FAT	9 g
17 g	SAT FAT	3 g
3 g	CARBS	4 g
1 g	FIBER	1 g
20 g	PROTEIN	20 g
594 mg	SODIUM	447 mg

Curb carbs: This breakfast is naturally low in carbohydrates, so go ahead and add a naturally wholesome slice or two of sprouted wheat bread.

Fill up on fiber: Green peppers and tomatoes are a great source of vitamin C and do add a bit of fiber. For the real fiber fill-up, be sure to accompany this yummy breakfast with your toast–ideally 3 grams of fiber per slice.

Favor fats: The canola oil in this recipe is a great source of monounsaturated fat, but since there is only a small amount, you can add 1 to 2 tablespoons of avocado to each serving to maximize MUFAs.

BEFORE		AFTER
340	CALORIES	283
19 g	FAT	8 g
8 g	SAT FAT	3 g
39 g	CARBS	35 g
1 g	FIBER	5 g
15 g	PROTEIN	21 g
590 mg	SODIUM	203 mg

Curb carbs: Substituting potatoes for the more typical biscuits in this dish reduces the carbs by 4 grams.

Fill up on fiber: The apples, onion, and potato skins all add fiber to this dish.

Favor fats: By combining whole eggs with egg whites, we can reduce the amount of saturated fat in this recipe.

APPLE, SAUSAGE, AND POTATO CASSEROLE

PREP TIME: **15 MINUTES** ■ TOTAL TIME: **1 HOUR 15 MINUTES + COOLING TIME**

Makes 6 servings

4 apples, cored and coarsely chopped

6 patties Homemade Breakfast Sausage (page 78), crumbled

2 red-skinned potatoes, cubed and steamed

1 yellow onion, chopped

¼ cup + 2 tablespoons shredded reduced-fat mild Cheddar cheese

2 cups 1% milk

4 whole eggs

4 egg whites

½ teaspoon dry mustard

¼ teaspoon ground black pepper

1. Preheat the oven to 375°F.

2. Coat a 2-quart (9" × 9") baking dish with cooking spray. Place the apples in a microwaveable bowl and cover. Microwave on high for 3 minutes. Uncover to cool.

3. In a medium nonstick skillet coated with cooking spray over medium-low heat, cook the sausage for 2 minutes, or until browned and cooked through.

4. Scatter the apples, sausage, potatoes, onion, and cheese in the bottom of the baking dish.

5. In a large bowl, whisk together the milk, eggs, egg whites, mustard, and pepper. Pour over the apple mixture in the baking dish. Bake for 50 minutes, or until a knife inserted in the center comes out clean. Let stand for 15 minutes and serve hot or warm.

SMARTSTART

Add salmon to this recipe for a source of omega-3 fatty acids.

GOOD MORNING "GRITS"

PREP TIME: **5 MINUTES** ■ TOTAL TIME: **10 MINUTES**

Makes 1 serving

3 tablespoons quinoa	¼ cup blackberries
¾ cup water	¼ teaspoon ground cinnamon

1. Combine the quinoa and water in a medium microwaveable bowl. Cover with vented plastic wrap or a loose lid and microwave on high for 3 minutes, stirring halfway through cooking. Reduce the power to 50% and microwave for another 4 minutes, or until the quinoa grains are tender.

2. Sprinkle with the berries and cinnamon.

Makeover Magic

BEFORE		AFTER
370	CALORIES	134
22 g	FAT	2 g
13 g	SAT FAT	0 g
33 g	CARBS	24 g
1 g	FIBER	4 g
11 g	PROTEIN	5 g
580 mg	SODIUM	588 mg

Curb carbs: Fresh fruit adds bulk and flavor to these "grits" without the added quantity of sugar that dried fruit such as raisins usually provides.

Fill up on fiber: While quinoa is higher in carbs than traditional grits, it's also higher in fiber and protein!

Favor fats: For a boost of omega-3s, sprinkle in some walnuts!

BEFORE		AFTER
347	CALORIES	121
39 g	FAT	3 g
13 g	SAT FAT	0.5 g
28 g	CARBS	23 g
1 g	FIBER	3 g
19 g	PROTEIN	3 g
1,257 mg	SODIUM	9 mg

Curb carbs: We added onions and peppers to our potatoes, creating a carbohydrate-friendly, portion-perfect side dish for Cheesy Scrambled Eggs and Ham (page 69) or another breakfast dish.

Fill up on fiber: They key to upping fiber in this recipe is to leave the vitamin-packed skins on the potatoes. Add extra bell peppers and onions for even more fiber and vitamins.

Favor fats: Olive oil and ground flaxseeds provide diabetes- and heart-friendly fat, while removing sausage and cheese cuts down on saturated fat.

COUNTRY-STYLE HASH BROWNS

PREP TIME: **10 MINUTES** ■ TOTAL TIME: **45 MINUTES**

Makes 4 servings

1 pound Yukon gold potatoes, cut into ¾" cubes

1 small onion, finely chopped

1 green bell pepper, finely chopped

2 teaspoons olive oil

2 teaspoons chopped fresh rosemary or ⅔ teaspoon dried

⅛ teaspoon ground black pepper

⅛ teaspoon ground red pepper

4 teaspoons ground flaxseeds (optional)

1. Place the potatoes in a large saucepan. Cover with cold water and bring to a boil over high heat. Reduce the heat to medium and simmer for 15 minutes, or until just tender when tested with a sharp knife. Drain.

2. Coat a large nonstick skillet with cooking spray and place over medium heat. Cook the onion and bell pepper, stirring occasionally, for 5 minutes, or until softened.

3. Add the oil, rosemary, black pepper, red pepper, flaxseeds (if using), and the cooked potatoes. Mix well, cover, and cook for 8 minutes, or until the underside is crispy and golden brown. Using a wide spatula, turn the potatoes over. Cover and cook for another 8 minutes, or until the potatoes are golden brown. (For extra-crispy hash browns, cook for an additional 5 to 10 minutes, turning the potatoes occasionally.)

ZUCCHINI AND SWEET POTATO LATKES

PREP TIME: **10 MINUTES** ▦ TOTAL TIME: **25 MINUTES**

Makes 6 servings

1 small zucchini, shredded

1 small onion, finely chopped

2 medium sweet potatoes, shredded

2 tablespoons whole wheat pastry flour

2 eggs, lightly beaten

1½ tablespoons canola oil, divided

1 teaspoon ground cinnamon

Vanilla or plain 0% Greek yogurt, for serving

2 tablespoons walnuts, for serving

1. In a large bowl, toss the zucchini, onion, potatoes, and flour to combine. Add the eggs to the mixture and stir gently until combined.

2. In a large skillet, heat 1 teaspoon oil over medium-high heat. Working in batches, spoon ¼ cup of the mixture to shape into 3"-diameter latkes.

3. Place a few latkes in the skillet and cook for 6 minutes, turning once, or until golden brown on the bottom. Repeat this process for additional batches, adding the remaining oil to the skillet as needed. You should have about 12 latkes. Sprinkle with cinnamon.

4. Serve with the yogurt and walnuts.

Makeover Magic

	BEFORE		AFTER
	250	CALORIES	126
	16 g	FAT	5 g
	5 g	SAT FAT	1 g
	22 g	CARBS	16 g
	2 g	FIBER	3 g
	5 g	PROTEIN	4 g
	40 mg	SODIUM	60 mg

Curb carbs: Sweet potatoes are nutrient-packed carbs that you want to include in your diet. Accompany your pancakes with a filling side of Greek yogurt rather than sour cream and applesauce. This really keeps carbs curbed and you happily full.

Fill up on fiber: The skins on the sweet potatoes are great forms of fiber.

Favor fats: Eliminating butter lowers saturated fat and calories for weight reduction. Favoring canola oil and walnuts gives you a dose of the omega-3 fatty acid ALA.

GOGREEK

Whether no fat or low fat, Greek yogurt is typically low in carbohydrates, containing only 7 to 14 grams of carbs per 6-ounce serving. Look for Greek yogurt with 20 to 50 percent of your daily value of calcium to help keep your bones strong.

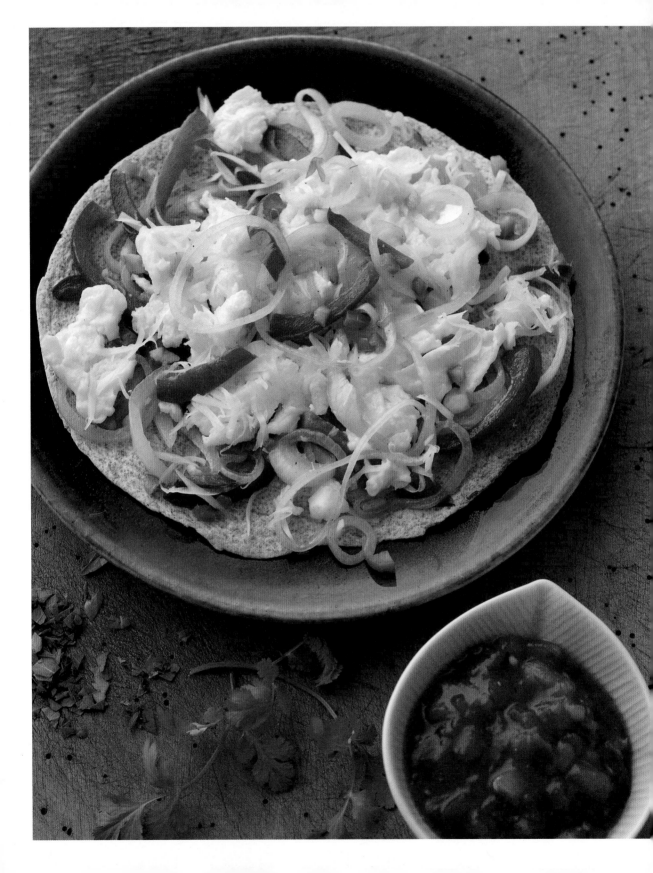

TEX-MEX BREAKFAST PIZZA

PREP TIME: **10 MINUTES** ■ TOTAL TIME: **25 MINUTES**

Makes 4 servings

4 low-carb whole wheat flour tortillas (6" diameter)

2 tablespoons olive oil

1 small onion, thinly sliced

1 red bell pepper, cut into thin strips

½ jalapeño chile pepper, finely chopped (wear plastic gloves when handling)

4 whole eggs

8 egg whites

2 teaspoons water

½ cup shredded reduced-fat provolone cheese

4 tablespoons salsa

¼ cup chopped fresh cilantro

1. Preheat the oven to 400°F.

2. Coat both sides of each tortilla with cooking spray and place on a baking sheet. Bake for 6 minutes, or until golden and crisp.

3. Meanwhile, heat the oil in a large nonstick skillet over medium heat. Cook the onion, bell pepper, and jalapeño pepper for 5 minutes, or until tender. Transfer to a plate.

4. In a mixing bowl, beat the eggs, egg whites, and water. Pour the eggs into the same skillet and cook over medium heat, stirring to scramble, for 2 minutes or until almost set, sprinkling the cheese onto the eggs halfway through cooking. Sprinkle two-thirds of the onion and peppers onto the tortillas. Top with the cooked eggs, remaining onion and peppers, and 1 tablespoon salsa per serving. Sprinkle cilantro onto each pizza.

Makeover Magic

BEFORE		AFTER
420	CALORIES	306
22 g	FAT	16 g
9 g	SAT FAT	4 g
37 g	CARBS	18 g
1 g	FIBER	9 g
19 g	PROTEIN	20 g
790 mg	SODIUM	667 mg

Note: This recipe is higher in sodium, so be sure to choose lower-sodium meals later in the day to ensure you don't go over the recommended daily allowance.

Curb carbs: A whole wheat tortilla is an easy way to control portion size rather than taking slices from a pizza.

Fill up on fiber: The whole wheat tortilla, onion, and pepper are packed with fiber and nutrients.

Favor fats: Egg yolks contain saturated fat, but they can be beneficial for their large dose of vitamin A. Choosing a harder cheese like Parmesan helps to decrease saturated fat and calories.

SMARTSTART

Add our favorite diabetes-friendly fat, avocado.

BEFORE		AFTER
200	CALORIES	124
15 g	FAT	5 g
0 g	SAT FAT	0.5 g
36 g	CARBS	5 g
0 g	FIBER	1 g
10 g	PROTEIN	17 g
324 mg	SODIUM	44 mg

Curb carbs: Maple syrup is naturally sweet, so you need only a small amount of syrup. This recipe is low in carbs and calories, so you can pair it with a higher-carb recipe like Zucchini and Sweet Potato Latkes (page 75) for a full breakfast.

Fill up on fiber: Be sure to serve a fiber-filled carbohydrate like fruit, veggies, or grains with these sausage patties.

Favor fats: The ground walnuts are a fantastic source of diabetes-friendly omega-3 fatty acids.

HOMEMADE BREAKFAST SAUSAGE

PREP TIME: **5 MINUTES** ■ TOTAL TIME: **20 MINUTES**

Makes 8 servings (2 patties each)

2 tablespoons maple syrup

2 tablespoons ground flaxseeds

2 tablespoons ground walnuts

1½ teaspoons ground black pepper

1½ teaspoons ground sage

½ teaspoon onion powder

¼ teaspoon salt

¾ pound extra-lean ground turkey

½ pound 96% lean ground pork

2 teaspoons canola oil, divided

1. In a large bowl, combine the syrup, flaxseeds, walnuts, pepper, sage, onion powder, and salt and mix with a fork until smooth. Add the turkey and pork and mix gently until the seasonings are evenly distributed. Divide the mixture into 16 small balls, approximately 1" in diameter each.

2. Heat 1 teaspoon of the oil in a skillet over medium-high heat. Place half of the balls in the skillet and flatten with a spatula. Cook for 6 minutes, turning once, or until no longer pink. Add the remaining 1 teaspoon oil and repeat with the remaining patties.

PB&J STUFFED FRENCH TOAST

PREP TIME: **5 MINUTES** ■ TOTAL TIME: **20 MINUTES**

Makes 4 servings

4 tablespoons all-natural creamy peanut butter, divided

2 tablespoons all-fruit strawberry jam, divided

8 slices thinly sliced sprouted whole grain bread

1 cup sliced strawberries, divided

2 large eggs

½ cup unsweetened almond milk

1 teaspoon vanilla extract

1 teaspoon ground cinnamon

1. Spread 1 tablespoon of the peanut butter and ½ tablespoon of the jam on 4 slices of the bread. Top each slice with ⅛ cup strawberries, evenly spread. Top with a second slice and press lightly to form a sandwich.

2. In a medium bowl, combine the eggs, milk, vanilla extract, and cinnamon. Working one sandwich at a time, dip both sides of each sandwich in the egg mixture and set on a plate.

3. Coat a large nonstick skillet with cooking spray and heat over medium heat. Cook the sandwiches for 8 minutes, turning once, until golden and cooked through. Serve hot, topped with the remaining strawberries.

Makeover Magic

BEFORE		AFTER
390	CALORIES	331
19 g	FAT	12 g
5 g	SAT FAT	2 g
43 g	CARBS	41 g
5 g	FIBER	9 g
15 g	PROTEIN	15 g
519 mg	SODIUM	209 mg

Curb carbs: Using slices of sprouted whole grain or oat bran bread makes each serving of stuffed French toast both bite-size and easy on your blood sugar! Look for bread that has 15 grams of carbs and 3 to 5 grams of fiber per slice. Decreasing jam and using real fruit also keeps carbs curbed.

Fill up on fiber: Fiber is found in fresh strawberries, especially the tiny seeds, and of course in the naturally higher-fiber bread.

Favor fats: Natural peanut butter is low sodium, low carb, and high in MUFAs.

SMARTSTART

Add 1 teaspoon of cinnamon to each sandwich for optimal glycemic control.

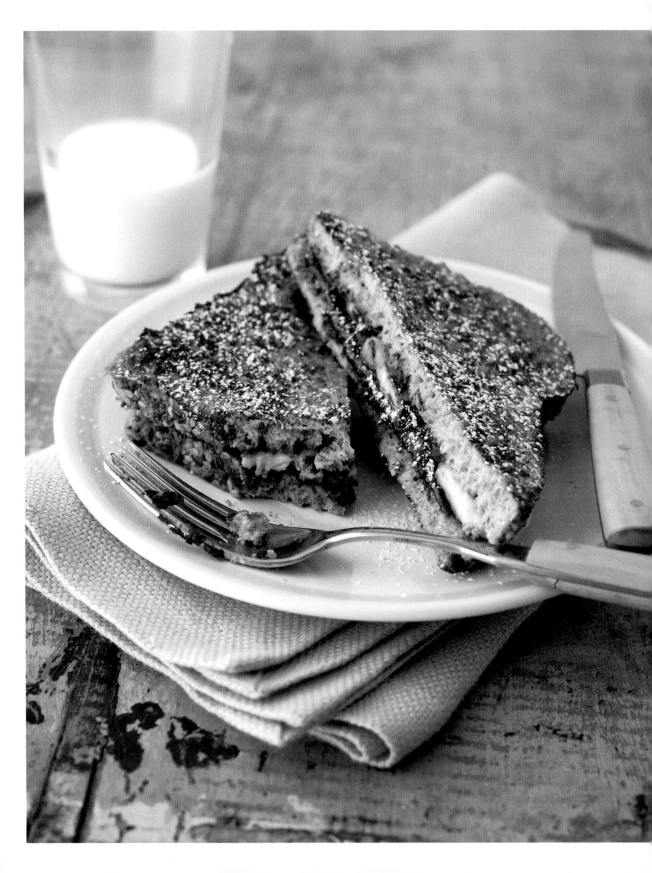

CHOCOLATE-BANANA-STUFFED FRENCH TOAST

PREP TIME: **5 MINUTES** ▪ TOTAL TIME: **20 MINUTES**

Makes 4 servings

FILLING

1 unripe banana, thinly sliced

2 tablespoons almond butter

2 tablespoons hazelnut spread

4 teaspoons dark chocolate chips

⅛ teaspoon ground nutmeg

⅛ teaspoon ground cinnamon

FRENCH TOAST

8 slices sprouted whole grain bread

½ cup unsweetened soy or almond milk

2 eggs

½ teaspoon vanilla extract

1 teaspoon ground cinnamon

Confectioners' sugar for dusting (optional)

1. **To make the filling:** Mash about one-quarter of the banana slices in a small bowl with the back of a spoon. (You should have about 2 tablespoons mashed.) Stir in the almond butter, chocolate hazelnut spread, chocolate chips, nutmeg, and cinnamon until smooth.

2. **To make the French toast:** Spread 4 slices of the bread with the banana filling, dividing evenly. Top with the remaining banana slices and bread slices to make 4 sandwiches.

3. In a shallow dish or pie plate, whisk together the milk, eggs, vanilla, and cinnamon until blended. Dip the sandwiches into the egg mixture, turning them over with a spatula to coat both sides, and set on a plate.

4. Heat a large nonstick skillet or griddle over medium-low heat and coat with cooking spray. Cook the sandwiches for 8 minutes, turning once, until golden and cooked through. Dust with confectioners' sugar, if using.

Makeover Magic

BEFORE		AFTER
660	CALORIES	367
34 g	FAT	13 g
24 g	SAT FAT	4 g
79 g	CARBS	50 g
4 g	FIBER	8 g
10 g	PROTEIN	15 g
460 mg	SODIUM	223 mg

Curb carbs: Out with the white and in with the wholesome grains, seeds, and nuts. This not only increases the firmness of the bread, but adds flavor and keeps carbs curbed.

Fill up on fiber: Both whole grain bread and banana slices boost the fiber in this old-time favorite. Using sprouted whole grain bread gives you the advantage of magic carbs.

Favor fats: Using cooking spray instead of butter to grease the pan decreases the saturated fat. Using almond butter and even hazelnut butter provides you with MUFAs.

BEFORE		AFTER
350	CALORIES	313
9 g	FAT	11 g
5 g	SAT FAT	1 g
60 g	CARBS	42 g
1 g	FIBER	10 g
5 g	PROTEIN	13 g
450 mg	SODIUM	26 mg

Curb carbs: Using a measuring cup helps you portion pancakes and serve yourself more so you feel psychologically satisfied while keeping carbs minimized and calories in check. Using unsweetened milks keeps your carbs in range.

Fill up on fiber: The fresh unpeeled apples, whole grain pastry flour, and wheat germ really make everyone's favorite flapjacks a great source of fiber for breakfast!

Favor fats: Using cooking spray instead of butter to coat the pan decreases the saturated fat. Walnuts and chia seeds provide a vegetarian source of omega-3 fatty acids.

SPICED APPLE PANCAKES

PREP TIME: **5 MINUTES** ■ TOTAL TIME: **15 MINUTES**

Makes 4 servings (3 pancakes each)

1 medium apple, unpeeled, cored, and thinly sliced

2 teaspoons ground cinnamon, divided

1½ cups whole grain pastry flour

1½ teaspoons baking powder

3 tablespoons wheat germ

½ teaspoon apple pie spice

1 egg, lightly beaten

1 teaspoon vanilla extract

1½ cups unsweetened soy, sunflower, or almond milk

3 tablespoons unsweetened applesauce

4 tablespoons chopped walnuts

2 tablespoons chia seeds

1. Heat a small skillet over medium heat. Lightly coat the pan with cooking spray and add the apple. Sprinkle 1 teaspoon cinnamon over the apple. Cover the pan and cook for 5 to 10 minutes, or until tender.

2. In a large bowl, whisk together the flour, baking powder, wheat germ, remaining teaspoon cinnamon, and apple pie spice. Add the egg, vanilla, milk, and applesauce. Mix well to combine.

3. Heat a large nonstick skillet or griddle pan coated with cooking spray over medium heat. Working in batches if necessary, scoop ¼-cup measures of batter onto the skillet or griddle. Sprinkle with the chopped walnuts and chia seeds. Cook for 2 minutes, or until bubbles appear on the edges of the pancakes. Flip with a spatula and cook for 2 minutes, or until cooked through. Top the pancakes with the cooked apple slices.

BELGIAN WAFFLES

PREP TIME: 5 MINUTES ▪ **TOTAL TIME: 20 MINUTES**

Makes 5 servings (1 waffle each)

1⅔ cups whole grain pastry flour

1 tablespoon wheat germ

1 tablespoon baking powder

¼ teaspoon salt

2 large eggs

1⅔ cups 1% milk

1 tablespoon maple syrup

2 tablespoons canola oil

¾ cup blueberries, sliced

1 cup strawberries, sliced

5 tablespoons slivered almonds

5 teaspoons chia seeds

1. Preheat the waffle iron.

2. In a large bowl, whisk together the flour, wheat germ, baking powder, and salt. In another bowl, whisk together the eggs, milk, maple syrup, and canola oil.

3. Add the wet ingredients into the dry ingredients and stir until combined. Mix in the blueberries.

4. Coat the waffle iron with cooking spray. For each waffle, use a full ½ cup of batter and cook according to manufacturer's directions.

5. Mix the strawberries, almonds, and chia seeds in a bowl.

6. Serve the waffles immediately, topped with the strawberry mixture.

Makeover Magic

BEFORE		AFTER
696	CALORIES	324
41 g	FAT	14 g
25 g	SAT FAT	2 g
72 g	CARBS	40 g
1 g	FIBER	7 g
10 g	PROTEIN	12 g
712 mg	SODIUM	182 mg

Curb carbs: Since whole grains make you feel fuller faster, you'll feel satisfied with just one of these decadent waffles. Add a side of protein and a calcium source such as Greek yogurt or low-fat cottage cheese for even better blood sugar control.

Fill up on fiber: Fiber up your morning with whole grain pastry flour, fresh fruit, nuts, and seeds.

Favor fats: Canola oil, chia seeds, and wheat germ pack the MUFAs and omega-3 fatty acids in this recipe.

Makeover Magic

BEFORE		AFTER
272	CALORIES	195
12 g	FAT	8 g
3 g	SAT FAT	2 g
37 g	CARBS	28 g
1 g	FIBER	6 g
4 g	PROTEIN	6 g
258 mg	SODIUM	25 mg

Curb carbs: Using honey or agave instead of white sugar keeps this recipe lower in carbs.

Fill up on fiber: The flours, fresh raspberries, and chia seeds in these muffins add over 2 grams of fiber per serving.

Favor fats: The olive oil is a healthy fat to use that provides for a moist muffin. Chia seeds add omega-3s, and you can add even more beneficial fats by spreading natural nut butter on half of the muffin.

RASPBERRY-LEMON MUFFINS

PREP TIME: **5 MINUTES** ■ TOTAL TIME: **30 MINUTES**

Makes 12 servings

1½ cups whole grain oat flour

1½ cups whole wheat flour

1 tablespoon baking powder

1 teaspoon ground cinnamon

2 eggs

1¼ cups 1% milk

3 tablespoons light olive oil

3 tablespoons honey (or 1½ tablespoons agave)

1 teaspoon lemon juice

1 tablespoon lemon zest

1 cup raspberries

¼ cup chia seeds

1. Preheat the oven to 400°F. Line a muffin pan with paper liners or coat with cooking spray.

2. In a large bowl, combine the flours, baking powder, and cinnamon.

3. In a small bowl, whisk together the eggs, milk, oil, honey, lemon juice, and lemon zest. Stir into the flour mixture just until blended. Gently stir in the raspberries and chia seeds.

4. Fill the muffin cups two-thirds full with the mixture. Bake for 20 minutes, or until a wooden pick inserted in the center comes out clean. Remove to a rack to cool.

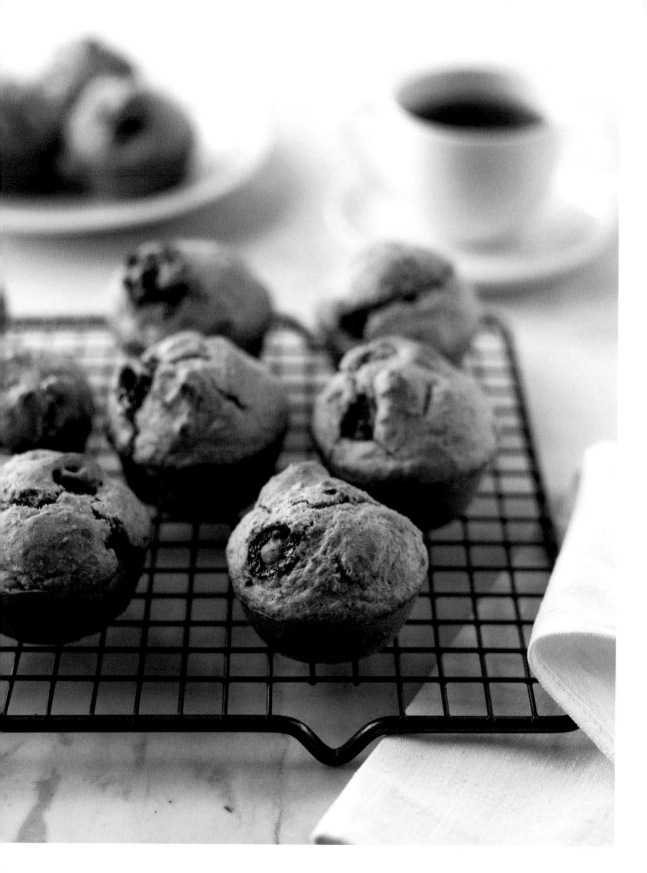

Makeover Magic

BEFORE		AFTER
510	CALORIES	204
27 g	FAT	9 g
16 g	SAT FAT	5 g
50 g	CARBS	25 g
2 g	FIBER	3 g
17 g	PROTEIN	8 g
2,680 mg	SODIUM	158 mg

Curb carbs: Keep carbs in check by filling up on higher-fiber grains like whole wheat flour and whole grain cornmeal.

Fill up on fiber: Whole wheat flour and whole grain cornmeal give these scones a huge kick of fiber to get you "moving" in the morning.

Favor fats: Opt for reduced-fat cheese when using butter to keep saturated fat at a minimum. Lox provides the omega-3 fatty acids you want to be including regularly.

LOX-CHEDDAR SCONES

PREP TIME: **10 MINUTES** ■ TOTAL TIME: **35 MINUTES**

Makes 8 servings

3 scallions, sliced

2 ounces smoked salmon (lox), chopped

1½ cups whole wheat flour

½ cup yellow cornmeal

1 tablespoon baking powder

4 tablespoons unsalted butter, cold, cut into small cubes

½ cup reduced-fat shredded Cheddar cheese

½ tablespoon agave syrup

1 cup 1% low-fat buttermilk

1. Preheat the oven to 425°F. Line a baking sheet with parchment paper.

2. Heat a large nonstick skillet coated with cooking spray over medium heat. Cook the scallions and salmon for 3 minutes, or until the scallions are softened.

3. In a large bowl, combine the flour, cornmeal, and baking powder. Cut in the butter with a pastry blender or fork until the mixture resembles small crumbles. Stir in the scallions and salmon and Cheddar.

4. In a small bowl, combine the agave and buttermilk. Pour this mixture into the large bowl with the flour mixture and stir until just combined and the dough comes together.

5. Pat the dough into an 8" circle, about ¾" thick. Transfer the disk to the prepared baking sheet, cut into 8 wedges, and separate the wedges on the pan. Bake the scones for 20 minutes, or until golden. Cool in the pan on a rack for 5 minutes. Remove from the rack and cool completely.

Breakfast

SUNRISE OATMEAL

PREP TIME: **5 MINUTES** ■ TOTAL TIME: **40 MINUTES**

Makes 4 servings

4 cups water

1 cup steel-cut oats

1 tablespoon flaxseeds

1 tablespoon wheat germ

2 tablespoons chopped pecans

½ teaspoon ground cinnamon

4 ounces vanilla 0% Greek yogurt

1 cup blueberries

1. In a medium saucepan, bring the water to a boil over high heat. Add the oats and stir until they begin to thicken. Reduce the heat and simmer for 30 minutes, or until the oatmeal is thick and creamy. Add the flaxseeds, wheat germ, and pecans to the saucepan and mix evenly.

2. Spoon the oatmeal into 4 bowls and sprinkle with the cinnamon. Top each with equal portions of the Greek yogurt and blueberries. Serve hot.

Makeover Magic

BEFORE		AFTER
340	CALORIES	214
10 g	FAT	5 g
6 g	SAT FAT	1 g
51 g	CARBS	36 g
5 g	FIBER	6 g
13 g	PROTEIN	10 g
380 mg	SODIUM	21 mg

Curb carbs: Freshly cooked steel-cut oats provide a healthy unrefined carbohydrate option just like your grandmother used to make! Using fat-free Greek yogurt keeps fat and carbs in range.

Fill up on fiber: Steel-cut oats are higher in fiber than instant or quick-cooking oatmeal.

Favor fats: Flaxseeds, wheat germ, and pecans add not only fiber but also essential fatty acids and a dose of vitamins B and E. Say good-bye to saturated fat when using naturally creamy steel-cut oats—there's no need for cream or even butter.

BEFORE		AFTER
308	CALORIES	194
15 g	FAT	7 g
2 g	SAT FAT	0.5 g
41 g	CARBS	27 g
4 g	FIBER	6 g
7 g	PROTEIN	7 g
70 mg	SODIUM	10 mg

Curb carbs: Adding nuts and seeds to an oatmeal-based granola can curb carbohydrates while still providing energy!

Fill up on fiber: The combination of oats, millet, and almonds makes an unstoppable fiber trio.

Favor fats: The nuts and seeds are jam-packed with beneficial fats.

HEARTY FRUIT AND NUT GRANOLA

PREP TIME: **5 MINUTES** ■ TOTAL TIME: **35 MINUTES + COOLING TIME**

Makes 6 servings

1½ cups old-fashioned rolled oats

¼ cup millet

¼ cup unsweetened dried cranberries

¼ cup ground flaxseeds

2 tablespoons unsalted sunflower seeds

¼ cup slivered almonds

3 tablespoons maple syrup

1 teaspoon ground cinnamon

½ teaspoon ground cardamom

1. Preheat the oven to 350°F. Coat a large baking sheet with sides with cooking spray. Set aside.

2. In a large bowl, add the oats, millet, cranberries, flaxseeds, sunflower seeds, almonds, maple syrup, cinnamon, and cardamom. Stir well to combine.

3. Spread evenly on the baking sheet and bake for 35 minutes, or until golden brown, stirring carefully once or twice. Remove from the oven and break up any large pieces of granola while it is still warm.

4. Cool completely before storing in an airtight container at room temperature for up to 1 week.

PEACH-BLUEBERRY YOGURT PARFAIT

PREP TIME: **10 MINUTES** ■ TOTAL TIME: **10 MINUTES**

Makes 4 servings

2 cups plain 0% Greek yogurt

2 teaspoons lemon juice

2 peaches, pitted and chopped

1 cup blueberries

⅔ cup (2 servings) Hearty Fruit and Nut Granola (opposite page)

2 tablespoons ground flaxseeds

1. In a small bowl, stir together the yogurt and lemon juice.

2. In 4 parfait glasses, layer the yogurt, peaches, blueberries, granola, and flaxseeds.

Makeover Magic

BEFORE		AFTER
330	CALORIES	218
10 g	FAT	5 g
2 g	SAT FAT	0.5 g
51 g	CARBS	29 g
3 g	FIBER	5 g
12 g	PROTEIN	15 g
170 mg	SODIUM	48 mg

Curb carbs: Adding a protein source like Greek yogurt means we can reduce carbs at breakfast. The carbs in this recipe come from granola and fresh fruit!

Fill up on fiber: Flaxseeds and sunflower seeds are an excellent source of fiber in this recipe.

Favor fats: Almonds are a delicious source of MUFAs.

Makeover Magic

BEFORE		AFTER
190	CALORIES	205
3 g	FAT	4 g
2 g	SAT FAT	0.5 g
36 g	CARBS	29 g
1 g	FIBER	3 g
6 g	PROTEIN	14 g
95 mg	SODIUM	36 mg

Curb carbs: Greek yogurt helps curb carbs in this smoothie.

Fill up on fiber: Bananas, cherries, and flaxseeds provide fiber in this delicious drink that won't make your blood sugar blast off.

Favor fats: Hemp or chia seeds give a morning dose of omegas, while choosing 0% Greek yogurt gives you a little bit of protein to help keep your blood sugar from peaking too fast.

SUNDAE BREAKFAST SMOOTHIE

PREP TIME: **5 MINUTES** ■ TOTAL TIME: **5 MINUTES**

Makes 4 servings

2   bananas, frozen

1   cup vanilla 0% Greek yogurt

½   cup fresh-squeezed orange juice

1   cup frozen cherries

1   scoop vanilla whey protein powder

2   tablespoons ground flaxseeds

2   tablespoons hemp or chia seeds

In a blender, combine the bananas, yogurt, orange juice, cherries, protein powder, flaxseeds, and chia seeds. Blend until smooth and creamy.

CHOCOLATE CAKE SMOOTHIE

PREP TIME: **5 MINUTES** ■ TOTAL TIME: **10 MINUTES**

Makes 2 servings

½ cup part-skim ricotta cheese

1½ cups unsweetened almond milk

1 scoop chocolate whey protein powder

2 tablespoons almond butter

¼ cup hazelnuts, chopped

2 tablespoons ground espresso (decaf or regular)

2 teaspoons vanilla extract

½ teaspoon ground cinnamon

8 ice cubes

In a blender, combine the ricotta, almond milk, protein powder, almond butter, hazelnuts, espresso, vanilla, cinnamon, and ice cubes. Blend until smooth and creamy.

Makeover Magic

BEFORE		AFTER
570	CALORIES	389
17 g	FAT	27 g
11 g	SAT FAT	5 g
91 g	CARBS	13 g
1 g	FIBER	3 g
12 g	PROTEIN	24 g
240 mg	SODIUM	313 mg

Curb carbs: Unsweetened almond milk and chocolate-flavored protein powder give you a sweet kickoff to your morning while keeping carbs naturally low.

Fill up on fiber: The hazelnuts create texture and provide fiber while enhancing the chocolate flavor.

Favor fats: This recipe may look high in fat, but that's because it's full of the good kind! The nuts and almond butter in this recipe are packed full of MUFAs.

SMARTSTART

Increase to 1 teaspoon cinnamon per smoothie to reduce your after-breakfast blood sugar.

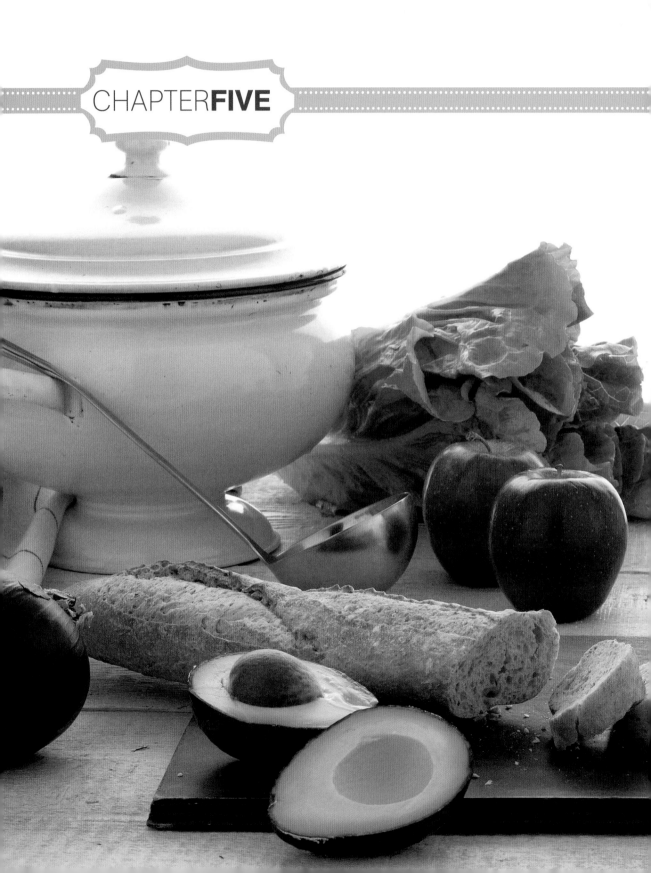

Soups, Salads & Sandwiches

Makeover Magic

BEFORE		AFTER
400	CALORIES	244
26 g	FAT	8 g
9 g	SAT FAT	2 g
26 g	CARBS	19 g
3 g	FIBER	5 g
20 g	PROTEIN	26 g
1,450 mg	SODIUM	152 mg

Curb carbs: There's no need for tortillas with this filling, veggie-packed soup. Save the carbs for the sandwich served on the side.

Fill up on fiber: Zucchini, corn, and the superstar beans are the major sources of fiber in this recipe.

Favor fats: The avocado topping adds healthy MUFAs.

FIESTA TURKEY SOUP

PREP TIME: **10 MINUTES** ■ TOTAL TIME: **50 MINUTES**

Makes 6 servings

1 tablespoon canola oil

1 onion, chopped

1 small jalapeño chile pepper, seeded and finely chopped (wear plastic gloves when handling)

1 zucchini, chopped

2 teaspoons ground cumin

½ teaspoon ancho chili powder

1 pound 99% fat-free ground turkey

1 package (32 ounces) low-sodium chicken broth

1 can (14.5 ounces) no-salt-added diced tomatoes

1 can (15 ounces) no-salt-added black beans, rinsed and drained

1 cup frozen corn kernels

½ cup chopped fresh cilantro

½ avocado, chopped

6 tablespoons shredded Cheddar cheese

1. In a large saucepan, heat the oil over medium-high heat. Cook the onion and pepper, stirring occasionally, for 5 minutes, or until lightly browned. Stir in the zucchini, cumin, and chili powder. Cook for 10 minutes, or until the zucchini is lightly browned. Add the turkey and cook, stirring to break up with a spoon, for 5 minutes, or until no longer pink.

2. Stir in the broth, tomatoes (with juice), beans, and corn. Bring to a boil over high heat. Reduce the heat to low and simmer for 20 minutes, or until the liquid has reduced by one-quarter. Remove from the heat.

3. Stir in the cilantro. Divide among 6 bowls. Sprinkle each serving with a spoonful of avocado and 1 tablespoon of shredded cheese.

Soups, Salads & Sandwiches

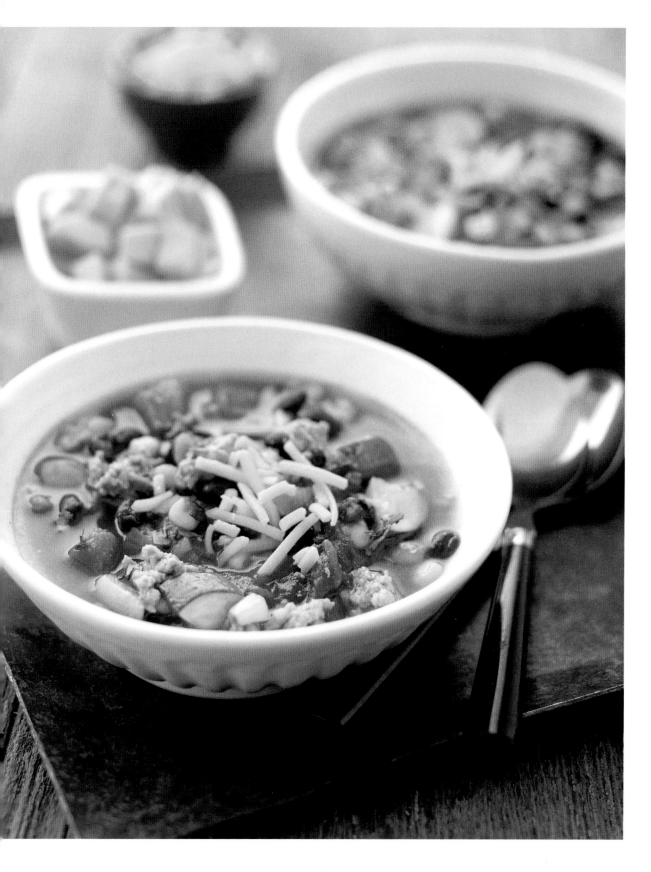

Makeover Magic

BEFORE		AFTER
588	CALORIES	229
19 g	FAT	5 g
9 g	SAT FAT	0.5 g
64 g	CARBS	33 g
6 g	FIBER	6 g
36 g	PROTEIN	14 g
2,164 mg	SODIUM	243 mg

Curb carbs: Instead of the traditional pasta in minestrone soup, we used wild rice, which is naturally lower in carbs.

Fill up on fiber: Cabbage, chickpeas, and wild rice are the key to a high fiber count.

Favor fats: Be sure to accompany this soup with a salad featuring sources of healthy fats such as olive oil and sunflower seeds.

MINESTRONE

PREP TIME: **10 MINUTES** ■ TOTAL TIME: **45 MINUTES**

Makes 6 servings

2¼ cups water

¾ cup wild rice

1 tablespoon canola oil

4 ounces Italian chicken or turkey sausage, thinly sliced

5 cups shredded green cabbage

1 medium zucchini, thinly sliced

2 cloves garlic, minced

1 rib celery, diced

1 can (14.5 ounces) no-salt-added diced tomatoes

1 can (15 ounces) no-salt-added chickpeas, rinsed and drained

8 cups (2 quarts) low-sodium chicken broth

2 sprigs parsley, finely chopped

1. In a microwaveable glass bowl, combine the water and the rice and cook on high in a microwave oven for 5 minutes. Set aside.

2. In a large soup pot, heat the oil over medium-high heat. Cook the sausage, stirring, for 4 minutes, or until no longer pink. Add the cabbage, zucchini, garlic, and celery and cook for 4 minutes, or until just tender.

3. Add the tomatoes (with juice), chickpeas, and broth. Bring to a boil over high heat, reduce the heat to medium, and simmer for 10 minutes. Stir in the rice and parsley, reduce the heat to low, and simmer for 10 minutes to blend the flavors.

BEEF BARLEY SOUP

PREP TIME: 15 MINUTES ■ **TOTAL TIME: 2 HOURS**

Makes 6 servings

1 tablespoon olive oil

1 pound well-trimmed lean boneless beef top sirloin, cut into ¾" cubes

2 onions, halved and thinly sliced

3 cloves garlic, minced

½ teaspoon dried thyme, crumbled

8 ounces cremini mushrooms, sliced

2 ribs celery, thinly sliced

3 carrots, sliced

1 parsnip, halved lengthwise and sliced

¼ cup no-salt-added tomato puree

3 cups water

3½ cups low-sodium beef broth

1 bay leaf

½ cup pearl barley

1. In a Dutch oven or a large, heavy saucepan, heat the oil over medium heat. Lightly brown the beef for 3 minutes, or until the liquid evaporates.

2. Add the onions and garlic and cook for 3 minutes, or until the onions soften. Add the thyme and cook for 1 minute. Add the mushrooms and cook for 3 minutes, or until the mushrooms begin to soften. Add the celery, carrots, and parsnip and stir for 2 minutes.

3. Reduce the heat to medium low. Add the puree, water, broth, and bay leaf and simmer for 45 minutes.

4. Stir in the barley and simmer for 45 minutes, or until the barley is soft. Discard the bay leaf before serving.

Makeover Magic

BEFORE		AFTER
332	CALORIES	229
11 g	FAT	5 g
5 g	SAT FAT	2 g
35 g	CARBS	28 g
6 g	FIBER	6 g
25 g	PROTEIN	18 g
1,681 mg	SODIUM	125 mg

Curb carbs: We used just a small amount of pearl barley, which cut the carbs but also added body to this hearty soup.

Fill up on fiber: Barley itself is full of fiber, but we've also added luscious, fiber-filled veggies.

Favor fats: We used a lean cut of beef for this soup to reduce saturated fat. Pair this soup with a salad or sandwich high in healthy fats.

Makeover Magic

BEFORE		AFTER
369	CALORIES	227
14 g	FAT	5 g
7 g	SAT FAT	2 g
47 g	CARBS	33 g
4 g	FIBER	5 g
11 g	PROTEIN	15 g
638 mg	SODIUM	337 mg

Curb carbs: We cut the potatoes in this traditional potato soup by adding lentils, which are higher in fiber and protein.

Fill up on fiber: Lentils are an added fiber source that sets this apart from the average potato soup!

Favor fats: Loaded baked potato soups are usually full of bacon, cheese, and heavy cream. We changed to 1% milk and ham to reduce saturated fat. For a dose of healthy fats, be sure to pair with a salad drizzled with olive oil and sliced olives.

CREAMY POTATO, LENTIL, AND HAM CHOWDER

PREP TIME: **10 MINUTES** ■ TOTAL TIME: **45 MINUTES**

Makes 8 servings

1 tablespoon olive oil

2 onions, chopped

2 tablespoons whole wheat flour

3 cups low-sodium chicken broth

2 cups water

4 red potatoes, cubed into ¾" pieces

1 rib celery, chopped

½ cup green lentils, rinsed

1 teaspoon mustard powder

1⅔ cups 1% milk

½ pound fully cooked lean, low-sodium ham, cut into ¾" pieces

1. In a large saucepan, heat the oil over medium-high heat. Cook the onions, stirring occasionally, for 5 minutes, or until translucent. Stir in the flour and cook for 1 minute. Gradually stir in the broth until well blended.

2. Add the water, potatoes, celery, lentils, and mustard. Bring to a boil. Reduce the heat to low, cover, and simmer for 20 minutes, or until the potatoes are tender.

3. Working in batches, transfer the vegetables to a blender or food processor and process until pureed. Return to the saucepan. Stir in the milk and ham. Gently simmer, stirring occasionally, for 5 minutes.

CHEESY VEGETABLE CHOWDER

PREP TIME: **10 MINUTES** ■ TOTAL TIME: **45 MINUTES**

Makes 6 servings

1 small red or green bell pepper, minced

1 small onion, minced

¼ cup apple juice

1 clove garlic, minced

¼ cup white whole wheat flour

2 cups low-sodium chicken broth

2 potatoes, diced

1¼ cups 1% milk

1 cup frozen chopped broccoli, thawed

½ cup frozen corn kernels, thawed

¾ cup shredded Cheddar cheese

¼ cup shredded Monterey Jack cheese

1. In a Dutch oven, combine the pepper, onion, apple juice, and garlic. Cook, stirring, over medium-high heat for 5 minutes. Add the flour and ½ cup of the broth. Cook, stirring, for 2 minutes. Add the potatoes and the remaining 1½ cups of broth. Bring to a boil. Reduce the heat to medium. Cover and cook for 20 minutes, or until the potatoes are tender. Check by inserting the tip of a sharp knife into 1 piece.

2. Transfer 1 cup of the soup to a blender or food processor. Process until smooth. Return to the pot. Add the milk, broccoli, corn, and cheeses. Stir to combine. Cook, stirring, for 3 minutes, or until the cheeses melt and the vegetables are heated through.

Makeover Magic

BEFORE		AFTER
270	CALORIES	198
7 g	FAT	7 g
2 g	SAT FAT	4 g
32 g	CARBS	25 g
2 g	FIBER	4 g
11 g	PROTEIN	10 g
1,490 mg	SODIUM	178 mg

Curb carbs: This soup cuts carbs by replacing gravy mix and other prepackaged ingredients with fresh whole foods such as whole wheat flour and apple juice.

Fill up on fiber: White whole wheat flour, potatoes (with the skin!), broccoli, and corn all add extra fiber compared to the traditional cheese chowder.

Favor fats: Instead of heavy cream and too much cheese, we used 1% milk and a minimal amount of cheese. Sneak a dose of healthy fats into this soup by adding ground flaxseeds.

BEFORE		AFTER
310	CALORIES	164
11 g	FAT	1 g
2 g	SAT FAT	0 g
46 g	CARBS	30 g
3 g	FIBER	4 g
10 g	PROTEIN	10 g
1,150 mg	SODIUM	574 mg

Curb carbs: The majority of the carbohydrates in this soup are from the potatoes. We cut the carbohydrates compared to our "before" chowder, because we added additional vegetables to add flavor and nutrients.

Fill up on fiber: All of the added vegetables boost the fiber compared to the original recipe.

Favor fats: We used turkey bacon as opposed to regular bacon, and we did not add any extra oil. This soup is almost fat free, so be sure to eat it with healthy fats.

MANHATTAN CLAM CHOWDER

PREP TIME: **10 MINUTES** ■ TOTAL TIME: **50 MINUTES**

Makes 6 servings

2   slices turkey bacon

2   ribs celery, thinly sliced

1   onion, finely chopped

1   green bell pepper, chopped

1   clove garlic, minced

2   cans (6.5 ounces each) chopped clams

¾   cup bottled clam juice

2   large potatoes, cubed

2   carrots, chopped

1   fresh thyme sprig

1   bay leaf

1   can (14.5 ounces) no-salt-added diced tomatoes

⅛   teaspoon ground red pepper

1. In a large saucepan over medium heat, cook the bacon until crisp. Transfer to a plate lined with paper towels. Crumble into a small bowl. Set aside.

2. Add the celery, onion, pepper, and garlic to the bacon drippings in the saucepan. Cook, stirring occasionally, for 5 minutes, or until the onion and celery are tender. Drain the juice from the clams into a small bowl. Set the clams aside.

3. Add the juice to the onion mixture. Stir in the bottled clam juice, potatoes, carrots, thyme, and bay leaf. Bring to a boil. Reduce the heat to low. Cover and simmer for 20 minutes. Stir in the tomatoes (with juice). Bring to a boil over high heat. Reduce the heat to low. Add the reserved clams. Cover and simmer for 8 minutes. Discard the bay leaf. Stir in the bacon and ground red pepper.

SMARTSTART

Serve with 1 slice toasted Vermont Bread Company Low Sodium Whole Wheat bread, covered with 1 to 2 tablespoons of low-sodium olive tapenade.

SOUTH-OF-THE-BORDER SHRIMP SOUP

PREP TIME: **10 MINUTES** ■ TOTAL TIME: **1 HOUR 15 MINUTES**

Makes 6 servings

1 bulb garlic

1 tablespoon olive oil

3 ribs celery, chopped

1 red bell pepper, chopped

1 green bell pepper, chopped

1 small leek, split, washed, and thinly sliced

1 serrano chile pepper, seeded and finely chopped (wear plastic gloves when handling)

2 cans (14.5 ounces each) no-salt-added diced tomatoes

3 cups low-sodium chicken broth

1 tablespoon Cajun seasoning mix

1 cup frozen corn kernels, thawed

1 pound medium shrimp, peeled and deveined

1. Preheat the oven to 350°F. Place the garlic bulb on a piece of foil, moisten it with water, and wrap it to seal. Bake for 45 minutes. When cool enough to handle, squeeze the garlic from the bulb.

2. Heat the oil in a large pot over medium-high heat. Cook the garlic, celery, bell peppers, leek, and serrano pepper for 10 minutes, or until soft. Add the tomatoes (with juice), broth, and seasoning mix and bring just to a boil. Add the corn and shrimp and cook for 5 minutes, or until the shrimp are opaque.

Makeover Magic

BEFORE		AFTER
317	CALORIES	185
13 g	FAT	4 g
4 g	SAT FAT	0.5 g
23 g	CARBS	18 g
2 g	FIBER	3 g
26 g	PROTEIN	19 g
689 mg	SODIUM	454 mg

Curb carbs: The carbs in this zesty soup come from the fresh vegetables like peppers and corn, leaving plenty of room for a slice of crusty bread or a half sandwich on the side.

Fill up on fiber: All of the vegetables in this soup provide 3 grams of fiber per serving. To boost the fiber even more, add whole grain pasta to the soup or a dinner roll and make it a meal.

Favor fats: Be sure to add a side high in healthy fats to this dish, like guacamole. Check out Wholly Guacamole single packs.

SMARTSTART

Get creative and fun: Savor this soup with a few blue corn chips and guacamole.

Makeover Magic

BEFORE		AFTER
305	CALORIES	136
23 g	FAT	3 g
14 g	SAT FAT	0.5 g
22 g	CARBS	22 g
4 g	FIBER	5 g
5 g	PROTEIN	6 g
1,131 mg	SODIUM	70 mg

Curb carbs: Instead of using flour and processed tomato puree as in a typical tomato soup, we thickened ours up with fresh vegetables, leaving plenty of room to add crunchy tortilla strips.

Fill up on fiber: This chunky tomato soup is full of high-fiber veggies, especially black beans, for a belly-filling meal!

Favor fats: Swap out heavy cream for a dollop of Greek yogurt to reduce saturated fat and pump up nutrition. To add healthy fat, try tossing in some kalamata olives or a bit of avocado.

KICKED-UP TOMATO SOUP

PREP TIME: **15 MINUTES** ■ TOTAL TIME: **50 MINUTES**

Makes 6 servings

2¼ cups water, divided

3 carrots, chopped

3 ribs celery, chopped

1 red bell pepper, chopped

1 tablespoon olive oil

1 small onion, chopped

1 jalapeño chile pepper, seeded and finely chopped (wear plastic gloves when handling)

1 can (28 ounces) no-salt-added diced tomatoes

1 can (15 ounces) no-salt-added black beans, rinsed and drained

½ cup chopped fresh cilantro

2 tablespoons lime juice

2 corn tortillas (6" diameter), sliced into ¼" strips

¼ cup + 2 tablespoons plain 0% Greek yogurt

1. In a large saucepan, heat ¼ cup of water over medium heat. Add the carrots, celery, and bell pepper and cook for 5 minutes, or until the vegetables are softened.

2. Add the oil to the saucepan and heat. Add the onion and jalapeño pepper. Cook, stirring occasionally, for 5 minutes, or until the vegetables are softened and golden.

3. Add the tomatoes (with juice) and the remaining 2 cups of water. Add the beans and cilantro and stir to blend. Bring to a simmer. Reduce the heat to low and cook for 25 minutes.

4. Add the lime juice. Ladle into 6 bowls and top with tortilla strips and a dollop of yogurt.

LENTIL–BROCCOLI RABE SOUP

PREP TIME: **10 MINUTES** ■ TOTAL TIME: **40 MINUTES**

Makes 6 servings

2 teaspoons olive oil

2 carrots, chopped

1 yellow onion, chopped

2 cloves garlic, minced

1 cup dried red lentils

4 cups low-sodium vegetable broth or water

2 tablespoons no-salt-added tomato paste

1 teaspoon ground cumin

½ pound broccoli rabe, rinsed, trimmed, and chopped

1 tablespoon finely chopped fresh oregano or 1 teaspoon dried

2 tablespoons grated Parmesan cheese

1. In a large saucepan, heat the oil over medium heat. Cook the carrots, onion, and garlic for 5 minutes, or until the vegetables start to soften. Stir in the lentils, broth or water, tomato paste, and cumin. Cover and bring to a brisk simmer.

2. Reduce the heat to low and simmer for 20 minutes. Stir in the broccoli rabe. Re-cover and simmer for 5 minutes, or until the lentils and broccoli rabe are tender. Add more water, if necessary, to thin the soup to the desired consistency. Serve garnished with the oregano and cheese.

Makeover Magic

BEFORE		AFTER
372	CALORIES	179
8 g	FAT	3 g
1 g	SAT FAT	0.5 g
55 g	CARBS	28 g
13 g	FIBER	7 g
24 g	PROTEIN	11 g
762 mg	SODIUM	154 mg

Curb carbs: Lentils are a major carb source, so instead of using a full pound of lentils for 6 servings as many lentil soups do, we replace some with broccoli rabe and other lower-carb veggies.

Fill up on fiber: Lentils *do* provide a lot of fiber, which is why our recipe has half as much as the comparison. To make up for lost fiber, add some crusty bread or a half sandwich to make a complete meal.

Favor fats: Olive oil is a source of healthy fats in this recipe, and using just a little grated Parmesan cheese gives the soup melty goodness without too much fat.

BEFORE		AFTER
390	CALORIES	99
20 g	FAT	0.5 g
11 g	SAT FAT	0 g
44 g	CARBS	23 g
4 g	FIBER	4 g
11 g	PROTEIN	2 g
930 mg	SODIUM	385 mg

Curb carbs: This dish uses fewer sweet potatoes than typical sweet potato soups and just enough apples to add a depth of flavor without piling on too many carbs.

Fill up on fiber: The fiber in this dish comes from the main ingredients—don't forget the apple skins!

Favor fats: This soup is still creamy even without added fat from butter, oils, and creams! Be sure to have a source of healthy fats on the side, or try sprinkling this soup with ground flaxseeds.

SMART**START**

Serve with 1 slice Ezekiel bread topped with 1 tablespoon natural almond butter or serve with fish and a green veggie for dinner.

APPLE–SWEET POTATO SOUP

PREP TIME: **10 MINUTES** ■ TOTAL TIME: **8 HOURS 20 MINUTES**

Makes 8 servings

4–5 sweet potatoes (2 pounds), peeled and cut into chunks

2 Granny Smith apples, cored and quartered

1 onion, finely chopped

3 cans (14.5 ounces each) low-sodium chicken broth

1 teaspoon chopped fresh thyme or ⅓ teaspoon dried

1. Place the sweet potatoes, apples, onion, broth, and thyme in a 4-quart or larger slow cooker and stir to combine. Cover and cook on low for 8 hours, or until the sweet potatoes are tender.

2. Let cool slightly, about 10 minutes. Puree the soup in a blender until smooth.

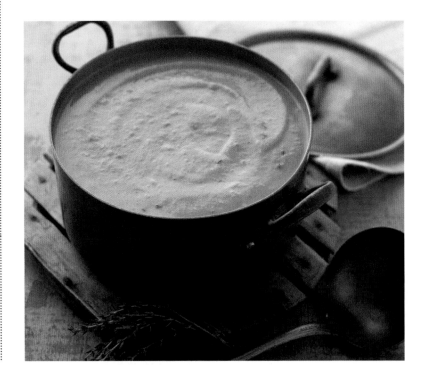

APPLE AND BLUE CHEESE SALAD

PREP TIME: 5 MINUTES ■ **TOTAL TIME: 10 MINUTES**

Makes 6 servings

2 tablespoons extra-virgin olive oil

3 tablespoons white distilled vinegar

2 tablespoons Dijon mustard

1 teaspoon lemon juice

10 ounces baby lettuce mix

Salt (optional)

Ground black pepper (optional)

3 firm-ripe Granny Smith apples, sliced

3 ounces reduced-fat blue cheese crumbles

⅓ cup walnut halves, chopped

1 tablespoon ground flaxseeds

1. In a small bowl, whisk together the oil, vinegar, mustard, and lemon juice.

2. Add the lettuce and toss gently to coat. Season with salt and pepper to taste, if using.

3. Divide the lettuce among 6 salad plates. Top each with apple slices, blue cheese, and walnuts and sprinkle with ground flaxseeds.

Makeover Magic

BEFORE		AFTER
330	CALORIES	170
24 g	FAT	11 g
5 g	SAT FAT	3 g
27 g	CARBS	14 g
4 g	FIBER	4 g
5 g	PROTEIN	5 g
630 mg	SODIUM	319 mg

Curb carbs: Many salads like this use added sweeteners such as maple syrup and brown sugar, but with ripe apples, this dish doesn't need them!

Fill up on fiber: The apples are the major source of fiber in this dish.

Favor fats: Ground flaxseeds and walnuts are our source of ALA omega-3 fatty acids, while olive oil provides additional MUFAs. To cut saturated fat, we made a light mustard vinaigrette in place of a sweet, creamy dressing.

Makeover Magic

BEFORE		AFTER
500	CALORIES	140
45 g	FAT	10 g
16 g	SAT FAT	3 g
10 g	CARBS	10 g
1 g	FIBER	4 g
15 g	PROTEIN	4 g
230 mg	SODIUM	160 mg

Curb carbs: Salads like this one are naturally low in carbs, meaning we have plenty of room to add a little carb-heavy dried fruit.

Fill up on fiber: Using spinach as a base and not spring greens makes the fiber and other nutrients shoot way up. Keep in mind that the fresh fruit is blended into the vinaigrette, so it does not pack as much fiber as the whole berries would.

Favor fats: Olive oil packs MUFAs, and walnuts pack the vegetarian source of omega-3 fatty acids known as ALA. And the goat cheese gives a creamy lift to this salad without going overboard on fat.

SPINACH-CRANBERRY SALAD

PREP TIME: **5 MINUTES** ■ TOTAL TIME: **10 MINUTES**

Makes 6 servings

VINAIGRETTE

¼ cup raspberries

¼ cup cranberries

2 tablespoons extra-virgin olive oil

1 tablespoon distilled white vinegar

1 teaspoon Dijon mustard

SALAD

12 ounces (2 bags) baby spinach

1 small red onion, thinly sliced

2 tablespoons unsweetened dried cranberries

2 ounces goat cheese, softened

¼ cup walnut halves

1. **To make the vinaigrette:** In a food processor, combine the raspberries, cranberries, oil, vinegar, and mustard and blend until smooth. Transfer to a small serving bowl.

2. **To make the salad:** In a large serving bowl, combine the spinach, onion, and cranberries. Drizzle the vinaigrette over the greens and toss to coat. Top with the goat cheese and walnuts.

Soups, Salads & Sandwiches

WARM ZUCCHINI SALAD

PREP TIME: **5 MINUTES** ■ TOTAL TIME: **15 MINUTES**

Makes 4 servings

3 zucchini

2 teaspoons canola oil

1 small red onion, thinly sliced

3 plum tomatoes, chopped

1 tablespoon lemon juice

¼ cup thinly sliced fresh basil

2 tablespoons grated Parmesan cheese

1. Using a vegetable peeler or mandoline, thinly slice the zucchini lengthwise, about ¹⁄₁₆" thick.

2. Heat the oil in a large nonstick skillet over medium-high heat. Cook the onion, stirring, for 3 minutes, or until soft. Add the tomatoes and zucchini and cook, stirring, for 5 minutes, or until tender.

3. Transfer the mixture to a serving bowl. Add the lemon juice and toss to coat. Sprinkle with the basil and cheese.

Makeover Magic

BEFORE		AFTER
150	CALORIES	73
10 g	FAT	4 g
5 g	SAT FAT	1 g
10 g	CARBS	8 g
1 g	FIBER	2 g
6 g	PROTEIN	3 g
200 mg	SODIUM	53 mg

Curb carbs: We swapped out corn for fresh tomatoes, which curbed the carbohydrates slightly. The thing we love about this salad is that the carbohydrates come from the vegetables, so it's all healthy! Plus, there's plenty of room to add more carbs to this meal.

Fill up on fiber: With just a few ingredients, this side salad serves up 2 grams of fiber, which makes a great addition to a main-course dish.

Favor fats: We think sometimes less really is more. In this case, smothering a salad in dressing is not going to help the freshness or flavor of the vegetables. We opted for a light drizzle of lemon juice and fresh herbs, which cut the fat back—the canola adds healthy fats, and a little Parmesan goes a long way to give this dish something special.

Makeover Magic

BEFORE		AFTER
280	CALORIES	175
23 g	FAT	7 g
3 g	SAT FAT	1 g
16 g	CARBS	12 g
6 g	FIBER	4 g
7 g	PROTEIN	17 g
1,990 mg	SODIUM	114 mg

Curb carbs: Many shrimp salads include noodles or rice, but this veggie version cuts carbs and adds crunch and flavor.

Fill up on fiber: Be sure to pair this salad with a half sandwich, a whole grain pita, or another good source of fiber.

Favor fats: Olive oil and flaxseeds in one recipe is a perfect way to boost the MUFAs and omega-3s!

CITRUS–GRILLED SHRIMP SALAD

PREP TIME: **5 MINUTES** ▪ TOTAL TIME: **45 MINUTES**

Makes 4 servings

3 tablespoons orange juice, divided

2 tablespoons lime juice, divided

½ teaspoon ground red pepper, divided

½ teaspoon ground cumin, divided

10 ounces peeled and deveined shrimp

1 red onion, cut into thick rounds

2 red bell peppers, sliced lengthwise

1 green bell pepper, sliced lengthwise

2 tablespoons ground flaxseeds

1 large tomato, cut into 8 wedges

1 tablespoon olive oil

1. In a medium bowl, combine 2 tablespoons of the orange juice, 1 tablespoon of the lime juice, ¼ teaspoon of the ground pepper, and ¼ teaspoon of the cumin. Add the shrimp and onion, turning to coat. Set aside to marinate for 30 minutes at room temperature.

2. Preheat the grill to medium. Oil a grill grate (and grill topper, if possible).

3. Place the onion and bell peppers (skin sides down) on the grill topper, cover, and grill, turning occasionally, for 7 minutes, or until the peppers are charred and the onion is crisp-tender. Transfer to a serving bowl.

4. In a small bowl, toss the shrimp with the ground flaxseeds until coated. Discard the remaining marinade. Place the shrimp on the grate, cover, and grill for 4 minutes, turning once, or until opaque.

5. In the serving bowl, toss together the bell peppers, onion, shrimp, tomato wedges, and oil. Add in the remaining 1 tablespoon of orange juice and lime juice and remaining ¼ teaspoon of ground pepper and cumin. Toss to coat.

Soups, Salads & Sandwiches

TRICOLOR SLAW AND POTATO SALAD

PREP TIME: **10 MINUTES** ▪ TOTAL TIME: **20 MINUTES**

Makes 6 servings

1½ pounds red potatoes, cut into ½" chunks

2 large red bell peppers, slivered

1½ cups frozen corn kernels, thawed

¼ cup distilled white vinegar

2 tablespoons olive oil

1 teaspoon paprika

½ teaspoon ground cumin

6 cups shredded cabbage

1. In a vegetable steamer, cook the potatoes for 8 minutes, or until firm-tender. Add the bell peppers for the last 2 minutes.

2. Transfer to a large bowl, along with the corn.

3. In a small bowl, whisk together the vinegar, oil, paprika, and cumin. Drizzle over the potatoes and peppers. Add the cabbage and toss to combine.

Makeover Magic

BEFORE		AFTER
320	CALORIES	185
17 g	FAT	5 g
3 g	SAT FAT	1 g
38 g	CARBS	32 g
4 g	FIBER	6 g
5 g	PROTEIN	5 g
1,200 mg	SODIUM	23 mg

Curb carbs: By replacing a portion of the potatoes in a traditional potato salad with peppers, cabbage, and corn, we curbed carbs while creating a salad that was both filling and delicious.

Fill up on fiber: This veggie-fied version has enough grams of fiber to take the "magic carbs" effect into account—this salad has just 26 grams of carbs once you do the math!

Favor fats: Mayonnaise is an obvious base for this type of salad, but by using vinegar we allow the ingredients to shine while cutting fat. Olive oil, meanwhile, provides healthy fats.

BEFORE		AFTER
566	CALORIES	165
36 g	FAT	3 g
12 g	SAT FAT	0.5 g
43 g	CARBS	29 g
4 g	FIBER	5 g
16 g	PROTEIN	7 g
1,226 mg	SODIUM	232 mg

Curb carbs: We used just enough potatoes to make the perfect serving size.

Fill up on fiber: Between the potatoes, celery, and flax-seeds, this salad is a fibrous side dish!

Favor fats: Instead of a heavy dressing of bacon and gorgon-zola, we went with a vinegar-based dressing and added ground flaxseeds, which adds healthy fats known as omega-3 fatty acids.

WARM GERMAN POTATO SALAD

PREP TIME: **5 MINUTES** ■ TOTAL TIME: **35 MINUTES**

Makes 6 servings

2 pounds red potatoes, unpeeled, cut into large chunks

3 ounces Canadian bacon, chopped

6 scallions, thinly sliced

5 ribs celery, sliced

3 tablespoons ground flaxseeds

3 tablespoons cider vinegar

3 tablespoons apple juice

2 tablespoons stone-ground mustard

3 sprigs parsley, finely chopped

1. Set a vegetable steamer in a medium saucepan. Fill with water to just below the steamer.

2. Place the potatoes on the steamer. Cover and bring to a boil over high heat. Reduce the heat to medium high. Cook for 15 minutes, or until tender. Transfer to a large bowl and allow to cool for 10 minutes.

3. In a medium nonstick skillet set over medium heat, cook the bacon for 3 minutes. Add the scallions and celery. Cook, stirring, for 3 minutes, or until the onion is soft and the bacon is browned. Reduce the heat to low. Add the flaxseeds and toss to coat. Add the vinegar, apple juice, mustard, and parsley. Cook for 2 minutes, or until heated through. Pour over the potatoes. Toss to evenly coat.

CORN, BLACK BEAN, AND EDAMAME SALAD

PREP TIME: **5 MINUTES** ■ TOTAL TIME: **10 MINUTES**

Makes 6 servings

2 cups frozen shelled edamame

1½ cups fresh corn kernels (from 2 large ears)

1½ cups canned black beans, rinsed and drained

3 plum tomatoes, chopped

1 small red onion, chopped

¼ cup chopped fresh cilantro

1 tablespoon extra-virgin olive oil

3 tablespoons freshly squeezed lime juice

½ teaspoon ground red pepper

1. Prepare the edamame according to package directions. Drain and rinse under cold water. Transfer to a large bowl.

2. Stir in the corn, beans, tomatoes, onion, cilantro, oil, lime juice, and pepper. Toss well.

Makeover Magic

BEFORE		AFTER
190	CALORIES	164
6 g	FAT	5 g
1 g	SAT FAT	0.5 g
33 g	CARBS	20 g
4 g	FIBER	6 g
5 g	PROTEIN	10 g
50 mg	SODIUM	141 mg

Curb carbs: The carbohydrates in this dish come from the various veggies and beans, leaving plenty of room for a half sandwich or another lunchtime treat.

Fill up on fiber: By adding a greater variety of fiber-packed ingredients to our corn salad, we not only double the fiber, but the flavor as well!

Favor fats: Instead of dousing the salad in mayo, we used a light coating of olive oil (our healthy fat!) and lime juice for a zesty, fresh flavor.

SMARTSTART

Check out our meal plan in Appendix A (page 328) to see what you can pair this salad with.

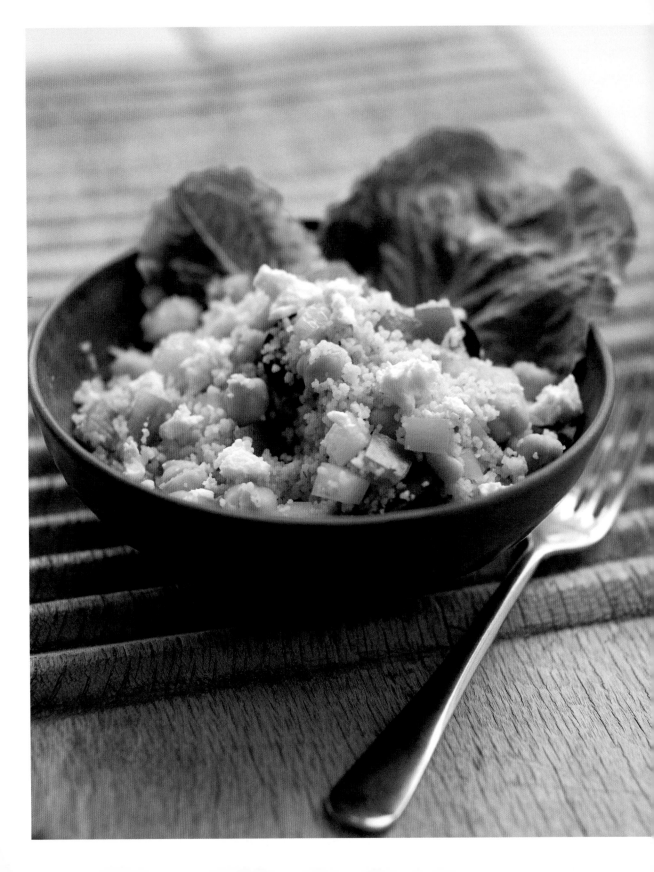

COUSCOUS AND CHICKPEA SALAD

PREP TIME: **10 MINUTES** ▪ TOTAL TIME: **50 MINUTES**

Makes 6 servings

1½ cups water

1 teaspoon + 1 tablespoon olive oil, divided

1 cup whole wheat couscous

1 can (15 ounces) chickpeas, rinsed and drained

1 plum tomato, chopped

1 red or yellow bell pepper, chopped

1 ounce pitted kalamata olives, sliced

1½ tablespoons pine nuts

1½ tablespoons lemon juice

⅓ cup crumbled feta cheese

1. In a medium saucepan over high heat, bring the water and 1 teaspoon of the oil to a boil. Stir in the couscous. Remove from the heat and cover. Let stand for 5 minutes, or until the liquid is absorbed. Fluff with a fork.

2. Transfer the couscous to a large bowl. Add the chickpeas, tomato, pepper, olives, and nuts. Toss gently until mixed.

3. In a small bowl, whisk together the lemon juice and remaining tablespoon of oil. Mix and pour over the salad. Toss to mix well. Cover and refrigerate for 30 minutes to blend the flavors. Top the salad with feta cheese.

Makeover Magic

BEFORE		AFTER
304	CALORIES	185
17 g	FAT	8 g
3 g	SAT FAT	2 g
31 g	CARBS	24 g
2 g	FIBER	4 g
8 g	PROTEIN	6 g
619 mg	SODIUM	235 mg

Curb carbs: Adding chickpeas to this couscous salad reduces the carbs while adding some fiber.

Fill up on fiber: In addition to the whole wheat couscous, chickpeas, peppers, tomatoes, and olives all boost the fiber.

Favor fats: Olives and olive oil both contribute to the fat in this dish, and best of all, they contribute healthy MUFAs.

Makeover Magic

BEFORE		AFTER
330	CALORIES	273
12 g	FAT	10 g
2 g	SAT FAT	1 g
48 g	CARBS	37 g
4 g	FIBER	4 g
9 g	PROTEIN	13 g
550 mg	SODIUM	436 mg

Curb carbs: A cup of soba noodles has nearly half as many carbs as a cup of spaghetti, making it a great alternative in pasta dishes.

Fill up on fiber: Both soba noodles and the beans in this salad provide fiber.

Favor fats: This salad is full of flavor, and much of it comes from the sesame oil, a great source of polyunsaturated fats!

CHILLED CILANTRO–SOBA NOODLE SALAD

PREP TIME: 5 MINUTES ■ **TOTAL TIME: 45 MINUTES**

Makes 6 servings

8 ounces soba noodles

2 cups frozen shelled edamame

1 red bell pepper, thinly sliced

1 green bell pepper, thinly sliced

3 scallions, thinly sliced

¼ cup thinly sliced fresh cilantro

3 tablespoons sesame oil

2 tablespoons low-sodium soy sauce

2 tablespoons orange juice

1 teaspoon orange zest

½ teaspoon crushed red-pepper flakes

1. Fill a 6-quart saucepan with water and bring to a boil. Cook the noodles and edamame for 6 minutes. Empty into a colander and rinse well with cold water. Drain and place in a serving bowl.

2. Stir in the bell peppers, scallions, and cilantro. Toss gently.

3. In a small bowl, whisk together the oil, soy sauce, orange juice, zest, and pepper flakes. Pour the dressing over the noodle mixture. Toss gently and refrigerate for 30 minutes to allow the flavors to blend. Serve cold or at room temperature.

Soups, Salads & Sandwiches

CREAMY PASTA SALAD

PREP TIME: **10 MINUTES** ■ TOTAL TIME: **25 MINUTES**

Makes 4 servings

6 ounces whole grain penne

½ cup plain 0% Greek yogurt

2 tablespoons grated Parmesan cheese

¼ cup finely chopped fresh basil

1 tablespoon red wine vinegar

½ teaspoon dried mustard

1 clove garlic, minced

1 green bell pepper, chopped

2 romaine hearts, chopped

1 cup cherry tomatoes, halved

1. Prepare the pasta according to package directions. Rinse under cold water and drain.

2. In a large bowl, stir together the yogurt, cheese, basil, vinegar, mustard, and garlic. Add the pepper, romaine, tomatoes, and pasta. Toss to coat well.

Makeover Magic

BEFORE		AFTER
282	CALORIES	210
6 g	FAT	2 g
2 g	SAT FAT	0.5 g
46 g	CARBS	39 g
3 g	FIBER	7 g
11 g	PROTEIN	11 g
200 mg	SODIUM	58 mg

Curb carbs: We cut the amount of penne in this pasta salad with peppers, tomatoes, and romaine hearts that add body without adding many carbs.

Fill up on fiber: Using whole grain pasta boosts the fiber.

Favor fats: To cut saturated fat, we used a lighter dressing made from Greek yogurt, vinegar, and seasonings instead of mayonnaise. Be sure to pair this dish with a healthy fat source.

SMARTSTART

Add 2 cans of tuna for a dose of DHA.

Makeover Magic

Curb carbs: This version has 6 grams of fiber, which can be subtracted from the carbs for a total of 34 grams of carbs– 11 grams fewer than the traditional version.

Fill up on fiber: By using whole wheat rolls and topping the steak with more vegetables than usual, you can really boost the fiber in this sandwich!

Favor fats: We used thin-sliced deli roast beef instead of chipped steak to cut down the saturated fat. For a dose of healthy fats, consider adding more olive oil, or a few sliced kalamata olives on top.

PHILLY CHEESE STEAKS

PREP TIME: **5 MINUTES** ▪ TOTAL TIME: **15 MINUTES**

Makes 4 servings

1½ teaspoons olive oil

1 onion, sliced

1 red bell pepper, sliced

1 green bell pepper, sliced

¾ pound thinly sliced low-sodium deli-style roast beef

¼ cup shredded Cheddar cheese

4 whole grain hoagie rolls

2 low-sodium dill pickle spears, halved, for garnish

1. In a large nonstick skillet, heat the oil over medium-high heat. Cook the onion and bell peppers for 5 minutes, or until tender. Transfer to a bowl.

2. Reduce the heat to medium. Cook the roast beef slices in the skillet for 1 minute, or until heated through. Top with the cheese and cook for 1 minute, or until the cheese is melted.

3. Divide the beef among the 4 rolls and top with the onion and peppers. Serve each sandwich with half a pickle.

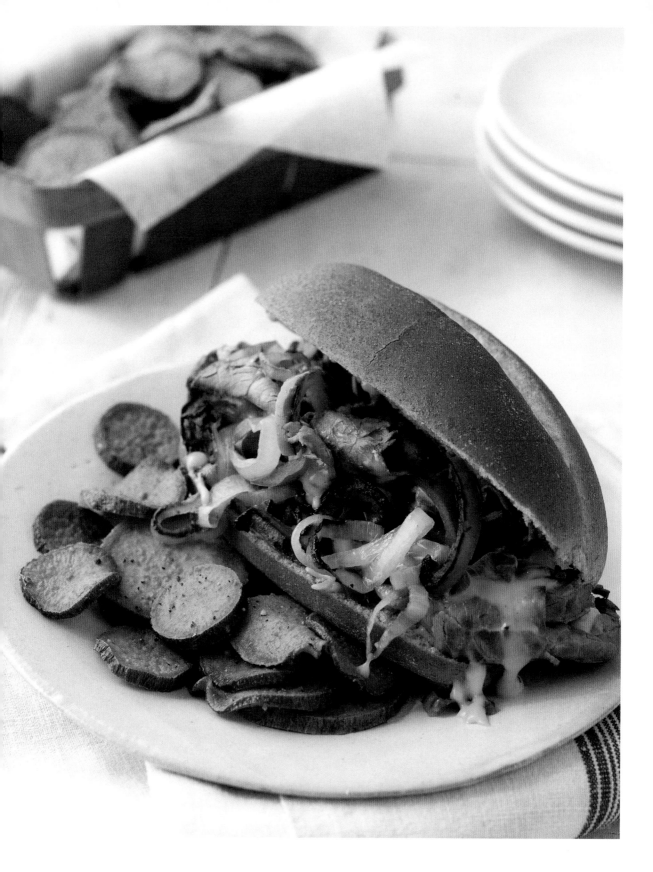

Makeover Magic

BEFORE		AFTER
470	CALORIES	197
31 g	FAT	8 g
11 g	SAT FAT	2 g
26 g	CARBS	22 g
2 g	FIBER	9 g
18 g	PROTEIN	17 g
1,100 mg	SODIUM	408 mg

Curb carbs: We turned the traditional sausage sandwich into a wrap, replacing the doughy bun with a tortilla to curb carbs.

Fill up on fiber: Use a whole wheat tortilla and pair the sausage with fiber-packed veggies. This dish has 9 grams of fiber, meaning with the magic carbs, you get just 13 grams!

Favor fats: To reduce saturated fat, opt for turkey sausage instead of pork. Be sure to pair this sandwich with a source of healthy fat, such as sliced olives.

SAUSAGE AND PEPPER WRAPS

PREP TIME: **5 MINUTES** ▪ TOTAL TIME: **20 MINUTES**

Makes 4 servings

½ pound sweet Italian turkey sausages, sliced

1 small onion, thinly sliced

1 green bell pepper, thinly sliced

2 cups low-sodium tomato-basil pasta sauce

4 whole wheat tortillas (6" diameter)

2 tablespoons grated Parmesan cheese

1. Line a baking sheet with aluminum foil. In a large nonstick skillet, cook the sausage over medium-high heat, stirring, for 5 minutes, or until no longer pink. Add the onion and pepper and cook for 3 minutes, or until slightly browned. Stir in the sauce and cook for 5 minutes, or until heated through and the flavors blend.

2. Preheat the broiler.

3. Stuff the tortillas with the sausage mixture and sprinkle 1½ teaspoons cheese on each tortilla. Put on the prepared baking sheet and place in the oven for 1 minute, or until the cheese is melted and golden.

Soups, Salads & Sandwiches

MONTE CRISTOS

PREP TIME: **5 MINUTES** ■ TOTAL TIME: **10 MINUTES**

Makes 2 servings

4 slices whole grain bread, toasted

¾ ounce low-sodium deli ham (about 2 slices)

¾ ounce low-sodium deli turkey (about 2 slices)

1 slice Gruyère cheese, halved

2 teaspoons Dijon mustard

2 egg whites

2 tablespoons 1% milk

1. On 2 slices of toast, layer the ham, turkey, and cheese.

2. Spread the mustard on the remaining 2 slices of toast and top the sandwiches.

3. Heat a cast-iron skillet over medium heat for 2 minutes.

4. In a shallow bowl, whisk the egg whites and milk together. Dip 1 side of a sandwich into the egg mixture and let the excess drip off. Repeat on the other side. Repeat with the other sandwich.

5. Coat the skillet with cooking spray. Cook the sandwiches for 6 minutes, turning once, until the meat is warmed through, the cheese is melting, and the egg is cooked.

Makeover Magic

BEFORE		AFTER
890	CALORIES	244
59 g	FAT	7 g
17 g	SAT FAT	3 g
65 g	CARBS	25 g
3 g	FIBER	4 g
26 g	PROTEIN	19 g
970 mg	SODIUM	598 mg

Curb carbs: Instead of using 3 slices of bread to make a club-style layered sandwich, we stuck with 2 slices and piled the filling high.

Fill up on fiber: Whole grain bread is versatile and works perfectly for this sandwich, providing 4 grams of fiber!

Favor fats: We cut the fat by not frying the sandwich in butter, and we used 1% milk and only egg whites, instead of 3 large eggs. Add healthy fats to this dish by substituting canola oil for cooking spray or adding olives or avocado slices into the sandwich.

Makeover Magic

Curb carbs: It's easy to curb the carbs on this sandwich by making it an open-faced version that uses just 1 slice of bread.

Fill up on fiber: Thanks to using whole grain bread, our open-faced sandwich has as much fiber as a regular *banh mi* sandwich that uses 2 slices.

Favor fats: Ground flaxseeds add healthy fats.

OPEN-FACED ASIAN CHICKEN SANDWICHES

PREP TIME: **15 MINUTES** ■ TOTAL TIME: **25 MINUTES**

Makes 4 servings

4 chicken cutlets (3 ounces each)

1 tablespoon + 2 teaspoons low-sodium soy sauce, divided

2 tablespoons seasoned rice vinegar

1 clove garlic, minced

¼ teaspoon red chile paste

1 tablespoon honey, divided

1 small cucumber, thinly sliced

1 cup shredded cabbage

¼ cup chopped fresh cilantro, divided

2 tablespoons ground flaxseeds

4 slices whole grain bread

½ cup plain 0% Greek yogurt

1. Coat a grill rack or broiler pan with cooking spray. Preheat the grill or broiler.

2. Brush each chicken cutlet with 1 teaspoon of the soy sauce and grill or broil the cutlets, turning once, for 10 minutes, or until no longer pink and the juices run clear.

3. Whisk together the vinegar, garlic, chile paste, and 2 teaspoons of the honey in a small bowl. Toss together the cucumber, cabbage, half of the cilantro, and the ground flaxseeds in a medium bowl. Toss with half of the vinegar mixture. Set aside.

4. Add the remaining 1 teaspoon soy sauce and 1 teaspoon honey to the remaining vinegar mixture. Place 1 bread slice on each of 4 plates. Top each with a chicken breast and one-quarter of the cabbage mixture. Drizzle with 2 tablespoons of the soy mixture. Top each with 2 tablespoons of the yogurt and sprinkle with the remaining cilantro.

SMARTSTART

Go ahead and use 2 slices of Ezekiel bread if you want a traditional sandwich.

SWEET TURKEY PANINIS

PREP TIME: **5 MINUTES** ■ TOTAL TIME: **15 MINUTES**

Makes 2 servings

1 tablespoon + 1 teaspoon olive oil mayonnaise	½ pound deli-sliced, no-salt turkey breast
2 teaspoons Dijon mustard	½ cup fresh arugula
4 whole wheat tortillas (6" diameter)	2 ounces Asiago cheese, shredded
1 pear, thinly sliced	

1. In a small bowl, whisk together the mayonnaise and mustard.

2. Lay the tortillas on a clean work surface. Divide the pear slices, turkey, arugula, and cheese among the top halves of the tortillas. Drizzle with the mayonnaise mixture. Fold over the other half of each tortilla.

3. Heat a nonstick skillet over medium heat. Add the sandwiches and place a second skillet on top, pressing down slightly. Cook for 6 minutes, turning once, until slightly flattened and toasted.

SMART START

Add 1 tablespoon pine nuts or walnuts for diabetes-friendly fats and more fiber.

Makeover Magic

BEFORE		AFTER
450	CALORIES	212
51 g	FAT	9 g
19 g	SAT FAT	3 g
41 g	CARBS	19 g
4 g	FIBER	9 g
25 g	PROTEIN	22 g
1,610 mg	SODIUM	293 mg

Curb carbs: Swap in a whole wheat tortilla for a white roll for instant carb control.

Fill up on fiber: At 9 grams of fiber, we can use magic carbs to bring the total carbs of this meal down to just 10 grams—plenty of room for a side of chips or pasta salad!

Favor fats: We used a lean cut of turkey and a small amount of olive oil–based mayo and cheese instead of tons of cheese, fatty spreads, and meat. For more healthy fats, add in some ground flaxseeds or drizzle each sandwich with a tablespoon of olive oil.

BUFFALO GRILLED CHEESE SANDWICHES

PREP TIME: **5 MINUTES** ■ TOTAL TIME: **10 MINUTES**

Makes 4 servings

1 tablespoon olive oil mayonnaise

1 tablespoon hot sauce

8 slices whole grain bread

4 thin slices red onion

2 ribs celery, sliced

4 slices Cheddar cheese

4 tablespoons reduced-fat blue cheese crumbles

1. In a small bowl, stir together the mayonnaise and hot sauce.

2. Place 4 bread slices on a work surface. Spread the mayonnaise on the bread slices. Layer with the onion, celery, and cheese and top with the remaining bread slices. Coat the top bread slice of each sandwich with cooking spray.

3. Place the coated side down on a grill pan or skillet. Coat the remaining bread slice of each sandwich with cooking spray. Place a heavy pan over the top of the sandwiches. Cook for 4 minutes, turning once, until lightly browned.

BACON AND APPLE GRILLED CHEESES

PREP TIME: **5 MINUTES** ■ TOTAL TIME: **20 MINUTES**

Makes 4 servings

4 strips turkey bacon, cut into small pieces

8 slices whole grain bread

1 tablespoon Dijon mustard

4 slices sharp Cheddar cheese

1 Granny Smith apple, peeled, cored, and sliced

1. Coat a large nonstick skillet with cooking spray. Cook the bacon strips over medium-low heat, turning once, for 2 minutes, or until golden brown. Transfer to a plate lined with paper towels. Reduce the heat to low.

2. Slather 4 slices of bread with the mustard and divide the cheese, apple, and bacon among them. Top with the other bread slices and add to the hot pan. Cook for 12 minutes, turning once, until each side is deep brown and crunchy.

Makeover Magic

BEFORE		AFTER
820	CALORIES	283
42 g	FAT	12 g
22 g	SAT FAT	6 g
75 g	CARBS	28 g
3 g	FIBER	5 g
37 g	PROTEIN	18 g
1,500 mg	SODIUM	658 mg

Curb carbs: Ditch the white bread and replace it with whole grain slices, which are lower in carbs thanks to magic carbs.

Fill up on fiber: The whole grain bread is also an excellent source of fiber.

Favor fats: We used turkey bacon instead of pork and a light mustard spread instead of a high-fat creamy dressing to moderate saturated fat. Add healthy fat to this meal by enjoying a handful of almonds on the side.

Makeover Magic

Curb carbs: Using 6" tortillas instead of the usual 10" or larger varieties is an easy way to cut carbs while getting more filling in every bite.

Fill up on fiber: These whole wheat tortillas are packed with fiber!

Favor fats: The walnuts in this wrap are a yummy source of ALA omega-3 fatty acids—plus the tuna packs DHA!

TUNA SALAD WRAPS

PREP TIME: **10 MINUTES** ■ TOTAL TIME: **10 MINUTES**

Makes 4 servings

2 tablespoons plain 0% Greek yogurt

1 teaspoon lemon juice

1 can (6 ounces) white tuna packed in water, drained

½ cup red grapes, halved

1 rib celery, chopped

¼ cup walnut halves, chopped

2 slices red onion, chopped

4 whole wheat tortillas (6" diameter)

2 cups arugula

1. In a bowl, stir together the yogurt and lemon juice. Add the tuna, grapes, celery, walnuts, and onion.

2. Lay the tortillas on a flat surface, top with the arugula and tuna mixture, and roll.

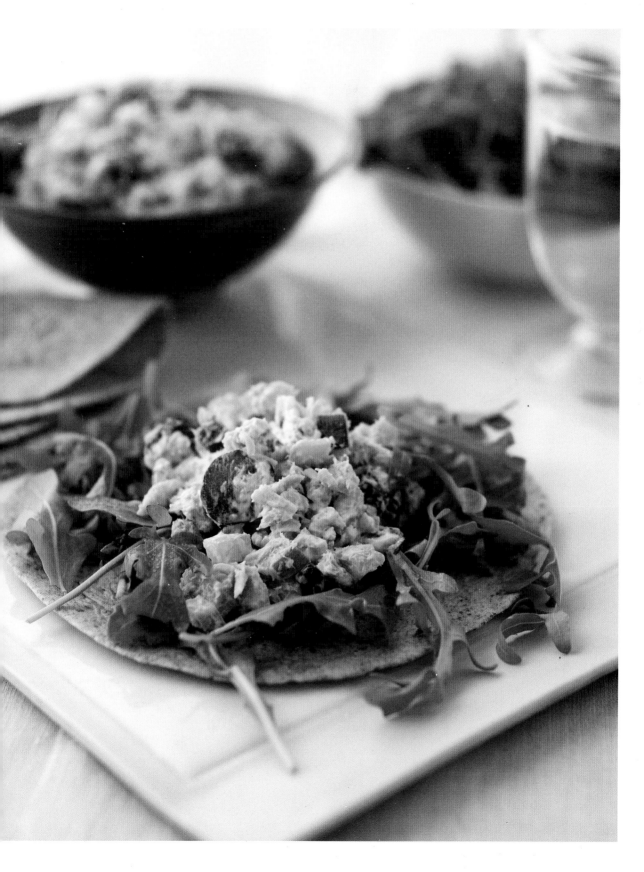

BEFORE		AFTER
440	CALORIES	230
16 g	FAT	11 g
3 g	SAT FAT	1 g
39 g	CARBS	21 g
3 g	FIBER	8 g
34 g	PROTEIN	19 g
1,850 mg	SODIUM	269 mg

Curb carbs: Substituting a whole wheat tortilla for 2 slices of bread is a surefire way to reduce the carbs. Look for tortillas with 20 grams of carbohydrates.

Fill up on fiber: Not only does the whole wheat tortilla have fiber, but lettuce and celery contribute an additional gram.

Favor fats: Thick, creamy dressings are usually filled with fat, so we opted for shrimp cooked in a small amount of oil, and a barbecue sauce to top! In this dish, cashews are our source of blood sugar–friendly MUFAs.

BARBECUE SHRIMP WRAPS

PREP TIME: **5 MINUTES** ■ TOTAL TIME: **10 MINUTES**

Makes 2 servings

2 teaspoons canola oil

2 cloves garlic, minced

4 ounces medium peeled and deveined shrimp

2 whole wheat tortillas (6" diameter)

2 ribs celery, chopped

2 tablespoons raw cashews

2 tablespoons barbecue sauce

1 cup shredded romaine lettuce

1. In a nonstick skillet, heat the oil over medium-high heat. Cook the garlic for 1 minute, or until fragrant. Add the shrimp and cook for 2 minutes, or until the shrimp are opaque.

2. Lay the tortillas on a clean work surface. Divide the shrimp mixture among the 2 tortillas. Add the celery and cashews. Drizzle 1 tablespoon barbecue sauce on each tortilla. Top with the lettuce and roll.

ROAST BEEF ROLLS

PREP TIME: **5 MINUTES** ■ TOTAL TIME: **5 MINUTES**

Makes 2 servings

1 cup cooked quinoa, chilled

1 pear, cored and finely chopped

1 tablespoon lemon juice

2 tablespoons chopped pine nuts

¼ small red onion, finely chopped

1 cup shredded romaine lettuce

8 slices low-sodium, lean deli roast beef, ¾ ounce each

1. In a medium bowl, combine the quinoa, pear, lemon juice, pine nuts, onion, and romaine. Stir to mix.

2. Fill the center of each roast beef slice with the mixture and roll up. Use a wooden pick to hold the roll together. Serve.

Makeover Magic

BEFORE		AFTER
810	CALORIES	288
74 g	FAT	4 g
12 g	SAT FAT	2 g
19 g	CARBS	40 g
1 g	FIBER	8 g
18 g	PROTEIN	24 g
590 mg	SODIUM	508 mg

Curb carbs: Quinoa is a carb that is higher in protein, so the perfect choice for someone eating to beat diabetes. Using roast beef as the roll instead of a wrap further curbs carbs.

Fill up on fiber: You can find fiber in grains like quinoa, chopped fresh fruits like the pear, and in the pine nuts.

Favor fats: By excluding cheese and adding nuts, you can decrease saturated fat and increase our favorite fats.

SMARTSTART

If eating this dish as an appetizer, serve 2 rolls per person. If eating this dish as an entrée, serve 4 rolls per person, with a side.

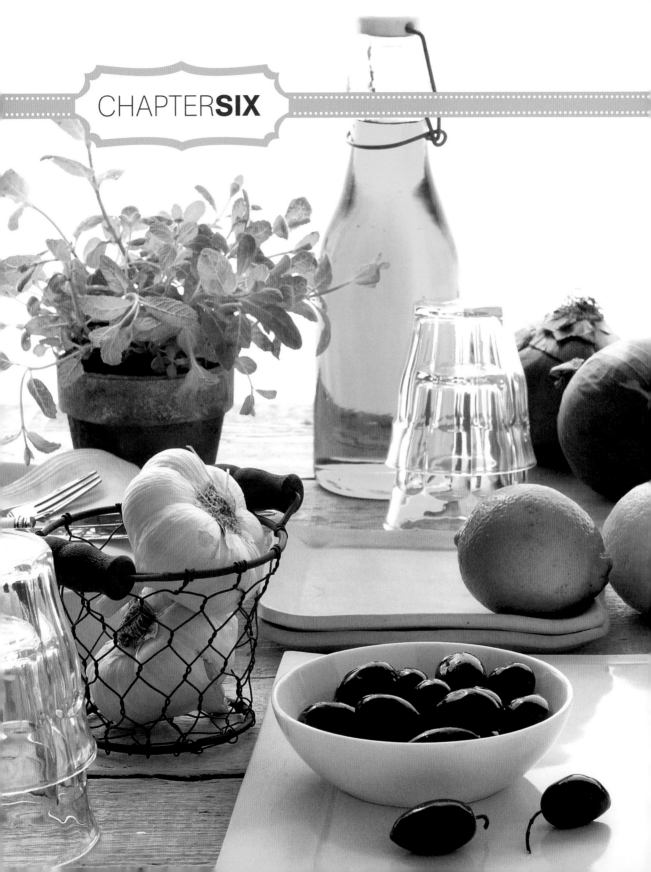

Appetizers & Snacks

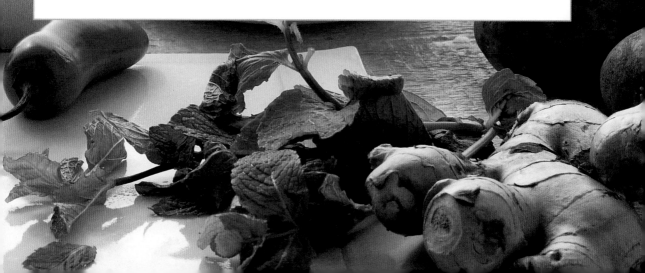

Makeover Magic

BEFORE		AFTER
230	CALORIES	112
13 g	FAT	2 g
3 g	SAT FAT	0.5 g
25 g	CARBS	21 g
2 g	FIBER	2 g
6 g	PROTEIN	3 g
450 mg	SODIUM	338 mg

Curb carbs: Swap a typical refined white bread for high-fiber, wholesome grains like this whole wheat baguette. Fresh fruit like papaya adds sweetness and antioxidants at the same time, but keep in mind that one serving has 21 grams of carbs, so you may need to choose a lower-carb entrée to complement the appetizer.

Fill up on fiber: Choosing whole wheat adds fiber to help make you feel full. If you can find a sprouted wheat baguette, choose that one for even more fiber.

Favor fats: Olive oil is chock-full of monounsaturated fats, making this the best oil for your bruschetta.

PAPAYA-TOMATO BRUSCHETTA

PREP TIME: **10 MINUTES** ■ TOTAL TIME: **20 MINUTES**

Makes 12 servings (2 slices each)

1 whole wheat baguette, cut into 24 slices (½" thick)

2 tablespoons olive oil, divided

1 clove garlic, halved

1 papaya, peeled, seeded, and chopped

4 plum tomatoes, finely chopped

½ small red onion, finely chopped

½ cup chopped fresh cilantro

1 teaspoon honey

½ teaspoon grated lemon zest

1. Preheat the oven to 450°F.

2. Brush the bread on both sides with 1 tablespoon of the oil. Place on a baking sheet and bake for 7 minutes, or until golden brown and crisp. Rub the toasted bread very lightly with the cut garlic clove.

3. In a medium bowl, combine the papaya, tomatoes, onion, cilantro, honey, lemon zest, and remaining 1 tablespoon oil. Spoon on top of the toasted garlic bread.

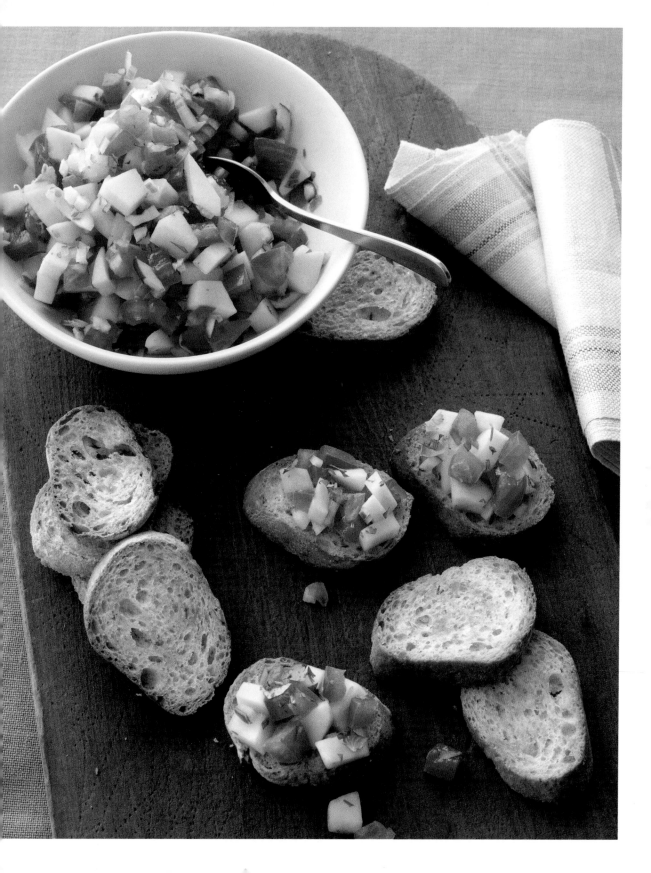

Makeover Magic

BEFORE		AFTER
240	CALORIES	112
10 g	FAT	2 g
4 g	SAT FAT	0.5 g
20 g	CARBS	12 g
<1 g	FIBER	1 g
17 g	PROTEIN	13 g
630 mg	SODIUM	121 mg

Curb carbs: This appetizer is surely friendly when curbing carbs!

Fill up on fiber: Low-carb apps are typically lower in fiber as well, since fiber comes from plant sources. Simply enjoy this healthy appetizer and choose a high-fiber entrée to accompany it.

Favor fats: Our marinade beats out bottled sauces that are high in saturated fat and processed ingredients. Serve with hawaiian cashews for a dose of healthy fats

HAWAIIAN CHICKEN SKEWERS

PREP TIME: **10 MINUTES** ■ TOTAL TIME: **1 HOUR 25 MINUTES**

Makes 6 servings

2 cloves garlic, minced

1 tablespoon grated fresh ginger or 1 teaspoon dried

1 jalapeño chile pepper, seeded and finely chopped (wear plastic gloves when handling)

2 tablespoons low-sodium soy sauce

2 tablespoons honey

2 tablespoons fresh lime juice (from 2 limes)

½ pineapple, cored, sliced, cut into 1" cubes

2 boneless, skinless chicken breasts, cut into 1" cubes

1 small red onion, cut into 8 wedges

1 tablespoon chopped fresh cilantro

1. In a small saucepan, combine the garlic, ginger, pepper, soy sauce, honey, and lime juice. Slowly bring to a boil over medium heat. Set aside and cool.

2. Toss the pineapple and chicken into the marinade and refrigerate. Let marinate for 1 to 2 hours.

3. Heat the grill over medium-high heat.

4. Thread the pineapple, chicken, and onion onto 6 metal skewers and grill for 10 minutes, turning once, until the chicken is browned and cooked through. Transfer to a serving platter and sprinkle with chopped cilantro.

Appetizers & Snacks

MEDITERRANEAN CHICKEN PINWHEELS

PREP TIME: **5 MINUTES** ■ TOTAL TIME: **55 MINUTES**

Makes 6 servings (3 pinwheels each)

2 cups packed baby spinach leaves

1 large boneless, skinless chicken breast (10 ounces)

2 tablespoons goat cheese, softened

2 tablespoons chopped, pitted kalamata olives

⅓ cup chopped sun-dried tomatoes

1. Preheat the oven to 375°F.

2. Coat a small baking sheet with canola cooking spray.

3. Heat a large nonstick skillet over medium heat. Place the spinach in the skillet, cover, and cook, tossing occasionally, for 2 minutes, or until wilted. Drain off any excess water. Pat dry with paper towels. Set aside.

4. Lay the chicken breast on a work surface. If the fillet is attached, open it away from the breast like opening a book. Using a sharp knife, cut through the thickest part of the chicken breast, without cutting through the edge. Open the breast like a book. With a heavy skillet or meat mallet, pound the chicken to ½" thickness. Spread the goat cheese evenly over the top side of the chicken. Scatter the reserved spinach, olives, and sun-dried tomatoes over the goat cheese. Starting with a long side of the chicken, roll the chicken horizontally, jelly-roll style. Using 2 pieces of cooking twine or string, tie the chicken to secure. Transfer the chicken to the small baking sheet. Bake for 40 minutes, or until an instant-read thermometer inserted in the center of the chicken pinwheel registers 165°F.

5. Remove and let stand for 10 minutes. Carefully unwrap the foil. Cut into 18 thin slices.

Makeover Magic

BEFORE		AFTER
400	CALORIES	98
20 g	FAT	4 g
6 g	SAT FAT	1 g
34 g	CARBS	3 g
1 g	FIBER	1 g
20 g	PROTEIN	12 g
1,230 mg	SODIUM	260 mg

Curb carbs: Unlike many pinwheel recipes, which use store-bought crescent roll dough, we opted to use a thin chicken fillet as our wrap.

Fill up on fiber: We snuck spinach into this recipe, which adds great flavor but also packs in many nutrients.

Favor fats: Pitted black olives serve up a dose of MUFAs.

BEFORE		AFTER
650	CALORIES	64
40 g	FAT	0 g
16 g	SAT FAT	0 g
48 g	CARBS	1 g
0 g	FIBER	0 g
28 g	PROTEIN	13 g
900 mg	SODIUM	326 mg

Curb carbs: These wings make a tasty pre-dinner low-carb snack with only 1 gram of carbs from the sauce!

Fill up on fiber: Pair this kickin' chicken with carrot sticks for vitamin A and fiber!

Favor fats: This recipe has almost no fat, so be sure to pump up your MUFAs and omega-3s with your entrée.

KICKIN' CHICKEN WINGS

PREP TIME: 5 MINUTES ■ TOTAL TIME: 40 MINUTES

Makes 6 servings (2 wings each)

3 tablespoons cayenne pepper sauce

2 tablespoons barbecue sauce

2 cloves garlic, minced

12 boneless, skinless chicken breast tenderloins (12 ounces)

2 tablespoons low-fat blue cheese dressing (optional)

1. In a large bowl, mix the pepper sauce, barbecue sauce, and garlic. Place the chicken and half of the sauce in a large resealable bag. Close and shake to coat each piece. Refrigerate and allow the chicken to marinate for 30 minutes.

2. Heat a large skillet over medium heat. Remove the chicken from the bag, with any extra sauce in the bag, and cook for 4 minutes, turning once, or until browned and the internal temperature reaches 165°F.

3. Add the chicken to a serving plate and drizzle with the remaining sauce. Serve with the dressing, if using.

GREEK MEATBALLS

PREP TIME: **5 MINUTES** ■ TOTAL TIME: **35 MINUTES**

Makes 8 servings (2 meatballs each)

1 package (10 ounces) frozen spinach, thawed and squeezed dry

1 pound 99% fat-free ground turkey

¾ cup whole wheat bread crumbs

2 tablespoons ground flaxseeds

2 cloves garlic, minced

1 teaspoon dried oregano

¼ cup crumbled feta cheese

1 egg, lightly beaten

1 cup no-sugar-added marinara sauce (optional)

1. Preheat the oven to 375°F.

2. Coat a large baking pan with cooking spray.

3. In a large bowl, combine the spinach, turkey, bread crumbs, flaxseeds, garlic, oregano, feta cheese, and egg. With clean hands, roll the mixture into 16 meatballs. Place on the prepared pan and bake for 15 minutes. Rotate the meatballs to ensure that they stay round. Bake for 15 minutes, or until the meatballs have reached an internal temperature of 165°F. Serve with marinara sauce, if using.

Makeover Magic

BEFORE		AFTER
540	CALORIES	125
32 g	FAT	4 g
11 g	SAT FAT	1 g
31 g	CARBS	6 g
2 g	FIBER	3 g
31 g	PROTEIN	18 g
900 mg	SODIUM	126 mg

Curb carbs: Use whole wheat bread crumbs to make these meatballs more wholesome.

Fill up on fiber: Pair with a dinner high in fiber to meet your fiber goals.

Favor fats: Be sure to serve these meatballs only with a tomato sauce made from pure olive oil, not vegetable oil. This will guarantee you are favoring MUFAs.

Makeover Magic

BEFORE		AFTER
520	CALORIES	124
37 g	FAT	4 g
14 g	SAT FAT	0.5 g
29 g	CARBS	8 g
2 g	FIBER	3 g
17 g	PROTEIN	5 g
1,250 mg	SODIUM	401 mg

Curb carbs: We swapped the average crescent roll dough for whole wheat pizza dough as the "blanket," to make this childhood favorite a blood-sugar-friendly option!

Fill up on fiber: The whole wheat pizza dough boosts the fiber to 3 grams, which is great for an appetizer!

Favor fats: Using lean, 100% beef hot dogs helps to guarantee you are eating real meat with no filler, plus it decreases the saturated fat. Olive oil is the favored fat in this recipe.

"PIGS" IN A BLANKET

PREP TIME: **5 MINUTES** ■ TOTAL TIME: **25 MINUTES**

Makes 6 servings (2 "pigs" each)

1 tablespoon whole wheat flour, for dusting

½ pound store-bought whole wheat pizza dough

3 extra-lean, nitrate-free, 100% beef hot dogs, each cut into 4 pieces

1 tablespoon olive oil

4 tablespoons unsalted stone-ground mustard

1. Preheat the oven to 375°F. Line a baking sheet with parchment paper.

2. Lightly dust a clean work surface with the flour. Using a rolling pin, roll the dough into a circle, about 12" in diameter.

3. Using a pizza cutter, slice the dough into 12 pizza-shaped slices.

4. Beginning at the base of each slice, add 1 piece of hot dog and roll up each triangle to the opposite point. Place on the prepared baking sheet. Repeat until all 12 slices have been filled. The ends of the hot dog may or may not be covered, depending on the size of each dough slice. Brush with the olive oil.

5. Bake for 12 minutes, or until the dough is golden brown and the hot dog is heated through.

6. Serve with the mustard for dipping.

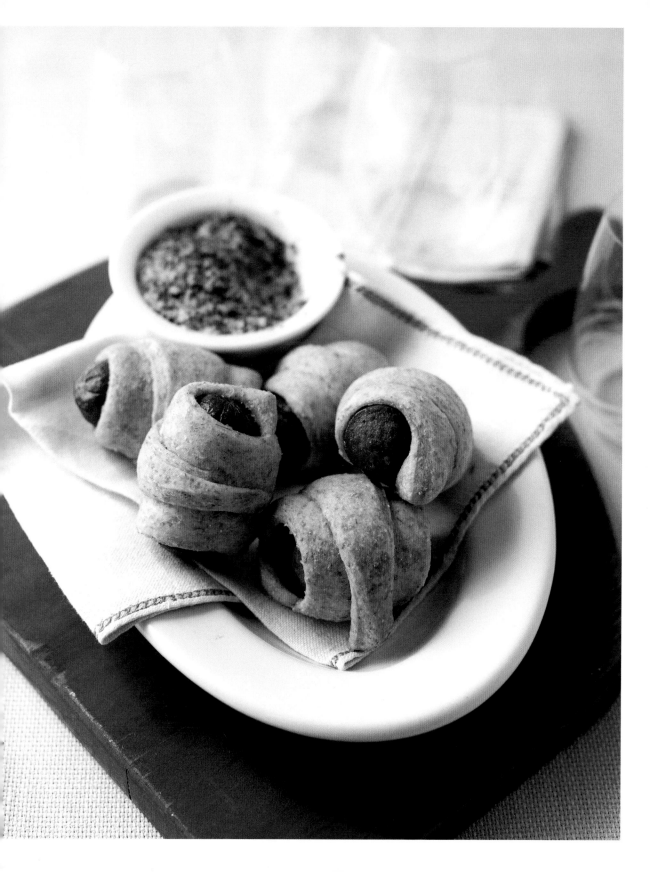

Makeover Magic

BEFORE		AFTER
630	CALORIES	131
21 g	FAT	3 g
7 g	SAT FAT	0.5 g
77 g	CARBS	22 g
3 g	FIBER	1 g
32 g	PROTEIN	5 g
980 mg	SODIUM	398 mg

Curb carbs: Who knew Chinese food could be healthy?

Fill up on fiber: Cruciferous vegetables like cabbage provide a great source of fiber. Serve over a bed of cabbage or broccoli slaw for even more filling fiber.

Favor fats: Peanut oil not only provides healthier fats than other oils, but it can be heated to a very high temperature without burning or smoking.

VEGETABLE-TOFU WONTONS

PREP TIME: **10 MINUTES** ■ TOTAL TIME: **40 MINUTES**

Makes 6 servings (4 wontons each)

SAUCE

2 tablespoons low-sodium soy sauce

2 teaspoons seasoned rice wine vinegar

⅛ teaspoon crushed red-pepper flakes

WONTONS

3 ounces firm tofu, drained and pressed dry

2 teaspoons grated fresh ginger or ⅔ teaspoon dried

1 clove garlic, minced

⅛ teaspoon ground black pepper

2 teaspoons peanut oil

3 shiitake mushrooms, trimmed and finely chopped

1 cup prepackaged shredded green cabbage or coleslaw mix, finely chopped

1 scallion, chopped

2 tablespoons chopped fresh cilantro

24 square wonton wrappers (3½" × 3½")

1. **To make the sauce:** In a small bowl, whisk together the soy sauce, vinegar, and red-pepper flakes. Set aside.

2. **To make the wontons:** Preheat the oven to 425°F. Coat a large baking sheet with cooking spray.

3. Place 1 folded-up paper towel on your work surface, place the tofu on it, and use another paper towel to gently press down on the tofu to release extra water. Do this on all sides of the tofu until much of the water has been released. You may need additional towels.

4. In a food processor, add the tofu, ginger, garlic, and pepper and pulse until the tofu is coarsely blended. There may be a few chunks in the mixture but not many. Set aside.

5. Heat the oil in a large nonstick skillet over medium-high heat. Cook the mushrooms for 4 minutes or until starting to brown. Stir in the cabbage and cook, stirring occasionally, for 4 minutes, or until wilted. Add the scallion and cook for 1 minute. Transfer to a mixing bowl. Stir in the cilantro. Add the tofu mixture and stir to combine all ingredients.

6. Arrange the wonton wrappers on a clean work surface. Place a rounded teaspoon of the tofu filling in the center of each wonton. Dampen the edges with water and fold over to form a triangle. Press the edges with your fingers to seal. Place the wontons on the prepared baking sheet and lightly coat with cooking spray.

7. Bake for 10 minutes, or until lightly golden and crisp. Serve with seasoned soy sauce.

Makeover Magic

BEFORE		AFTER
220	CALORIES	133
7 g	FAT	6 g
2 g	SAT FAT	1 g
28 g	CARBS	6 g
4 g	FIBER	1 g
11 g	PROTEIN	14 g
470 mg	SODIUM	184 mg

Curb carbs: Instead of serving the traditional slider on a bun, we chose to do without—fancy this dish up by serving it over a bed of greens drizzled with balsamic vinegar. Now you can get most of your 45 grams of carbs from your entrée.

Fill up on fiber: These tasty sliders are mostly protein, so get your fiber with your entrée.

Favor fats: Ground flaxseeds provide your daily dose of ALA omega-3s, while wild salmon is super rich in DHA omega-3s.

SALMON SLIDER BITES

PREP TIME: **5 MINUTES** ■ TOTAL TIME: **15 MINUTES**

Makes 6 servings (1 slider each)

1 egg

⅛ teaspoon salt

⅛ teaspoon ground black pepper

1 tablespoon Dijon mustard

2 tablespoons finely chopped fresh dill

½ red onion, finely chopped

12 ounces wild salmon fillet, skin removed, finely chopped

⅓ cup whole wheat bread crumbs

2 tablespoons ground flaxseeds

1. In a bowl, whisk the egg until lightly beaten. Stir in the salt, pepper, and mustard. Add the dill, onion, salmon, bread crumbs, and flaxseeds and gently fold just until combined.

2. Divide the mixture into 6 parts. Roll into balls and press slightly to form 6 small patties in all.

3. Heat a large skillet over medium-high heat and coat with cooking spray. Cook for 8 minutes, turning once, or until the fish is opaque.

Appetizers & Snacks

SWEET-N-SPICY GRILLED SHRIMP

PREP TIME: **10 MINUTES** ■ TOTAL TIME: **20 MINUTES**

Makes 4 servings

SAUCE

2   tablespoons olive oil mayonnaise

¼   cup plain 0% Greek yogurt

2   tablespoons lime juice

2   tablespoons chopped fresh cilantro leaves

SHRIMP

1   tablespoon brown sugar

½   teaspoon ground cumin

¼   teaspoon garlic powder

¼   teaspoon ground black pepper

¼   teaspoon ground red pepper

1   tablespoon olive oil

12 ounces shrimp, peeled and deveined, patted dry

1. **To make the sauce:** In a small bowl, whisk together the mayonnaise, Greek yogurt, lime juice, and cilantro leaves. Refrigerate.

2. **To make the shrimp:** In a small bowl, combine the brown sugar, ground cumin, garlic powder, black pepper, and red pepper. Add the oil and mix. Add the shrimp and toss to coat.

3. Preheat the grill to medium-high heat. Thread the shrimp onto 4 metal skewers, leaving ¼" between the pieces. Grill for 4 minutes, turning once, or until opaque. Serve with the dipping sauce.

Makeover Magic

BEFORE		AFTER
560	CALORIES	165
29 g	FAT	7 g
6 g	SAT FAT	1 g
47 g	CARBS	6 g
4 g	FIBER	0 g
28 g	PROTEIN	19 g
3,040 mg	SODIUM	191 mg

Curb carbs: We want the delicious flame-grilled shrimp flavor, so we opted to use real brown sugar and no breading on our shrimp, which curbs carbohydrates.

Fill up on fiber: To add fiber and vitamins to this protein-based dish, we recommend adding ½ cup steamed broccoli on the side.

Favor fats: Shrimp is a marine source of DHA, and using olive oil and olive oil–based mayonnaise gives this recipe a heart-healthy flair.

Makeover Magic

BEFORE		AFTER
330	CALORIES	194
18 g	FAT	8 g
3 g	SAT FAT	1 g
20 g	CARBS	11 g
0 g	FIBER	2 g
22 g	PROTEIN	19 g
690 mg	SODIUM	407 mg

Curb carbs: We added just enough whole wheat bread crumbs to act as a binder, leaving more room for the meaty crab and carbs with your entrée!

Fill up on fiber: The bread crumbs in the cakes provide the fiber in this recipe. To turn this appetizer into a meal, add fiber-full grilled veggies and spicy baked sweet potato fries on the side.

Favor fats: Choosing a canola oil–based mayonnaise keeps the dip healthy. A crab contains omegas!

CRAB CAKES WITH LEMON-DIJON SAUCE

PREP TIME: **15 MINUTES** ■ TOTAL TIME: **30 MINUTES**

Makes 4 servings (2 cakes each)

LEMON-DIJON SAUCE

2 tablespoons canola oil mayonnaise

1 tablespoon Dijon mustard

1 tablespoon lemon juice

1 clove garlic, minced

CRAB CAKES

12 ounces lump crabmeat

2 scallions, chopped

½ red bell pepper, finely chopped

¼ cup plain 0% Greek yogurt

1 egg, lightly beaten

2 tablespoons lemon juice

¼ teaspoon Old Bay seasoning

½ cup whole wheat panko bread crumbs, divided

1. **To make the lemon-Dijon sauce:** In a small bowl, whisk together the mayonnaise, mustard, lemon juice, and garlic. Refrigerate.

2. **To make the crab cakes:** Preheat the oven to 425°F.

3. In a large bowl, combine the crabmeat, scallions, pepper, yogurt, egg, lemon juice, Old Bay seasoning, and ¼ cup of the bread crumbs.

4. Using your hands, loosely form the crab mixture into 8 patties.

5. Spread the remaining bread crumbs on a plate and roll each crab cake over the crumbs to lightly coat. As the cakes are formed, place them on a nonstick baking sheet coated with canola cooking spray. If the patties are misshaped, use the palm of your hand to press them down into an evenly shaped circle, the size of a small hockey puck. Bake for 12 minutes, or until golden brown on the outside.

6. Top each crab cake with a heaping teaspoon of sauce.

BUFFALO CHICKEN QUESADILLAS

PREP TIME: **10 MINUTES** ■ TOTAL TIME: **25 MINUTES**

Makes 4 servings (3 wedges each)

4 whole wheat tortillas (8" diameter)

2 scallions, thinly sliced

1 rib celery, finely chopped

1 cooked boneless, skinless chicken breast (6 ounces), finely shredded or chopped

1 tablespoon cayenne pepper sauce

1 cup no-salt-added canned black beans, rinsed and drained

⅓ cup blue cheese crumbles

½ cup blue cheese dressing (optional)

1. Arrange the tortillas on a work surface.

2. In a small bowl, combine the scallions, celery, chicken, pepper sauce, beans, and cheese crumbles. Spread the mixture over the lower half of each tortilla. Fold the plain half over the filling to form a semicircle.

3. Heat a large nonstick skillet over medium heat until hot. Cook 2 of the tortillas for 8 minutes, turning once, until lightly browned and heated through. Transfer to a cutting board and repeat with the remaining tortillas. Cut each into 3 wedges and serve with blue cheese dressing, if using.

Makeover Magic

BEFORE		AFTER
250	CALORIES	175
10 g	FAT	6 g
5 g	SAT FAT	3 g
27 g	CARBS	14 g
5 g	FIBER	2 g
13 g	PROTEIN	16 g
590 mg	SODIUM	389 mg

Curb carbs: Use whole wheat wraps instead of refined wheat. Look for wraps that have about 20 grams of carbs and 3 grams of fiber.

Fill up on fiber: Adding fiber with beans is easy! Remember, beans offer both carbs and protein.

Favor fats: To make this dish truly comforting to your health, serve with guacamole.

SMARTSTART

If eating this dish as an appetizer, serve 2 wedges per person. If eating as an entrée, serve 3 to 4 wedges each, with a side.

BEFORE		AFTER
210	CALORIES	108
6 g	FAT	1 g
0.5 g	SAT FAT	0 g
29 g	CARBS	16 g
1 g	FIBER	1 g
8 g	PROTEIN	10 g
360 mg	SODIUM	238 mg

Curb carbs: Rice paper wrappers are naturally low in carbohydrates.

Fill up on fiber: Choose a high-fiber dinner entrée to meet your fiber goals.

Favor fats: Tuna is an outstanding source of omega-3 fatty acids. And while many spring rolls are fried, these are not! Instead they are packed full of fresh flavor.

MANGO-TUNA SPRING ROLLS

PREP TIME: **10 MINUTES** ■ TOTAL TIME: **45 MINUTES**

Makes 8 servings

DIPPING SAUCE

1 tablespoon lime juice

3 tablespoons low-sodium soy sauce

1 tablespoon honey

1 teaspoon Sriracha chili sauce

1 clove garlic, minced

SPRING ROLLS

8 rice paper wrappers (8" round)

8 leaves Bibb lettuce

24 fresh mint leaves

2 cooked wild tuna steaks (5 ounces each), sliced very thin

1 red bell pepper, thinly sliced

1 mango, peeled, pitted, and thinly sliced

2 scallions, thinly sliced

1. **To make the dipping sauce:** In a small dish, stir together the lime juice, soy sauce, honey, chili sauce, and garlic. Let stand at least 20 minutes for the flavors to blend.

2. **To make the spring rolls:** Fill a large pie plate with very warm water. Set a clean towel nearby. Add 1 rice paper wrapper at a time and soak each for 30 to 45 seconds, or until softened. Place the wontons in a stack on the towel and let stand for 2 minutes, or until soft and pliable.

3. Layer the ingredients in a 4" line in the center of the rice paper, starting 3" up from the edge closest to you. On each wrapper, arrange 1 leaf lettuce, 3 mint leaves, and one-eighth of the slices of tuna, pepper, mango, and scallions. Drizzle each spring roll with 1 teaspoon sauce. Fold in the sides and roll up, envelope-style. Set seam side down on a plate. Repeat with the remaining ingredients.

4. To serve, cut each roll in half on the diagonal and serve with the remaining dipping sauce.

SPICED SWEET POTATO CHIPS

PREP TIME: **5 MINUTES** ■ TOTAL TIME: **25 MINUTES**

Makes 4 servings

2 sweet potatoes, cut into ⅛" slices

1 tablespoon olive oil

1 tablespoon maple syrup

1 teaspoon ground cumin

⅛ teaspoon ground black pepper

⅛ teaspoon salt

1. Preheat the oven to 375°F.

2. Line 2 large baking sheets with parchment paper.

3. In a large bowl, toss the potato slices with the olive oil and maple syrup until coated. Add the cumin, pepper, and salt and toss again to coat.

4. Arrange the potato slices in a single layer on the baking sheets. Bake for 20 minutes, turning once, or until golden and crisp.

Makeover Magic

BEFORE		AFTER
283	CALORIES	101
20 g	FAT	4 g
3 g	SAT FAT	0.5 g
25 g	CARBS	17 g
2 g	FIBER	2 g
3 g	PROTEIN	1 g
1,283 mg	SODIUM	110 mg

Curb carbs: Did you know sweet potatoes have the same amount of carbs as white potatoes? Yes, they do! Our secret is leaving the skins on to get more fiber–plus, sweet potatoes are high in antioxidants that help prevent disease.

Fill up on fiber: Just 1 serving of these sweet potato chips packs 2 grams of fiber.

Favor fats: Olive oil is an easy way to sneak in the day's worth of healthy fats–and baking these chips in the oven makes this a snack you can eat daily.

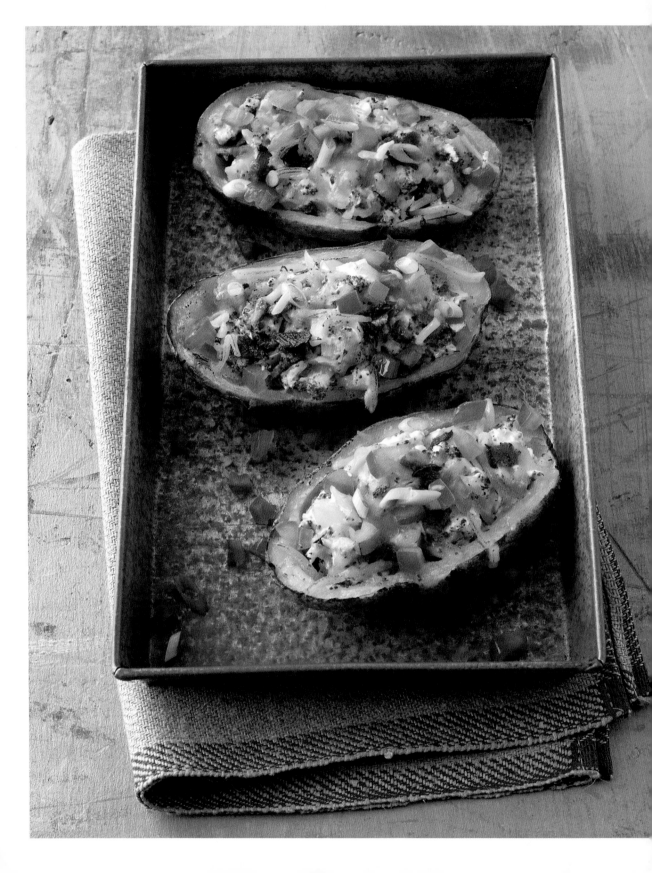

STUFFED POTATO SKINS

PREP TIME: **5 MINUTES** ■ TOTAL TIME: **1 HOUR 20 MINUTES**

Makes 6 servings

3 potatoes, scrubbed

3 slices turkey bacon, halved

2 tablespoons olive oil

1 cup frozen broccoli florets, thawed, finely chopped

¼ cup shredded Cheddar cheese

¼ cup plain 0% Greek yogurt

1 plum tomato, finely chopped

1 scallion, thinly sliced

1. Preheat the oven to 400°F.

2. Cover a baking sheet with foil. Prick the potatoes with a fork several times and place on a baking sheet. Bake for 45 minutes, or until the potatoes are cooked through and soft.

3. In a medium skillet over low heat, cook the bacon for 3 minutes, turning once, or until cooked through. Transfer to a paper towel–lined plate to drain. Crumble into small pieces. Set aside.

4. When the potatoes are done, transfer to a cooling rack for 10 minutes, or until cool enough to handle.

5. Increase the oven temperature to 450°F.

6. Cut each potato in half lengthwise. Using a spoon, scoop out the flesh, leaving ¼" of flesh in the skin. Reserve the flesh for another use.

7. Brush both sides of the potato skin halves with olive oil, place on the baking sheet, and bake for 10 minutes, or until golden and crisp.

8. In a small bowl, mix the bacon, broccoli, cheese, and yogurt. Remove the potato skins from the oven and fill each potato skin with the bacon mixture. Bake for 5 minutes, until the cheese is melted.

9. Top each with tomato and scallion.

Makeover Magic

BEFORE		AFTER
338	CALORIES	229
17 g	FAT	6 g
8 g	SAT FAT	1 g
35 g	CARBS	35 g
3 g	FIBER	3 g
11 g	PROTEIN	9 g
408 mg	SODIUM	157 mg

Curb carbs: By removing some of the flesh and filling the potato with protein and healthy fats, you can easily curb the carbs, leaving plenty of room for carbs with your entrée!

Fill up on fiber: In addition to the broccoli florets, the nutrient-dense skin of the potato packs a wallop of fiber.

Favor fats: Top each potato with pine nuts or guacamole to keep your blood sugar balanced.

BEFORE		AFTER
193	CALORIES	116
9 g	FAT	4 g
1 g	SAT FAT	0.5 g
26 g	CARBS	19 g
3 g	FIBER	1 g
3 g	PROTEIN	2 g
299 mg	SODIUM	300 mg

Curb carbs: The key to curbing carbs here is portion control. This recipe makes a perfect snack or accompaniment to your sandwich at lunch!

Fill up on fiber: Keeping the skin on these potatoes is important, as the skin provides the bulk of the fiber.

Favor fats: The olive oil coating douses the chips in healthy fats, and baking means no deep-frying in saturated fat.

SALT-N-VINEGAR POTATO CHIPS

PREP TIME: **10 MINUTES** ■ TOTAL TIME: **1 HOUR 25 MINUTES**

Makes 4 servings

2 russet potatoes, thinly sliced using a mandoline or vegetable peeler

2½ cups white vinegar

1 tablespoon olive oil

½ teaspoon sea salt

1. Lightly coat 2 large baking sheets with cooking spray.

2. In a large bowl, add the potatoes and vinegar and cover for 1 hour.

3. After 50 minutes have passed, preheat the oven to 400°F.

4. Drain the potatoes and transfer to the baking sheets. Drizzle with the oil and toss to coat. Arrange in a single layer. Sprinkle with the salt.

5. Bake for 8 minutes, turning once, or until the chips are golden and crisp.

GRAND SLAM NACHOS

PREP TIME: **10 MINUTES** ■ TOTAL TIME: **25 MINUTES**

Makes 6 servings

4 ounces unsalted blue corn tortilla chips

½ tablespoon olive oil

½ red onion, diced

½ red bell pepper, finely chopped

1 jalapeño chile pepper, seeded and finely chopped (wear plastic gloves when handling)

¼ cup sliced pitted kalamata olives

1 cup canned black beans, drained and rinsed (reserve remaining beans for another use)

1 cup frozen corn kernels, thawed

½ teaspoon ground cumin

⅔ cup shredded Cheddar cheese

½ cup plain 0% Greek yogurt

2 tablespoons lime juice

¼ cup finely chopped fresh cilantro

⅔ cup salsa

1. Preheat the oven to 425°F.

2. Arrange the chips in a single layer on a large baking sheet. Set aside.

3. In a large skillet over medium-high heat, heat the oil. Cook the onion and bell and jalapeño peppers for 5 minutes, or until softened.

4. In a bowl, combine the pepper mixture, olives, black beans, corn, and cumin.

5. Scatter the mixture over the tortilla chips evenly. Sprinkle with the cheese.

6. Bake for 10 minutes, or until the cheese is melted and bubbling.

7. In a small bowl, combine the Greek yogurt, lime juice, and cilantro. Spoon over the nachos evenly. Top with salsa.

Makeover Magic

BEFORE		AFTER
610	CALORIES	234
21 g	FAT	10 g
8 g	SAT FAT	3 g
76 g	CARBS	28 g
4 g	FIBER	4 g
30 g	PROTEIN	9 g
1,240 mg	SODIUM	396 mg

Curb carbs: Beans provide complex carbs, making this dish blood sugar friendly!

Fill up on fiber: You'll find fiber in the tortillas, beans, and corn.

Favor fats: This is a lower-saturated-fat nacho recipe compared to most because beans replace meat, and olives contribute our favored fats. Serve with 1 tablespoon of guacamole to make this dish even higher in monoun-saturated fatty acids.

FRESH GUACAMOLE WITH VEGETABLES

PREP TIME: **10 MINUTES** ■ TOTAL TIME: **10 MINUTES**

Makes 6 servings

6 ribs celery, trimmed, halved lengthwise, and cut into 2" pieces

3 green bell peppers, cut into 1" slices

2 ripe avocados, pitted and peeled

1 tablespoon lemon juice

2 plum tomatoes, seeded and finely chopped

1 jalapeño chile pepper, seeded and finely chopped (wear plastic gloves when handling)

½ red bell pepper, finely chopped

½ small red onion, finely chopped

1 tablespoon finely chopped fresh cilantro

1. Arrange the celery and green bell pepper slices on a serving plate.

2. In a large bowl, mash the avocados with a fork until chunky. Add the lemon juice, tomatoes, jalapeño and red bell peppers, onion, and cilantro and stir until all ingredients are combined.

3. Serve with the celery and peppers for dipping.

MEXICAN DIP

PREP TIME: **10 MINUTES** ■ TOTAL TIME: **35 MINUTES**

Makes 12 servings

½ package (4 ounces) Neufchâtel cheese, softened

1 cup plain 0% Greek yogurt

½ cup shredded Cheddar cheese

1 red bell pepper, finely chopped

1 jalapeño chile pepper, seeded and finely chopped (wear plastic gloves when handling)

2 cloves garlic, minced

¾ cup frozen corn kernels, thawed

1 can (14.5 ounces) black beans, drained and rinsed

2 scallions, thinly sliced

2 plum tomatoes, chopped

¼ cup chopped fresh cilantro

1. Preheat the oven to 350°F. Lightly coat an 8" x 8" baking dish with cooking spray.

2. In a large bowl, stir the Neufchâtel cheese, yogurt, and Cheddar cheese to combine. Stir in the bell and jalapeño peppers, garlic, corn, and black beans and stir until blended.

3. Transfer to the baking dish. Bake for 15 minutes, or until bubbling.

4. Sprinkle with the scallions, tomatoes, and cilantro. Serve with bell pepper slices, cucumber slices, or whole grain tortilla chips.

Makeover Magic

BEFORE		AFTER
230	CALORIES	83
12 g	FAT	5 g
7 g	SAT FAT	2 g
24 g	CARBS	7 g
4 g	FIBER	2 g
9 g	PROTEIN	5 g
1,200 mg	SODIUM	140 mg

Curb carbs: Blood sugar–friendly carbs come mainly from the corn and beans.

Fill up on fiber: Beans and corn are the fiber-boosting ingredients in this creamy dip!

Favor fats: Top this dish with sliced avocado for healthy fats galore!

Makeover Magic

BEFORE		AFTER
160	CALORIES	78
12 g	FAT	4 g
4 g	SAT FAT	2 g
5 g	CARBS	5 g
2 g	FIBER	2 g
7 g	PROTEIN	5 g
300 mg	SODIUM	189 mg

Curb carbs: Choose to eat this dip with high-fiber vegetables and you'll save plenty of carbs for dinner and dessert!

Fill up on fiber: Artichokes are packed with fiber—as much as 2 grams per serving!

Favor fats: Be sure to eat a dinner entrée high in MUFAs or omega-3s to get your daily dose of favored fats. Think fish fajitas!

GUILT-FREE SPINACH-ARTICHOKE DIP

PREP TIME: **10 MINUTES** ■ TOTAL TIME: **40 MINUTES**

Makes 12 servings

1 cup plain 0% Greek yogurt

¾ package (6 ounces) Neufchâtel cheese, softened

¼ cup grated Parmesan cheese, divided

3 cloves garlic, minced

2 tablespoons Dijon mustard

⅛ teaspoon paprika

1 small red onion, finely chopped

1 package (9 ounces) frozen artichoke hearts, thawed, squeezed dry, and chopped

1 package (10 ounces) frozen chopped spinach, thawed and squeezed dry

1. Preheat the oven to 350°F.

2. In a large bowl, stir the yogurt, Neufchâtel cheese, ⅛ cup of the Parmesan cheese, garlic, mustard, and paprika to combine. Add the onion, artichoke hearts, and spinach to the mixture and stir to combine.

3. Pour into an 8" × 8" baking dish. Top with the remaining ⅛ cup Parmesan cheese.

4. Bake for 20 minutes, or until bubbling hot. Serve with veggies or unsalted tortilla chips.

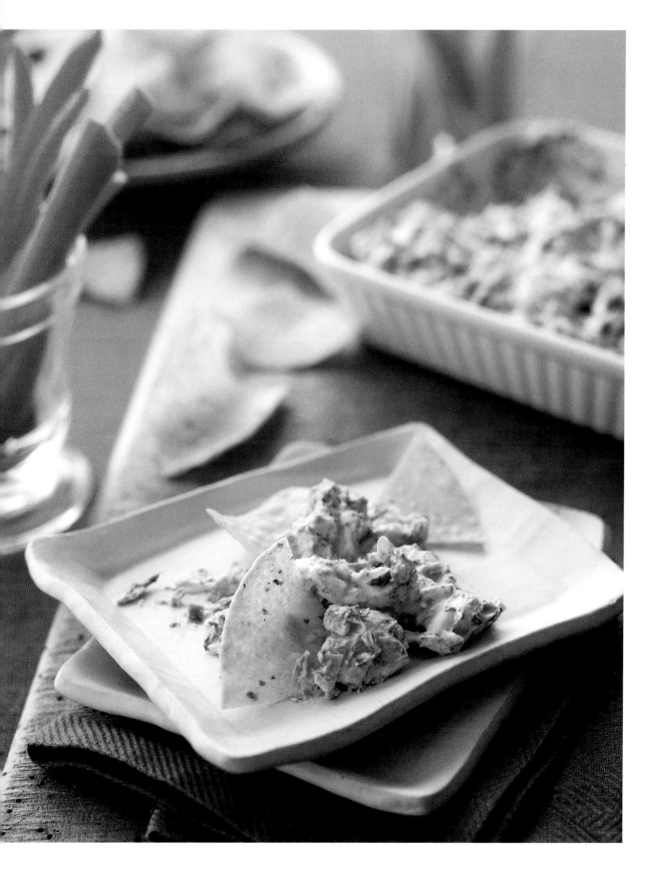

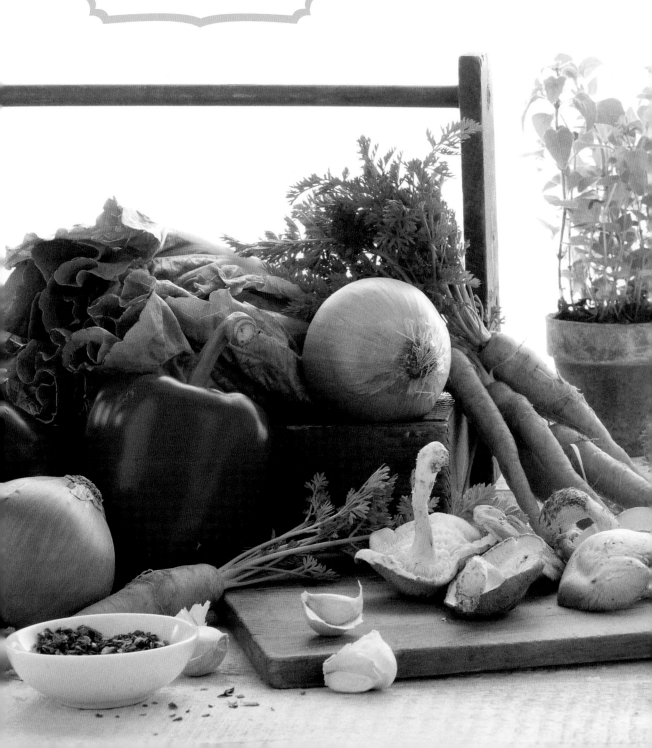

CHAPTERSEVEN

Meat

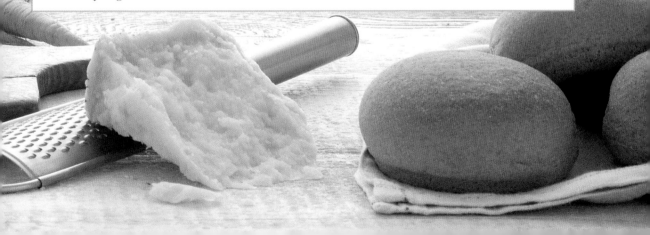

Makeover Magic

BEFORE		AFTER
630	CALORIES	298
40 g	FAT	13 g
13 g	SAT FAT	3 g
32 g	CARBS	13 g
1 g	FIBER	2 g
34 g	PROTEIN	31 g
670 mg	SODIUM	183 mg

Curb carbs: Just coat the steaks once with whole wheat flour—it curbs carbs *and* gives the dish a slightly different look that sets it apart from the classic fried steak.

Fill up on fiber: Pair this recipe with a small baked sweet potato and 1 cup of steamed broccoli to add 4 grams of fiber.

Favor fats: Instead of frying in oil that is nearly 2" deep in the pan, we simply pan-fried our steaks in a small amount of canola oil, a source of MUFAs.

COUNTRY-FRIED STEAK

PREP TIME: **5 MINUTES** ■ TOTAL TIME: **25 MINUTES**

Makes 4 servings

STEAK

½ cup whole wheat flour

½ teaspoon ground black pepper

¼ teaspoon ground red pepper

¼ teaspoon garlic powder

⅛ teaspoon salt

2 egg whites

2 tablespoons 1% milk

4 lean, top round steaks (4 ounces each)

2 tablespoons canola oil

SAUCE

¾ cup low-sodium beef broth

2 teaspoons cornstarch

⅛ teaspoon ground black pepper

1. Preheat the oven to 350°F. Line a baking sheet with foil.

2. **To make the steak:** In a shallow bowl, combine the flour, black and red pepper, garlic powder, and salt.

3. In another shallow bowl, whisk the egg whites and milk together.

4. On a cutting board, pound the steaks to ¼" thickness using a meat mallet.

5. Dredge each steak in the flour mixture, then in the egg mixture, shaking off the excess, and back in the flour mixture to fully coat the steak. Transfer to a plate.

6. In a large nonstick skillet, heat the oil over medium-high heat. Cook the steaks, in batches if needed, for 4 minutes, turning once, or until golden brown and crisp. Set aside the skillet and juices.

7. Transfer the steaks to the prepared baking sheet and place in the oven to bake for 10 minutes, or until a thermometer inserted in the center registers 145°F for medium-rare.

8. **To make the sauce:** In the same skillet over medium-high heat, heat the broth for 30 seconds. In a small bowl, whisk together ¼ cup of the warmed broth and the cornstarch. Add the mixture into the skillet and whisk for 2 minutes, or until thickened. Stir in the black pepper. Serve the sauce over the steaks.

Curb carbs: We kept the car-bohydrates low by making a low-sugar red wine sauce instead of a heavier sauce.

Fill up on fiber: Artichokes are full of fiber, a great ingredient for balancing blood sugar.

Favor fats: This dish often has bacon, but we were able to cut that out, along with using a lean cut of beef to reduce sat-urated fat. Olive oil provides flavor and monounsaturated fats in this savory recipe.

STEAK WITH MUSHROOM SAUCE AND ROASTED ARTICHOKES

PREP TIME: **5 MINUTES** ■ TOTAL TIME: **1 HOUR 5 MINUTES**

Makes 4 servings

ARTICHOKES

4 artichokes, stems and tips removed

1 tablespoon olive oil

1 tablespoon lemon juice

2 cloves garlic, minced

STEAK AND SAUCE

1 tablespoon olive oil, divided

1 pound lean flank steak

⅛ teaspoon salt

⅛ teaspoon ground black pepper

4 ounces cremini mushrooms, thinly sliced

¾ cup dry red wine

¼ cup balsamic vinegar

2 tablespoons low-sodium beef broth

2 teaspoons chopped fresh thyme or ⅔ teaspoon dried

1 tablespoon finely chopped fresh rosemary or 1 teaspoon dried

1. **To make the artichokes:** Preheat the oven to 425°F. Line a baking sheet with foil and lightly coat with cooking spray. Place the artichokes on the baking sheet and drizzle with the oil and lemon juice. Sprinkle with the garlic. Bake for 1 hour, or until fork-tender and lightly golden.

2. **To make the steak and sauce:** After 30 minutes, in a large nonstick griddle or skillet, heat $\frac{1}{2}$ tablespoon of the oil over medium heat. Season the steak with the salt and pepper. Cook the steak on the griddle, turning once, for 10 minutes, or until a thermometer inserted in the center registers 145°F for medium-rare. Transfer the steak to a plate and cover.

3. In the same skillet, heat the remaining oil over medium-high heat. Add the mushrooms and cook for 3 minutes, or until golden brown. Add the wine, vinegar, and broth, stirring constantly, and bring to a boil. Reduce the heat to medium low, add the thyme and rosemary, and simmer for 10 minutes, or until the sauce reduces and thickens, stirring occasionally.

4. On a clean cutting board, slice the steak into $\frac{1}{2}$" slices and divide among 4 serving plates. Top with the sauce and serve with the artichokes.

Makeover Magic

BEFORE		AFTER
595	CALORIES	279
29 g	FAT	9 g
11 g	SAT FAT	2 g
34 g	CARBS	24 g
4 g	FIBER	5 g
50 g	PROTEIN	27 g
1,100 mg	SODIUM	446 mg

Curb carbs: We love that the carbohydrate sources in this recipe are the vegetables. Vegetables provide healthy, energizing carbs while keeping this recipe comforting.

Fill up on fiber: Carrots and celery pumped up this recipe, taking it up to 5 grams of fiber per serving, which is great!

Favor fats: Using broth with canola oil allows for a recipe with low saturated fat and more healthy fats.

TRADITIONAL SLOW-COOKER POT ROAST

PREP TIME: **10 MINUTES** ■ TOTAL TIME: **8 HOURS 25 MINUTES**

Makes 4 servings

- 6 carrots, cut into 1" pieces
- 1 onion, sliced lengthwise
- 3 ribs celery, coarsely chopped
- 1 small potato, cut into 1" pieces
- ½ cup no-salt-added tomato puree or sauce
- 1 cup low-sodium beef broth
- 2 teaspoons chopped fresh thyme or 1 teaspoon dried
- 1 tablespoon canola oil
- 1 pound boneless beef chuck roast, trimmed of all visible fat
- ½ teaspoon salt
- 1 teaspoon paprika

1. In a 4- to 6-quart slow cooker, combine the carrots, onion, celery, potato, tomato puree or sauce, broth, and thyme.

2. In a large nonstick skillet, heat the oil over medium-high heat. Season the beef with the salt and paprika. Cook the beef for 4 minutes, turning occasionally, or until browned on all sides. Place on the vegetables. Cover and cook on low for 8 hours, or until the beef is fork-tender.

3. Remove the beef to a cutting board. Allow to sit for 10 minutes. Slice.

Meat

SIZZLIN' BEEF FAJITAS

PREP TIME: **10 MINUTES** ■ TOTAL TIME: **4 HOURS 35 MINUTES**
(MARINATING TIME INCLUDED)

Makes 4 servings

1   tablespoon olive oil

4   cloves garlic, minced

2   tablespoons lime juice

1   teaspoon ground cumin

¾   pound lean flank steak, trimmed of all visible fat

1   green bell pepper, seeded and cut into ¼"-wide strips

1   red bell pepper, seeded and cut into ¼"-wide strips

1   small onion, cut into ¼"-wide slices

4   whole wheat tortillas (6" diameter)

¼   cup salsa

1. In a resealable plastic bag, combine the oil, garlic, lime juice, and cumin. Add the steak and toss well to coat. Refrigerate for 4 hours or overnight.

2. Coat a grill rack or broiler pan rack with cooking spray. Preheat the grill or broiler to medium high. Remove the steak from the marinade. Grill or broil 4" from the heat for 12 minutes, turning once, until a thermometer inserted in the center registers 145°F for medium-rare. Transfer to a cutting board and cover loosely with foil.

3. Heat a nonstick skillet, coated with cooking spray, over medium-high heat. Cook the bell peppers and onion, stirring often, for 9 minutes, or until the vegetables are softened. Warm the tortillas according to the package directions. Thinly slice the steak across the grain on a slight angle.

4. To assemble a fajita, place 1 tortilla on a plate and top with one-quarter of the steak, one-quarter of the vegetable mixture, and 1 tablespoon of the salsa.

Makeover Magic

BEFORE		AFTER
1,433	CALORIES	261
73 g	FAT	9 g
26 g	SAT FAT	3 g
119 g	CARBS	22 g
13 g	FIBER	10 g
73 g	PROTEIN	23 g
3,062 mg	SODIUM	357 mg

Curb carbs: We opted for a 6" whole wheat tortilla instead of the traditional 8" white flour tortilla. Your fajita will be packed full with flavorful, juicy ingredients.

Fill up on fiber: We stuffed these whole wheat fajitas with more veggies than meat, a smart fiber-full move.

Favor fats: Although the Before figure above represent a restaurant-size portion that may actually be 2 servings' worth, you can see the high amount of fat, calories, and carbs in the dish. Our home-made version is so delicious and so healthy. For more healthy fats, add a dollop of guacamole to your fajita or opt for fish instead of beef.

Makeover Magic

BEFORE		AFTER
554	CALORIES	330
28 g	FAT	9 g
14 g	SAT FAT	4 g
44 g	CARBS	28 g
3 g	FIBER	4 g
26 g	PROTEIN	35 g
797 mg	SODIUM	229 mg

Curb carbs: Who would have thought whole wheat egg noodles could be this good? As with all pasta-based dishes, keep an eye on the portions. We use just an ounce of egg noodles per person, but you can increase it depending on your individual needs.

Fill up on fiber: Whole wheat egg noodles, mushrooms, and asparagus provide us with 4 grams of fiber per serving and will keep you satisfied.

Favor fats: This dish gets its creaminess from Greek yogurt and reduced-fat sour cream, decreasing the fat without taking away the creaminess. Be sure to start with an appetizer high in healthy fats like Mediterranean Chicken Pinwheels on page 131.

BEEF STROGANOFF

PREP TIME: **10 MINUTES** ■ TOTAL TIME: **45 MINUTES**

Makes 4 servings

4 ounces whole wheat egg noodles

1 tablespoon canola oil

5 ounces white or cremini mushrooms, stems removed, halved

8 ounces asparagus, trimmed and cut into 1" pieces

1 pound lean sirloin steak, trimmed of visible fat, cut into thin strips

⅛ teaspoon salt

1 yellow onion, finely chopped

2 cloves garlic, minced

½ cup low-sodium beef broth

2 teaspoons cornstarch

1 tablespoon tomato paste

2 tablespoons plain 0% Greek yogurt

¼ cup reduced-fat sour cream

2 sprigs fresh parsley, chopped

Meat

1. Prepare the noodles according to package directions. Drain and set aside.

2. In a large nonstick skillet, heat the oil over medium heat. Cook the mushrooms and asparagus for 5 minutes, or until the asparagus is lightly golden and the mushrooms are caramelized. Remove to a large bowl and set aside.

3. Season the steak with salt. In the same skillet, adding more oil if necessary, cook the steak for 5 minutes, until browned. Remove and set aside.

4. In the same skillet, cook the onion and garlic for 5 minutes, or until softened. Stir in the broth, scraping the pan to release any browned bits. Transfer ¼ cup of the broth into a small measuring cup and stir in the cornstarch until smooth. Add the tomato paste and broth mixture and stir until combined. Reduce the heat to low and simmer for 12 minutes, or until the liquid thickens and reduces by half.

5. Return the asparagus, mushrooms, and steak to the skillet and cook for 2 minutes or until heated through.

6. After the liquid cools just slightly, stir in the yogurt and sour cream. (If the heat is too high, the yogurt will separate.) Serve over the noodles and sprinkle with the parsley.

BEFORE		AFTER
670	CALORIES	272
35 g	FAT	9 g
8 g	SAT FAT	3 g
33 g	CARBS	19 g
4 g	FIBER	6 g
56 g	PROTEIN	30 g
3,260 mg	SODIUM	504 mg

Curb carbs: Often the take-out or premade sauces in Asian cuisine are loaded with sugar. Here, we let the plentiful amount of vegetables be the main source of carbohydrates in this dish.

Fill up on fiber: The fibrous vegetables add bulk to this dish, making us full without loading on extra calories or carbs.

Favor fats: We used just enough peanut oil, a source of MUFAs, to coat the vegetables for stir-frying, making this a dish that focuses on just the right kinds of fats.

CHINESE BEEF AND VEGETABLES

PREP TIME: **10 MINUTES** ■ TOTAL TIME: **20 MINUTES**

Makes 4 servings

SAUCE

3 tablespoons low-sodium soy sauce, divided

1 tablespoon brown sugar

3 tablespoons low-sodium chicken broth

½ teaspoon cornstarch

STIR-FRY

2 teaspoons peanut oil

1 pound lean flank steak, thinly sliced

4 stalks broccoli, chopped into bite-size pieces

2 tablespoons water

1 onion, halved and sliced

1 green bell pepper, sliced

1 red bell pepper, sliced

4 ounces cremini mushrooms, trimmed and sliced

1 tablespoon finely chopped fresh ginger or 1 teaspoon dried

1 clove garlic, minced

1. **To make the sauce:** In a small saucepan over medium heat, combine the soy sauce and brown sugar.

2. In a small bowl, whisk together the broth and cornstarch until the cornstarch is dissolved. Whisk into the soy sauce. Cook for 2 minutes, or until the sauce begins to thicken. Set aside.

3. **To make the stir-fry:** Heat a wok or large skillet over high heat for 1 minute. Add the oil. Cook the steak, stirring often, for 2 minutes, or until no longer pink. With a slotted spoon or tongs, transfer the meat to a plate and set aside. Reduce the heat to medium high.

4. Add the broccoli and water. Cover and cook for 3 minutes, or until tender-crisp. Add the onion, peppers, and mushrooms. Cook, stirring, for 5 minutes, or until the vegetables are tender-crisp.

5. Add the ginger and garlic. Cook for 30 seconds. Add the reserved meat and sauce. Cook for 2 minutes, or until heated through.

Makeover Magic

Curb carbs: The trick to this dish is balancing the rice with all the other ingredients. Add just enough brown rice to give bulk to the dish, but leave most of the bowl for everything else.

Fill up on fiber: Between the beans, brown rice, and vegetables in this dish, you won't be surprised that each serving has 5 grams of fiber.

Favor fats: Once again, guacamole is our star source of healthy fats. Using lean flank steak and reduced-fat cheese keeps the saturated fat within a reasonable range.

STEAK BURRITO BOWL

PREP TIME: **5 MINUTES** ▪ TOTAL TIME: **25 MINUTES**

Makes 6 servings

1¼ cups instant brown rice

12 ounces lean flank steak, trimmed

1 teaspoon chipotle seasoning

½ teaspoon ground black pepper

1 teaspoon olive oil

1 can (15 ounces) black beans, rinsed and drained

3 hearts romaine lettuce, shredded

¼ cup salsa

¼ cup guacamole

¼ cup reduced-fat shredded Cheddar cheese

1. Prepare the rice according to package directions, omitting the salt. Set aside.

2. In a 13" × 9" baking dish, place the steak and rub it with the chipotle seasoning and pepper on both sides. Rub the oil onto the steak.

3. Coat a grill rack with cooking spray. Heat the grill over medium-high heat. Grill the steak for 12 minutes, turning once, or until a thermometer inserted in the center registers 145°F for medium-rare.

4. Transfer the steak to a cutting board and let sit for 5 minutes. Slice into thin strips.

5. Evenly divide the rice, steak, beans, lettuce, salsa, guacamole, and cheese among 6 bowls.

SMARTSTART

If desired, another option to keep saturated fat low would be to use a leaner cut of steak while enjoying full-fat cheese.

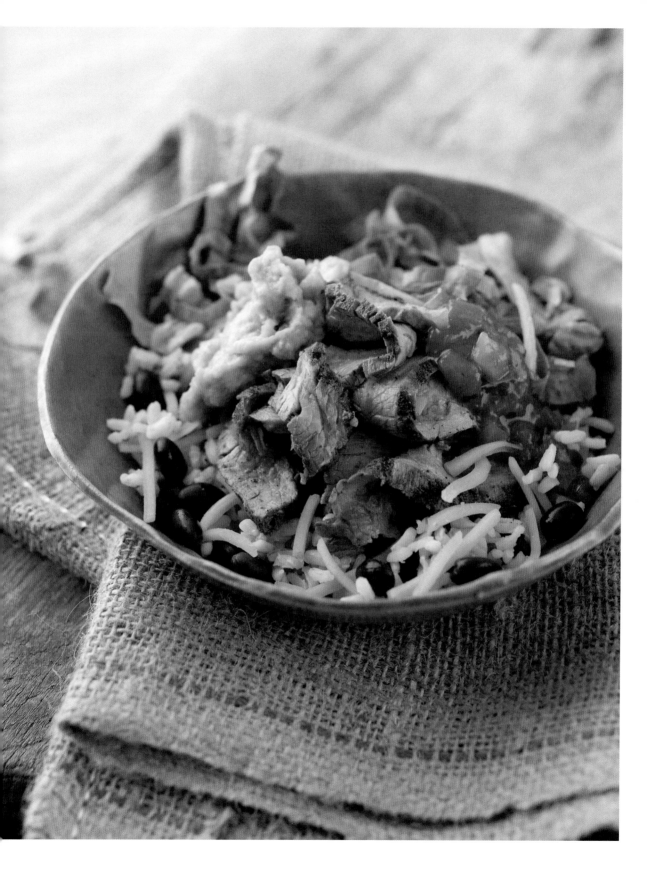

Makeover Magic

BEFORE		AFTER
548	CALORIES	252
30 g	FAT	5 g
14 g	SAT FAT	2 g
40 g	CARBS	33 g
4 g	FIBER	5 g
30 g	PROTEIN	21 g
850 mg	SODIUM	185 mg

Curb carbs: The carbohydrates in this recipe come from all the veggies. We reduced the potatoes and filled the rest of the crust mixture with delicious cauliflower.

Fill up on fiber: Shepherd's pie is such a classic recipe, and the basic contents of the recipe do not change much. There will always be meat, veggies, and potatoes to top a traditional shepherd's pie. We boosted the fiber of this dish by leaving the skins on our potatoes, and packing in extra peas and adding carrots.

Favor fats: The comparison shepherd's pie uses canned cream of mushroom soup as its gravy, but we opted for the lighter version, using cornstarch to thicken beef broth for a flavorful bite. Be sure to serve a side high in healthy fats!

SHEPHERD'S PIE

PREP TIME: **10 MINUTES** ■ TOTAL TIME: **1 HOUR 25 MINUTES**

Makes 6 servings

8 ounces russet potatoes, cubed

2 cups fresh cauliflower florets

3 tablespoons low-fat buttermilk

¼ cup reduced-fat shredded Cheddar cheese

¾ pound top round steak, cut into thin strips

3 carrots, chopped

2 cloves garlic, minced

1 can (14.5 ounces) no-salt-added diced tomatoes

1 onion, chopped

1½ cups frozen peas, thawed

2 teaspoons low-sodium Worcestershire sauce

2 teaspoons cornstarch

¼ cup low-sodium beef broth

1. Preheat the oven to 350°F. Coat an 11" × 8" baking dish with cooking spray.

2. Place the potatoes and cauliflower in a large saucepan. Add enough cold water to cover. Bring to a boil over high heat. Reduce the heat to medium and cook for 15 minutes, or until very tender. Drain and place in a medium bowl.

3. Mash well with an electric mixer, adding the buttermilk and cheese.

4. Heat a large nonstick skillet coated with cooking spray over medium-high heat. Cook the steak, carrots, and garlic for 5 minutes, stirring, until the steak is browned. Add the tomatoes (with juice), onion, peas, and Worcestershire sauce. Bring to a boil.

5. In a small bowl, whisk together the cornstarch and broth. Add to the skillet and cook, stirring, for 3 minutes, or until the sauce thickens.

6. Spoon the mixture into the baking dish. Top with the mashed potato mixture. Bake for 40 minutes, or until the top is golden brown. Let stand for 10 minutes before serving.

MOM'S MEAT LOAF

PREP TIME: **10 MINUTES** ■ TOTAL TIME: **1 HOUR 25 MINUTES**

Makes 8 servings

GLAZE

⅓ cup ketchup

2 cloves garlic, minced

1 teaspoon mustard powder

2 tablespoons low-sodium Worcestershire sauce

MEAT LOAF

1½ pounds 95% lean ground beef

½ cup ground flaxseeds

1 teaspoon dried oregano

1 tablespoon low-sodium Worcestershire sauce

1 small onion, finely chopped

1 egg

1. Preheat the oven to 350°F. Coat a 9" × 5" loaf pan with cooking spray.

2. **To make the glaze:** In a small bowl, mix together the ketchup, garlic, mustard powder, and Worcestershire sauce. Set aside.

3. **To make the meat loaf:** In a bowl, mix together the ground beef, flaxseeds, oregano, Worcestershire sauce, onion, egg, and 2 tablespoons of the reserved ketchup mixture. Press the mixture into the loaf pan. Bake for 1 hour, or until a thermometer inserted in the center registers 160°F and the meat is no longer pink.

4. Coat the top with the remaining ketchup mixture and bake for 10 additional minutes.

SMARTSTART

Add 2 tablespoons of wheat germ to this dish for a boost in B vitamins, fiber, protein, and MUFAs.

Makeover Magic

BEFORE		AFTER
394	CALORIES	205
23 g	FAT	7 g
9 g	SAT FAT	3 g
17 g	CARBS	8 g
1 g	FIBER	1 g
28 g	PROTEIN	26 g
1,094 mg	SODIUM	307 mg

Curb carbs: Many meat loaves are full of carbohydrates not only from extra bread crumbs, but also from the sauces used for the glaze. We used flaxseeds and a thin glaze of ketchup, Worcestershire sauce, and spices to keep this a low-carb dinner option.

Fill up on fiber: The key to making a meat loaf dinner high in fiber is to pair it with tons of veggies! Check Appendix B for some high-fiber ideas. Or add oats, wheat germ, and chia seeds to your meat mixture.

Favor fats: Flaxseeds are our healthy fat source in this dish. We're able to cut saturated fats by using extra-lean ground beef.

BEFORE		AFTER
458	CALORIES	375
18 g	FAT	15 g
6 g	SAT FAT	5 g
42 g	CARBS	29 g
2 g	FIBER	6 g
31 g	PROTEIN	31 g
767 mg	SODIUM	300 mg

Curb carbs: Instead of egg noodles, we served our steak with half of a baked potato per serving to cut the carbs.

Fill up on fiber: The skin of the baked potato packs a wallop of fiber.

Favor fats: Ground flaxseeds add ALA omega-3 fatty acids to this dish. To reduce the saturated fat, we used only egg whites and opted for lightly greasing the pan instead of using extra oil.

SALISBURY STEAK

PREP TIME: **5 MINUTES** ■ TOTAL TIME: **35 MINUTES**

Makes 4 servings

STEAKS

1 pound 95% lean ground beef	1 tablespoon Worcestershire sauce
⅓ cup ground flaxseeds	1 tablespoon tomato paste
1 clove garlic, minced	2 egg whites
½ teaspoon onion powder	

GRAVY

½ onion, halved and thinly sliced	1½ tablespoons cornstarch
4 ounces cremini mushrooms, sliced	2 tablespoons Worcestershire sauce
1½ cups low-sodium beef broth, divided	2 baked potatoes, halved

1. **To make the steaks:** In a large bowl, combine the beef, flaxseeds, garlic, onion powder, Worcestershire sauce, tomato paste, and egg whites and mix well. Form into 4 patties.

2. Heat a large nonstick skillet coated with cooking spray over medium-high heat. Cook the patties for 8 minutes, turning once, until browned. Transfer to a plate.

3. **To make the gravy:** In the same skillet over medium-high heat, cook the onion and mushrooms for 5 minutes, or until tender and golden brown. Add 1¼ cups broth and stir.

4. In a small bowl, whisk the remaining ¼ cup broth and the cornstarch until the cornstarch has dissolved. Add to the skillet and bring the mixture to a boil, whisking continuously. Reduce the heat to a simmer and whisk for 5 minutes, or until the gravy has reduced and thickened. Stir in the Worcestershire sauce.

5. In the skillet with the gravy, cook the patties for 5 minutes, or until a thermometer inserted in the center registers 160°F and the meat is no longer pink.

6. Transfer to serving plates and top with gravy. Serve each with half of a baked potato.

UN-STUFFED PEPPERS

PREP TIME: **5 MINUTES** ■ TOTAL TIME: **30 MINUTES**

Makes 4 servings

⅔ cup water

⅓ cup quinoa, rinsed well

1 teaspoon olive oil

1 pound 95% lean ground beef

2 cups low-sodium marinara sauce, divided

2 green bell peppers, sliced

2 red bell peppers, sliced

1 onion, halved and sliced

1 clove garlic, minced

1. Preheat the oven to 350°F.

2. In a saucepan, bring the water and quinoa to a boil over high heat. Reduce the heat to low, cover, and simmer for 15 minutes. Remove from the heat and cool for 5 minutes. Fluff the quinoa with a fork and set aside.

3. In a large nonstick skillet, heat the oil over medium heat. Cook the ground beef for 5 minutes, or until lightly browned, stirring occasionally.

4. Add ½ cup of the sauce, the peppers, onion, and garlic and cook for 5 minutes or until the peppers begin to soften.

5. Spoon ½ cup of the sauce on the bottom of a 13" × 9" baking dish and add the beef mixture, quinoa, and remaining sauce. Mix until all ingredients are incorporated.

6. Bake for 10 minutes, or until heated through.

SMARTSTART

If available, choose grass-fed beef. In addition to being lower in fat than grain-fed beef, your choice helps to support sustainable agriculture.

Makeover Magic

BEFORE		AFTER
390	CALORIES	275
17 g	FAT	8 g
7 g	SAT FAT	3 g
29 g	CARBS	25 g
4 g	FIBER	5 g
29 g	PROTEIN	26 g
1,470 mg	SODIUM	173 mg

Curb carbs: Whole grain quinoa adds protein and fiber naturally lacking in white rice.

Fill up on fiber: The quinoa is a source of fiber, as are the peppers. Go ahead and add more quinoa on the side.

Favor fats: Using 95% lean ground beef keeps saturated fat down while we include healthy fats like olive oil in the marinara sauce. Quinoa gives a small dose of favored fats, too.

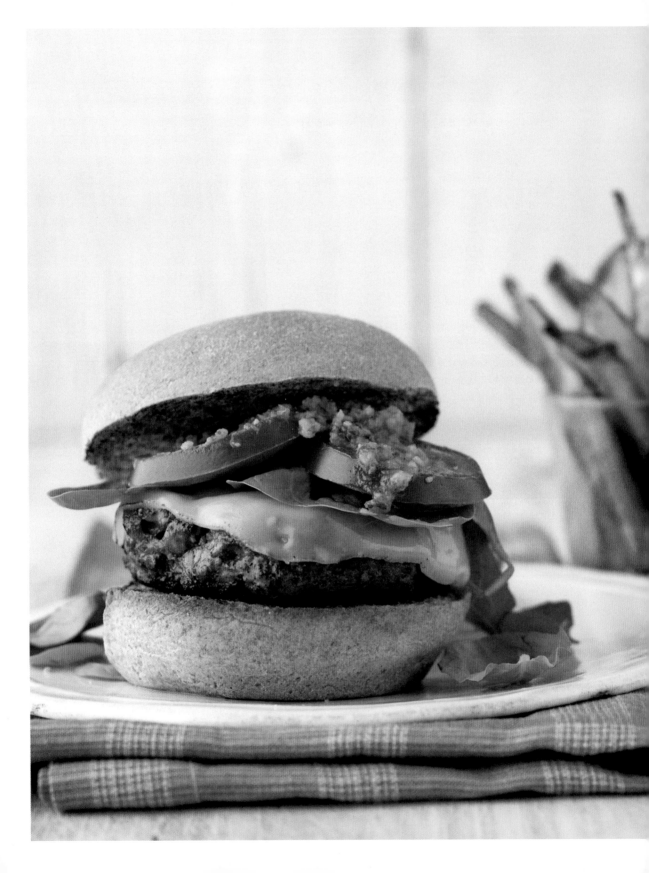

ZESTY ITALIAN CHEESEBURGERS

PREP TIME: **5 MINUTES** ■ TOTAL TIME: **22 MINUTES**

Makes 4 servings

1 egg

1 pound ground beef

2 cloves garlic, minced

¼ cup no-salt-added tomato sauce

1 teaspoon dried basil

⅛ teaspoon salt

4 whole wheat hamburger buns

4 slices part-skim mozzarella cheese

2 cups fresh spinach

1 plum tomato, sliced

2 tablespoons store-bought pesto

1. In a large bowl, whisk the egg. Add the beef, garlic, tomato sauce, basil, and salt, mixing with your hands until all ingredients are combined.

2. Form into 4 patties.

3. Heat a grill pan or large nonstick skillet coated with cooking spray over medium-high heat. Cook the patties for 10 minutes, turning once, until a thermometer inserted in the center registers 145°F for medium-rare.

4. Place each burger on a bun and top each with 1 slice of cheese, ½ cup of spinach, tomato slices, and ½ tablespoon of pesto.

Makeover Magic

BEFORE		AFTER
490	CALORIES	328
23 g	FAT	12 g
11 g	SAT FAT	4 g
37 g	CARBS	22 g
2 g	FIBER	3 g
32 g	PROTEIN	33 g
785 mg	SODIUM	476 mg

Curb carbs: Adding a whole wheat hamburger bun instead of Italian bread, which is popular with melts, worked wonders. With only 18 grams of carbs per bun, you can still add Spiced Sweet Potato Chips (page 143).

Fill up on fiber: Fresh vegetables boost the fiber in this juicy burger! Pair with a side of baked beans or sweet potato fries for a fiber-packed meal.

Favor fats: Topping this burger with pesto not only adds Italian flair, but also provides healthy fats in the form of MUFAs. We love pesto for its olive oil and pine nuts.

Makeover Magic

BEFORE		AFTER
680	CALORIES	446
30 g	FAT	12 g
12 g	SAT FAT	4 g
63 g	CARBS	54 g
6 g	FIBER	9 g
39 g	PROTEIN	36 g
1,320 mg	SODIUM	393 mg

Curb carbs: Be careful to use just 8 ounces of whole wheat spaghetti in this dish—the key to curbing carbs with a pasta dish is always portion control!

Fill up on fiber: The spinach in the sauce boosts the fiber, and using whole wheat pasta instead of white spaghetti helps, too. Thanks to the magic carbs in this dish, we can serve more pasta per person than the usual 6 ounces.

Favor fats: Packed with omega-3 fatty acids, flaxseeds are an easy substitute for bread crumbs in meat dishes including meat loaf, meatballs, and breaded cutlets.

GO-TO SPAGHETTI AND MEATBALLS

PREP TIME: **5 MINUTES** ■ TOTAL TIME: **35 MINUTES**

Makes 4 servings

8 ounces whole wheat spaghetti

¼ cup ground flaxseeds

¾ pound 95% lean ground beef

2 cloves garlic, minced

2 tablespoons grated Parmesan cheese

½ teaspoon dried oregano

1 egg

1 small onion, chopped

1½ cups low-sodium pasta sauce with olive oil

6 cups fresh spinach

1. Prepare the spaghetti according to package directions, omitting the salt.

2. In a large bowl, mix the flaxseeds, beef, garlic, cheese, and oregano with your hands until all ingredients are combined. Add the egg and mix until all ingredients are again combined. Form into 16 meatballs.

3. Heat a large nonstick skillet coated with cooking spray over medium heat. Cook the meatballs for 6 minutes, turning often, or until browned. Transfer to a clean platter and set aside.

4. Return the skillet to medium-high heat and add the chopped onion. Cook for 5 minutes, stirring often, or until softened. Add the pasta sauce. Bring to a boil, reduce the heat to medium low, cover, and simmer for 5 minutes, stirring often. Add the meatballs and cook for 8 minutes, or until a thermometer inserted in the center registers 160°F. Add the spinach to the sauce mixture, stir, and cook for 2 minutes.

5. Divide the spaghetti among 4 plates and top with the meatballs and sauce.

BEEF GOULASH

PREP TIME: **10 MINUTES** ■ TOTAL TIME: **55 MINUTES**

Makes 4 servings

1 package (8 ounces) shirataki noodles

1 tablespoon canola oil

1 onion, chopped

1 red bell pepper, chopped

1 green bell pepper, chopped

1¼ teaspoons paprika

¾ pound 95% lean ground beef

1 can (14.5 ounces) no-salt-added petite diced tomatoes

½ cup fat-free reduced-sodium beef broth

¼ teaspoon salt

¼ cup plain 0% Greek yogurt

1½ tablespoons all-purpose flour

1. Preheat the oven to 350°F. Prepare the noodles according to package directions and drain.

2. In an ovenproof Dutch oven, warm the oil over medium-high heat. Cook the onion, peppers, and paprika, stirring, for 3 minutes. Crumble the beef into the pan. Cook, stirring, for 4 minutes, or until the beef is no longer pink. Stir in the tomatoes (with juice), noodles, broth, and salt. Bring to a simmer.

3. Whisk the yogurt and flour in a small bowl. Whisk into the casserole. Stir over low heat for 2 minutes, or until thickened.

4. Cover tightly and bake for 15 minutes. Carefully remove the cover and stir. Bake, uncovered, for 10 minutes.

Makeover Magic

BEFORE		AFTER
510	CALORIES	242
18 g	FAT	9 g
6 g	SAT FAT	2 g
53 g	CARBS	17 g
3 g	FIBER	5 g
33 g	PROTEIN	23 g
850 mg	SODIUM	307 mg

Curb carbs: Choose shirataki noodles, a widely available Japanese noodle made from yams, for a naturally low-carb alternative to the white pasta found in most goulashes.

Fill up on fiber: The veggies make this a really great fibrous meal to maximize that filling feeling while not raising your blood sugar. Feel free to add beans for more fiber and protein—just be sure to stay within your allotted grams of carbs.

Favor fats: Personalize this dish by tossing in your favorite healthy fat source such as veggies in an olive oil and garlic sauce.

BEFORE		AFTER
695	CALORIES	410
24 g	FAT	10 g
7 g	SAT FAT	3 g
84 g	CARBS	44 g
6 g	FIBER	6 g
34	PROTEIN	29 g
736 mg	SODIUM	391 mg

Curb carbs: Serving our ragù with an appropriate amount of higher-fiber polenta makes for a filling meal while meeting the goal of 45 to 60 grams of carbs per meal.

Fill up on fiber: With so many vegetables in the ragù, we aren't surprised that it has 6 grams of fiber.

Favor fats: Olive oil is the favored fat in this cozy comfort dish.

BEEF RAGÙ OVER POLENTA

PREP TIME: **5 MINUTES** ■ TOTAL TIME: **1 HOUR 10 MINUTES**

Makes 4 servings

2 teaspoons olive oil, divided

1 pound 95% lean ground beef

2 zucchini, halved lengthwise and sliced

1 onion, chopped

3 carrots, sliced

2 cloves garlic, minced

4 tablespoons tomato paste

1 cup dry red wine

1 can (14.5 ounces) no-salt-added diced tomatoes

¾ cup low-sodium chicken broth

1½ teaspoons Italian seasoning

4 cups water

1 cup cornmeal

⅛ teaspoon salt

¼ teaspoon ground black pepper

2 tablespoons grated Parmesan cheese

1. In a large, heavy saucepan or Dutch oven, heat 1 teaspoon of the oil over medium heat. Cook the beef, stirring, for 5 minutes, or until lightly browned.

2. Add the remaining teaspoon of oil, zucchini, onion, carrots, and garlic, and cook for 5 minutes, or until the onion softens. Stir in the tomato paste and wine and cook for 2 minutes, or until the wine has reduced by half.

3. Add the tomatoes, broth, and Italian seasoning, stir to combine, and bring the mixture to a simmer. Reduce the heat to low, cover, and cook for 50 minutes, stirring occasionally, or until the sauce has thickened.

4. Meanwhile, in a saucepan, bring the water to a boil over high heat.

5. Add the cornmeal and salt, whisking constantly until the mixture comes to a boil. Reduce the heat to low and cover partially, allowing the steam to escape. Cook for 30 minutes, stirring every few minutes to avoid burning and clumps. Once thickened, stir in the pepper and cheese, cover, remove from the heat, and keep warm.

6. When the ragù is finished, serve over the polenta.

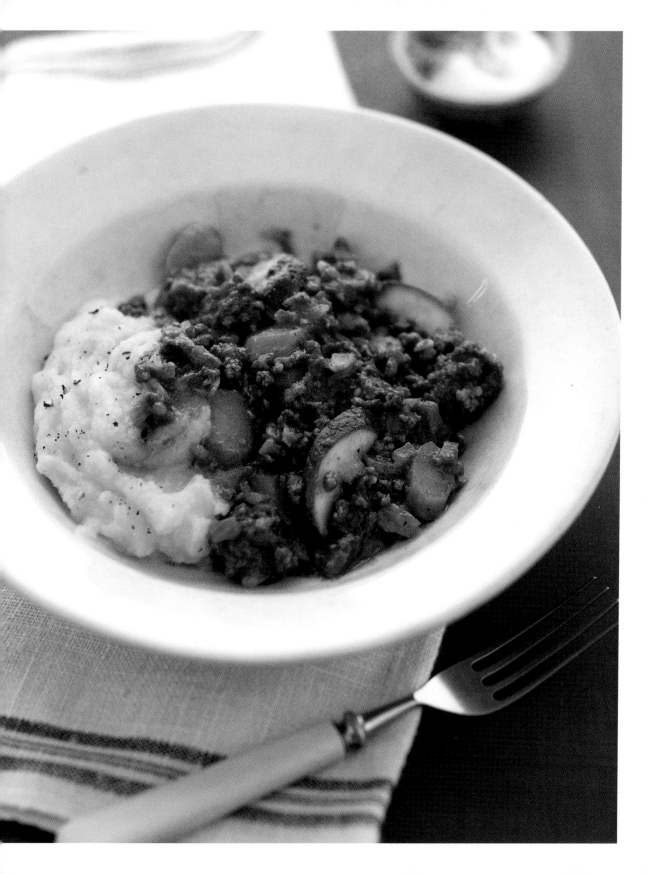

Makeover Magic

BEFORE		AFTER
390	CALORIES	165
23 g	FAT	10 g
10 g	SAT FAT	3 g
31 g	CARBS	12 g
3 g	FIBER	8 g
15 g	PROTEIN	15 g
1,020 mg	SODIUM	303 mg

Curb carbs: With a different spin on the average hot dog, we ran with the "wrap" craze and rested our dogs in a naturally lower-carb whole wheat tortilla. Our comparison recipe used a hearty sandwich roll, but we wanted minimal bread and lots of hot dog.

Fill up on fiber: Between the whole wheat wraps, lettuce, and tomatoes, this is an insanely high-fiber lunch!

Favor fats: Buffalo hot dogs aren't a concession-stand staple, but they are so much better! Avocado is the source of healthy fats in this dish.

COBB SALAD–STYLE BUFFALO DOGS

PREP TIME: **5 MINUTES** ■ TOTAL TIME: **12 MINUTES**

Makes 4 servings

4 buffalo hot dogs or 97% fat-free beef hot dogs

4 whole wheat tortillas (8" diameter)

1 cup shredded romaine lettuce

¼ small onion, chopped

½ avocado, thinly sliced

1 plum tomato, chopped

¼ cup reduced-fat blue cheese crumbles

2 slices low-sodium bacon, cooked and crumbled

1. Coat a grill rack with cooking spray. Heat the grill to high.

2. Grill the hot dogs, turning occasionally , for 7 minutes, or until browned.

3. Put 1 hot dog in each tortilla and divide the lettuce, onion, avocado, tomato, cheese crumbles, and bacon crumbles among the wraps.

Meat

GROUND BISON WITH SPAGHETTI SQUASH

PREP TIME: **5 MINUTES** ■ TOTAL TIME: **60 MINUTES**

Makes 4 servings

1 medium (3–4 pound) spaghetti squash

2 teaspoons canola oil, divided

1 pound 90% lean ground bison or beef

1 small onion, finely chopped

1 green bell pepper, sliced ¼" thick

1 red bell pepper, sliced ¼" thick

4 ounces cremini or white mushrooms, sliced

4 cups fresh spinach leaves

¼ cup water

4 tablespoons no-salt-added tomato paste

1 can (14.5 ounces) no-salt-added diced tomatoes

3 cloves garlic, minced

6 fresh basil leaves, finely chopped

1 teaspoon dried oregano

¾ teaspoon ground black pepper, divided

¼ teaspoon salt

¼ cup grated Parmesan cheese

1. Preheat the oven to 400°F. Pierce the squash with a fork. Place in a roasting pan. Bake for 55 minutes, or until fork-tender. When cool enough to handle, cut the squash in half, scoop it out, and discard the seeds. Scrape the flesh crosswise with a fork to separate the spaghetti-like strands. Place in a large serving bowl.

2. Meanwhile, in a Dutch oven, heat 1 teaspoon of the oil over medium-high heat. Cook the bison for 5 minutes, or until browned. Add the remaining teaspoon of oil and the onion, peppers, and mushrooms and cook for 3 minutes, or until the vegetables are lightly golden. Add the spinach, water, tomato paste, diced tomatoes, garlic, basil, oregano, pepper, and salt, and stir to combine. Reduce the heat to low and cook for 30 minutes, or until the sauce thickens and the vegetables are soft.

3. Divide the squash and sauce among 4 plates. Sprinkle with Parmesan cheese.

Makeover Magic

BEFORE		AFTER
510	CALORIES	360
22 g	FAT	16 g
9 g	SAT FAT	5 g
42 g	CARBS	28 g
5	FIBER	7 g
38 g	PROTEIN	27 g
1,552 mg	SODIUM	364 mg

Curb carbs: Spaghetti squash looks similar to pasta but is lower in carbs when compared serving for serving.

Fill up on fiber: The squash happens to be full of fiber, and all of the additional vegetables in the sauce add fiber as well.

Favor fats: Bison is not very common, but we wanted to use it because it is lean and the flavor is so unique. Add healthy fats to this dish by tossing in ground flaxseeds or adding more canola oil to the meat sauce.

LEMON-ROSEMARY LAMB CHOPS

PREP TIME: **5 MINUTES** ▪ TOTAL TIME: **1 HOUR 20 MINUTES**

Makes 4 servings

8 ounces whole wheat orzo	8 lamb loin chops
4 tablespoons lemon juice	½ cucumber, chopped
2 cloves garlic, minced	2 plum tomatoes, chopped
1 tablespoon finely chopped fresh rosemary or 1 teaspoon dried	1 teaspoon olive oil
	2 teaspoons balsamic vinegar

1. Prepare the orzo according to package directions.

2. In a small bowl, combine the lemon juice, garlic, and rosemary.

3. In an 11" × 8" baking dish, place the lamb chops and drizzle with the lemon mixture, massaging it into the meat. Cover the dish with plastic wrap and refrigerate for 40 minutes. Remove for 20 minutes before grilling to allow to come up to room temperature.

4. In a serving bowl, whisk together the orzo, cucumber, tomatoes, oil, and vinegar. Refrigerate.

5. Coat a grill rack with cooking spray. Preheat the grill to medium high.

6. Grill the lamb chops for 10 minutes, or until browned and a thermometer inserted in the center registers 145°F for medium-rare. Discard the remaining marinade from the baking dish. Serve with the cucumber salad.

LAMB BURGERS WITH LEMON-YOGURT SAUCE

PREP TIME: **5 MINUTES** ■ TOTAL TIME: **20 MINUTES**

Makes 4 servings

SAUCE

¼ cup plain 0% Greek yogurt

2 tablespoons lemon juice

5 mint leaves, finely chopped

½ teaspoon honey

BURGERS

1 pound lean ground lamb

1 cup fresh spinach leaves, chopped

1 small red onion, finely chopped

⅓ cup crumbled feta cheese

¼ teaspoon ground cumin

1 egg white

2 whole wheat pita breads, halved

2 cups fresh spinach leaves

1 plum tomato, thinly sliced

1. **To make the sauce:** In a small bowl, whisk together the yogurt, lemon juice, mint, and honey. Set aside.

2. **To make the burgers:** In a large bowl, mix together the lamb, chopped spinach, onion, cheese, cumin, and egg white. Form into 4 burgers.

3. In a large nonstick skillet over medium-high heat, cook the burgers for 10 minutes, turning once, or until a thermometer inserted in the center registers 160°F and the meat is no longer pink.

4. Open a pita pocket and spread a spoonful of sauce inside. Cut each burger in half and place 2 halves into each pita pocket half. Fill each with ½ cup spinach leaves and a few tomato slices.

Makeover Magic

BEFORE		AFTER
712	CALORIES	270
42 g	FAT	8 g
17 g	SAT FAT	3 g
43 g	CARBS	19 g
3 g	FIBER	3 g
40 g	PROTEIN	32 g
1,150 mg	SODIUM	414 mg

Curb carbs: We chose to serve this Mediterranean burger in a heart-healthy whole wheat pita instead of a higher-carb bun. We also used honey in place of regular sugar. Since honey is sweeter, we're able to use less of it.

Fill up on fiber: The pita bread and fresh spinach add fiber here! Pair with a side salad and boost the fiber even more.

Favor fats: We kept the oils and extra fat sources to a minimum because ground lamb is naturally fattier than other ground meats. For added healthy fats, smear on some olive tapenade, but watch your overall saturated fat intake for the entire day.

Makeover Magic

BEFORE		AFTER
470	CALORIES	312
19 g	FAT	5 g
7 g	SAT FAT	2 g
43 g	CARBS	26 g
2 g	FIBER	3 g
32 g	PROTEIN	38 g
870 mg	SODIUM	494 mg

Note: To allow the spices to penetrate the pork, if time permits, rub the spice mixture over the pork and refrigerate for 4 to 8 hours before placing in the slow cooker.

Curb carbs: Replace bottled barbecue sauce with our simple vinegar- and tomato-based sauce to curb carbs deliciously.

Fill up on fiber: We added coleslaw to this sandwich, which boosted the fiber. If we could fit more coleslaw on top, we would. Whole wheat buns also add fiber.

Favor fats: We used a lean pork tenderloin instead of pork shoulder, which cut the saturated fat. Add chia seeds to the coleslaw for a small helping of omega-3 fatty acids and fiber.

SLOW-COOKER PORK BARBECUE

PREP TIME: **15 MINUTES** ■ TOTAL TIME: **5 HOURS 15 MINUTES**

Makes 6 servings

½ teaspoon salt

½ teaspoon chili powder

2 tablespoons honey

1 teaspoon olive oil

2 pounds lean pork tenderloin

1 onion, chopped

2 cloves garlic, minced

½ cup apple cider vinegar

3 tablespoons tomato paste

4 whole wheat hamburger buns, split and toasted

1½ cups store-bought fresh coleslaw mix

1 tablespoon lemon juice

1 teaspoon Dijon mustard

¼ cup plain 0% Greek yogurt

1. In a small bowl, combine the salt, chili powder, honey, and oil.

2. In a 13" × 9" baking dish, place the pork and rub the spice mixture on it.

3. Lightly coat a 5- or 6-quart slow cooker with cooking spray and add the pork. Add the onion, garlic, vinegar, and tomato paste, spreading over the pork to cover. Cover and cook on high for 5 hours (or low for 8 hours), or until a thermometer inserted in the center reaches 145°F and the juices run clear.

4. Meanwhile, in a bowl, stir together the coleslaw, lemon juice, mustard, and yogurt. Refrigerate.

5. When the pork is done, transfer it to a bowl and shred it. Stir in the juices from the pan and divide among the hamburger buns. Top the sandwiches with coleslaw.

PORK CHOPS WITH APPLE SALAD

PREP TIME: **10 MINUTES** ■ TOTAL TIME: **25 MINUTES**

Makes 4 servings

APPLE SALAD

2 tablespoons balsamic vinegar

1 tablespoon Dijon mustard

2 apples, cored and thinly sliced lengthwise

1 head Bibb lettuce, chopped

2 cups fresh spinach

1 rib celery, sliced

½ small onion, sliced

¼ cup reduced-fat blue cheese crumbles

PORK CHOPS

4 pork chops (6 ounces each)

⅛ teaspoon salt

1 tablespoon chopped fresh thyme or 1 teaspoon dried

1 clove garlic, minced

1. **To make the apple salad:** In a large bowl, whisk together the vinegar and mustard. Add the apples, lettuce, spinach, celery, and onion. Toss to coat. Sprinkle with the blue cheese. Set aside.

2. **To make the pork chops:** Season each pork chop with the salt, thyme, and garlic.

3. Heat a large nonstick skillet coated with cooking spray over medium heat. Cook the pork chops for 8 minutes, turning once, or until lightly browned and a thermometer inserted in the center of a chop registers 145°F and the juices run clear. Serve with the apple salad.

Makeover Magic

BEFORE		AFTER
410	CALORIES	319
21 g	FAT	8 g
5 g	SAT FAT	3 g
21 g	CARBS	18 g
3 g	FIBER	4 g
35 g	PROTEIN	42 g
860 mg	SODIUM	381 mg

Curb carbs: We decided not to bread our pork chops. We just wanted to get a great sear on them to serve with our salad.

Fill up on fiber: Apples and all of the greens make this a really sweet and satisfying meal.

Favor fats: Toss some flax-seeds or another nut or seed of your choice into the apple salad for a dose of healthy fats.

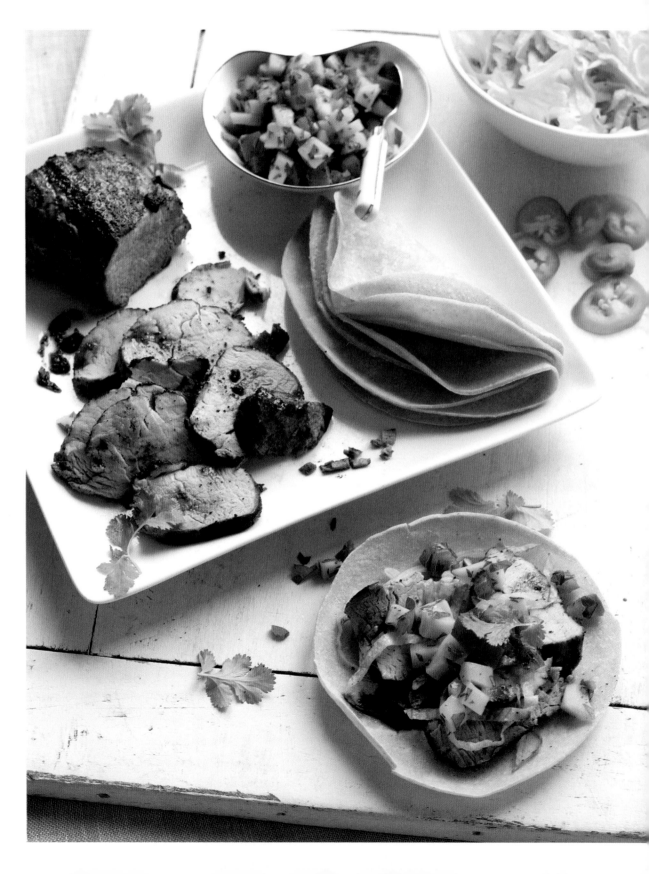

GRILLED PORK TACOS WITH MANGO SALSA

PREP TIME: **10 MINUTES** ■ TOTAL TIME: **50 MINUTES**

Makes 4 servings (2 tacos each)

1 mango, peeled, pitted, and diced

2 plum tomatoes, diced

¼ cup diced fresh cilantro

1 jalapeño chile pepper, seeded and finely chopped (wear plastic gloves when handling)

½ teaspoon paprika

¼ teaspoon salt

2 cloves garlic, minced

1½ teaspoons chipotle seasoning

1¼ pounds trimmed pork tenderloin

1 tablespoon olive oil

8 soft corn tortillas (6" diameter)

1 cup shredded lettuce

1. In a bowl, stir together the mango, tomatoes, cilantro, and pepper. Set aside.

2. Coat a grill rack with cooking spray. Heat the grill to medium.

3. In a cup, mix the paprika, salt, garlic, and chipotle seasoning. Rub all over the pork and drizzle with the oil.

4. Grill the pork for 25 minutes, turning occasionally, or until a thermometer inserted in the center reaches 145°F and the juices run clear. Let stand for 10 minutes before slicing. Cut the pork into thin slices.

5. Stack the tortillas and wrap them in foil.

6. Place the tortillas on a cool corner of the grill to warm for 10 minutes.

7. Place the tortillas on a work surface. Arrange pork in the center of each tortilla. Top with lettuce and salsa.

SMARTSTART

For a bigger dose of healthy fats, try adding avocado to the mango salsa.

Makeover Magic

BEFORE		AFTER
420	CALORIES	307
21 g	FAT	8 g
10 g	SAT FAT	2 g
38 g	CARBS	27 g
4 g	FIBER	4 g
21 g	PROTEIN	32 g
900 mg	SODIUM	211 mg

Curb carbs: These tacos are packed with enough ingredients to be double-deckers, but instead of using 2 taco shells, we used just 1.

Fill up on fiber: Shredded lettuce is key in a good taco, but the mango salsa really boosts the fiber this time.

Favor fats: We ditched cheese and sour cream to let the naturally low-fat mango salsa shine through. Remember, fats are key in balancing blood sugar, so be sure to pair with a side dish high in healthy fats.

BEFORE		AFTER
890	CALORIES	389
62 g	FAT	17 g
23 g	SAT FAT	4 g
30 g	CARBS	9 g
1 g	FIBER	1 g
52 g	PROTEIN	48 g
1,975 mg	SODIUM	303 mg

Curb carbs: Instead of a thick, saucy glaze, we opted for a flavorful dry rub. The thick glazes often have many carbohydrates because of the barbecue sauce in them.

Fill up on fiber: This dish, while hearty, is naturally low in fiber, so be sure to pair it with a salad of greens, or steamed veggies drizzled with lemon juice.

Favor fats: There's enough olive oil in this dish to provide plentiful MUFAs.

MARINATED GRILLED BONELESS PORK RIBS

PREP TIME: **5 MINUTES** ■ TOTAL TIME: **4 HOURS 25 MINUTES**

Makes 4 servings

2 tablespoons brown sugar

1 tablespoon ground cumin

1 tablespoon chili powder

1 teaspoon ground red pepper

1 teaspoon garlic powder

¼ teaspoon salt + additional to taste

2 pounds lean country-style boneless loin pork ribs

4 tablespoons olive oil, divided

Ground black pepper, to taste

1. In a small bowl, combine the sugar, cumin, chili powder, pepper, garlic powder, and ¼ teaspoon salt.

2. Place the ribs on a large baking sheet. Make crosswise slits halfway through the meat, without slicing through it completely. Rub 1 tablespoon of oil in the meat of the ribs and the dry rub all over the ribs on all sides, including into the cuts you made. Cover the baking sheet with plastic wrap and refrigerate at least 4 hours or up to 8 hours, turning occasionally.

3. Coat a grill rack with cooking spray. Preheat the grill to medium high. Sprinkle the ribs with salt and pepper. Grill the ribs for 20 minutes, turning once, or until a thermometer inserted in the center of a rib registers 145°F and the juices run clear. Brush the ribs with the remaining 3 tablespoons of the oil and grill for 2 minutes.

SWEET PORK TAGINE

PREP TIME: **10 MINUTES** ▪ TOTAL TIME: **7 HOURS 10 MINUTES**

Makes 6 servings

⅔ cup apple juice

½ cup low-sodium chicken broth

3 tablespoons olive oil

1 tablespoon cornstarch

¼ teaspoon salt

1 teaspoon ground cumin

1 teaspoon ground cinnamon

1 pound lean pork tenderloin, cut into 1" cubes

4 Granny Smith apples, cored and cut into eighths

6 carrots, cut into 1" pieces

1 small onion, chopped

⅓ cup pine nuts

2 tablespoons raisins

2 cloves garlic, minced

1 teaspoon grated fresh ginger

½ cup chopped fresh cilantro (optional)

1. In a 5- to 6-quart slow cooker coated with cooking spray, whisk together the juice, broth, olive oil, cornstarch, salt, cumin, and cinnamon until smooth. Add the pork, apples, carrots, onion, pine nuts, raisins, garlic, and ginger. Cover and cook on low for 7 to 8 hours (or on high for 3 to 4 hours), or until a thermometer inserted in the center reaches 145°F and the juices run clear.

2. Stir in the cilantro, if using.

Makeover Magic

BEFORE		AFTER
560	CALORIES	392
24 g	FAT	15 g
7 g	SAT FAT	2 g
51 g	CARBS	31 g
5 g	FIBER	5 g
35 g	PROTEIN	34 g
1,850 mg	SODIUM	229 mg

Curb carbs: Dried fruit adds flavor but also adds carbs. We use just enough dried fruit to add flavor without causing blood sugar to skyrocket.

Fill up on fiber: Dried fruits, fresh fruits, and vegetables provide 5 grams of fiber to this filling dish. Serve with whole wheat couscous, and the fiber will increase even more.

Favor fats: Pine nuts and olive oil are the healthy fat sources in this succulent dish.

BEFORE		AFTER
589	CALORIES	329
24 g	FAT	7 g
4 g	SAT FAT	2 g
59 g	CARBS	37 g
5 g	FIBER	6 g
35 g	PROTEIN	30 g
1,493 mg	SODIUM	590 mg

Curb carbs: The carbohydrates in our dish are primarily from the healthy brown rice, which we use less of thanks to bulky, delicious veggies.

Fill up on fiber: Using brown rice instead of white rice increases the fiber, as do the broccoli, pepper, and peas.

Favor fats: This dish is low in fat compared to many similar dishes because we chose to use a minimal amount of oil and low-fat add-ins for flavor, such as the lime juice and a lean cut of meat.

PORK AND BROCCOLI STIR-FRY

PREP TIME: **10 MINUTES** ■ TOTAL TIME: **20 MINUTES**

Makes 4 servings

SAUCE

3 tablespoons low-sodium soy sauce

2 tablespoons lime juice

1 tablespoon Asian chili paste

1 teaspoon honey

STIR-FRY

1 tablespoon sesame oil, divided

1 pound pork tenderloin, cut into ¼" strips

1 tablespoon grated fresh ginger or 1 teaspoon dried

1 clove garlic, minced

3 cups broccoli florets

2 carrots, sliced

1 red bell pepper, thinly sliced

3 tablespoons water

½ cup (1 ounce) snap peas

2 cups cooked brown rice

SMARTSTART

Add ¼ cup crushed peanuts to this Asian favorite to get MUFAs!

1. **To make the sauce:** In a small bowl, combine the soy sauce, lime juice, chili paste, and honey. Set aside.

2. **To make the stir-fry:** In a large nonstick skillet, heat 1 teaspoon of the oil over medium-high heat. Cook the pork, in batches if necessary so as not to overcrowd the skillet, stirring often, for 3 minutes, or until lightly browned. Transfer to a plate and set aside.

3. Return the skillet to medium-high heat and stir in the remaining 2 teaspoons oil. Cook the ginger and garlic for 30 seconds, or until fragrant. Stir in the broccoli and cook for 1 minute. Add the carrots, peppers, and water. Cover and simmer for 3 minutes, or until tender-crisp. Uncover and stir in the peas, reserved soy sauce mixture, and pork.

4. Cook, stirring, for 2 minutes, or until the sauce reduces and flavors blend. Remove from the heat and serve over the rice.

BEFORE		AFTER
520	CALORIES	321
15 g	FAT	7 g
6 g	SAT FAT	2 g
53 g	CARBS	34 g
4 g	FIBER	6 g
41 g	PROTEIN	29 g
1,310 mg	SODIUM	249 mg

Curb carbs: We curbed the carbs in this recipe by not using breading or barbecue sauce on our pork. Potatoes and turnips are starchy vegetables that you can absolutely enjoy as part of a healthy, balanced diet for diabetes.

Fill up on fiber: We kept the skins on our mashed potatoes and added an extra kick with turnips in our vegetable mixture to top the pork.

Favor fats: We used lean pork tenderloin, minimal oil, and a vegetable mixture instead of cheese. The olive oil used in our recipe adds MUFA power. For even more MUFAs, serve this dish with roasted asparagus drizzled with olive oil.

ROSEMARY PORK MEDALLIONS AND MASHED POTATOES

PREP TIME: **10 MINUTES** ■ TOTAL TIME: **45 MINUTES**

Makes 4 servings

¾ pound Yukon gold potatoes, cut into 2" cubes

¾ pound turnips, peeled and cut into 2" cubes

1 tablespoon + 1 teaspoon olive oil, divided

2 tablespoons plain 0% Greek yogurt

⅛ teaspoon salt

1 pound well-trimmed pork tenderloin, cut into 1" thick medallions

1½ teaspoons cornstarch

½ cup low-sodium chicken broth, divided

2 tablespoons fresh rosemary or 1 teaspoon dried

2 cloves garlic, minced

1 small red onion, sliced

1. In a large saucepan, add the potatoes and turnips and fill with enough water to cover. Bring to a boil over medium-high heat, reduce the heat to a simmer, and cook for 15 minutes, or until the turnips and potatoes are fork-tender.

2. Remove from the heat and drain. With a potato masher, mash the potatoes and turnips. Add 1 teaspoon of the olive oil, the yogurt, and the salt and continue to mash until well blended. Cover and keep warm.

3. In a large nonstick skillet, heat 1 teaspoon of the oil over medium-high heat. Cook the pork for 8 minutes, turning once, or until a thermometer inserted in the center reaches 145°F and the juices run clear. Transfer to a plate and set aside.

4. In a small bowl, whisk together the cornstarch and ¼ cup of the chicken broth.

5. In the same skillet over medium-high heat, add the remaining oil, rosemary, garlic, onion, and remaining chicken broth. Whisk in the cornstarch mixture until combined and cook for 5 minutes, or until the broth is reduced by half and thickened and the onions are softened. Return the pork to the skillet and toss to combine. Serve the pork over the mashed potatoes and top with the herbed onion mixture and juices.

Makeover Magic

BEFORE		AFTER
410	CALORIES	297
9 g	FAT	5 g
4 g	SAT FAT	1 g
68 g	CARBS	34 g
4 g	FIBER	5 g
17 g	PROTEIN	30 g
1,045 mg	SODIUM	149 mg

Curb carbs: Our recipe has just enough carbohydrates to satisfy you without going overboard. The grilled potatoes provide much of the carbohydrates.

Fill up on fiber: Along with this flavorful rubbed pork, we added bell pepper, mushrooms, and potatoes, with the skins, to make the dish fiber-full.

Favor fats: The saturated fat in this recipe is so low thanks to the lean pork tenderloin we use. The olive oil contains MUFAs, but we suggest adding more healthy fats with a side dish like Quinoa Pilaf with Pistachios (page 290).

TANGY PORK KABOBS

PREP TIME: **10 MINUTES** ■ TOTAL TIME: **1 HOUR 5 MINUTES**

Makes 4 servings (2 skewers each)

1 tablespoon brown sugar

½ teaspoon garlic powder

½ teaspoon chili powder

½ teaspoon onion powder

¼ teaspoon dry mustard

⅛ teaspoon salt

1¼ pounds red potatoes, cut into 1" pieces

1 pound lean pork tenderloin, cut into 1" pieces

2 teaspoons olive oil, divided

1 onion, cut into 1" pieces

1 green bell pepper, cut into 1" pieces

12 ounces (¾ pound) cremini mushrooms, halved

8 metal skewers (7"–8" each), or wooden skewers soaked in water 30 minutes before cooking

1. In a small bowl, combine the sugar, garlic, chili and onion powders, mustard, and salt.

2. In a large saucepan, add the potatoes and fill with enough water to cover. Bring to a boil over high heat and cook for 10 minutes, until nearly tender. Drain.

3. Coat a grill rack with cooking spray. Preheat the grill to medium high.

4. In an 8" × 8" baking dish, toss the pork, 1 teaspoon olive oil, and 1½ tablespoons of the sugar mixture. Rub into the pork and allow to sit for 30 minutes.

5. In a large bowl, toss the cooked potatoes, onion, pepper, and mushrooms with the remaining olive oil and remaining sugar mixture until coated.

6. Thread the skewers with pork, onion, potatoes, pepper, and mushrooms. Grill for 10 minutes, turning once, or until the vegetables have softened and a thermometer inserted in the center of the pork reaches 145°F and the juices run clear.

ITALIAN SAUSAGE AND LINGUINE

PREP TIME: **10 MINUTES** ■ TOTAL TIME: **35 MINUTES**

Makes 4 servings

8 ounces whole grain linguine

½ teaspoon olive oil

8 ounces sweet Italian sausage, sliced

6 cloves garlic, sliced

1 red bell pepper, thinly sliced

1 bag (10 ounces) frozen chopped broccoli, thawed

1 cup reduced-sodium, fat-free chicken broth

1 teaspoon crushed red-pepper flakes

4 tablespoons grated Parmesan cheese

1. Prepare the pasta according to package directions. Drain and set aside.

2. Meanwhile, in a large nonstick skillet, heat the oil over medium-high heat. Cook the sausage for 6 minutes, stirring and breaking it into smaller pieces with a wooden spoon, until no longer pink. Reduce the heat to medium. Cook the garlic, bell pepper, and broccoli for 4 minutes, or until lightly golden and softened. Add the broth and bring to a boil. Cook for 4 minutes, or until reduced by half. Stir in the pepper flakes and cook for 2 minutes, stirring, until hot. Add the pasta and cheese and toss well.

Makeover Magic

BEFORE		AFTER
488	CALORIES	348
21 g	FAT	9 g
8 g	SAT FAT	3 g
55 g	CARBS	49 g
4 g	FIBER	9 g
22 g	PROTEIN	20 g
694 mg	SODIUM	541 mg

Curb carbs: Eight ounces of whole grain linguine is a perfect portion for four people. This will keep within the recommended 45 grams of carbs.

Fill up on fiber: Whole grain linguine, peppers, and broccoli provide 9 grams of fiber per serving. We like this dish because it has more going on than the average sausage and pasta dish.

Favor fats: We reduced the amount of sausage in this recipe till it is just enough to enjoy with the pasta. We also used a light sauce made from chicken broth instead of heavy cream.

SMARTSTART

If you are in the Repeating or Time stage (see page 7), swap the broth for a healthy fat source like pesto sauce, which is packed with MUFAs!

Makeover Magic

BEFORE		AFTER
354	CALORIES	241
12 g	FAT	8 g
3 g	SAT FAT	2 g
43 g	CARBS	17 g
1 g	FIBER	3 g
20 g	PROTEIN	27 g
1,025 mg	SODIUM	517 mg

Curb carbs: We used just enough brown rice to add bulk to these lettuce cups to make them a satisfying, heart-healthy meal.

Fill up on fiber: All of the vegetables in this dish as well as the rice pack fiber.

Favor fats: To reduce saturated fat, we chose lean ground pork and used a small amount of oil, unlike many stir-fry-style dishes. Peanut oil is a great source of MUFAs and is best used when cooking over high heat.

ASIAN LETTUCE CUPS

PREP TIME: **5 MINUTES** ■ TOTAL TIME: **20 MINUTES**

Makes 4 servings (3 wraps each)

2 teaspoons peanut oil, divided

1 pound lean ground pork

1 clove garlic, minced

1 red bell pepper, thinly sliced

4 ounces shiitake mushrooms, trimmed, thinly sliced

2 tablespoons low-sodium soy sauce

2 tablespoons Asian chili paste

4 scallions, thinly sliced

1 cup cooked brown rice

12 leaves Bibb lettuce (1–2 large heads)

¼ cup chopped fresh cilantro

1. In a large nonstick skillet, heat 1 teaspoon of the oil over medium heat. Cook the pork for 5 minutes, stirring often, or until browned and cooked through. Add the remaining oil, garlic, pepper, and mushrooms and cook for 5 minutes, stirring often. Stir in the soy sauce, chili paste, scallions, and brown rice and cook for 2 minutes, or until heated through.

2. Arrange the lettuce leaves on a serving platter. Fill the leaves with the pork mixture evenly. Sprinkle with cilantro leaves.

SMARTSTART

Try wild rice for even more fiber and flavor. And add ¼ cup chopped cashews for your favorite source of fat, MUFAs, and even more fiber.

Meat

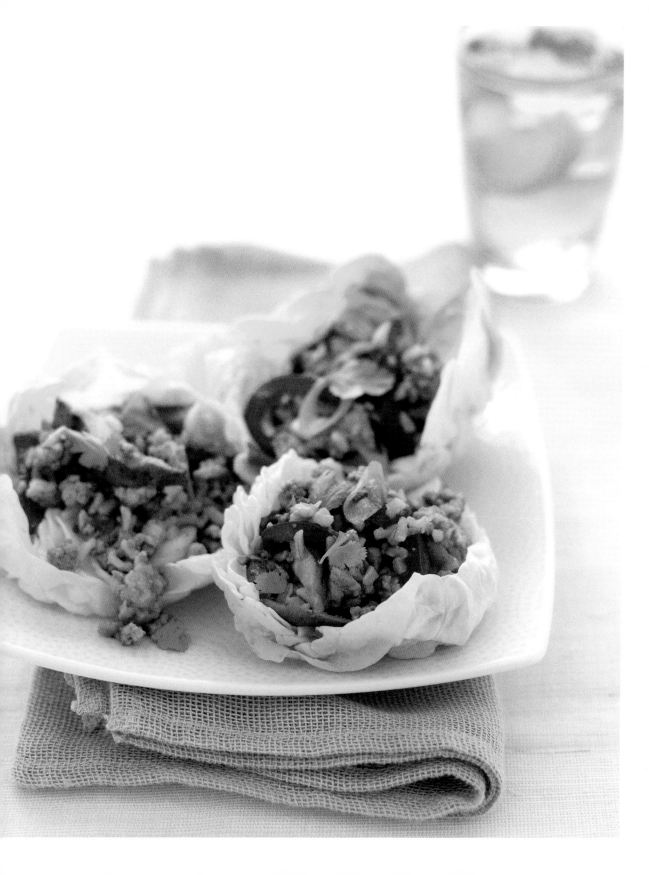

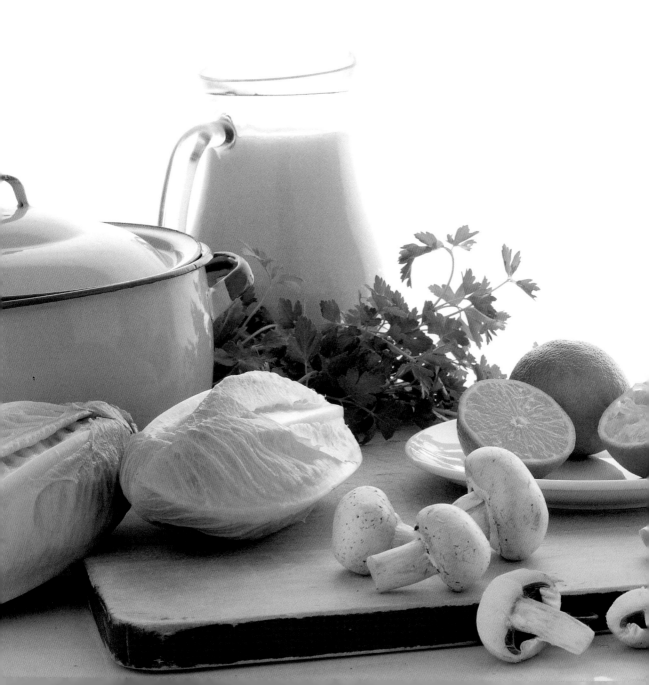

Poultry

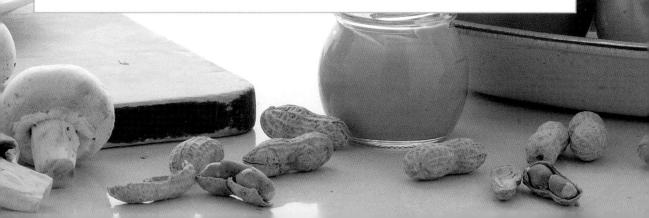

Makeover Magic

BEFORE		AFTER
500	CALORIES	282
30 g	FAT	17 g
12 g	SAT FAT	2.5 g
15 g	CARBS	7 g
1 g	FIBER	1 g
40 g	PROTEIN	25 g
980 mg	SODIUM	178 mg

Curb carbs: We cut the carbohydrates by using less flour and swapping out all-purpose flour for white whole wheat flour.

Fill up on fiber: The white whole wheat flour has a good amount of fiber, but since we are using such a small amount, pair this dish with steamed vegetables or a salad to boost the fiber even more!

Favor fats: We used our favorite heart-healthy olive oil and removed saturated fat by trading full-fat cream sauce for the flavorful lemon-caper broth.

CHICKEN PICCATA

PREP TIME: **5 MINUTES** ■ TOTAL TIME: **15 MINUTES**

Makes 4 servings

1 pound boneless, skinless chicken breast tenderloins

4 tablespoons white whole wheat flour, divided

4 tablespoons olive oil

3 tablespoons low-sodium chicken broth

2 tablespoons freshly squeezed lemon juice

1 sprig fresh parsley, finely chopped

2 teaspoons capers

1. Lay the tenderloins on a work surface. With a smooth meat mallet or a rolling pin, flatten to ¼" thickness. Dredge the cutlets lightly in 2 tablespoons of the flour.

2. In a large skillet over medium heat, heat the oil. Cook the chicken for 4 minutes, turning once, or until no longer pink and the juices run clear.

3. In a small bowl, whisk together the chicken broth and the remaining 2 tablespoons flour until a smooth paste forms.

4. Add the lemon juice, parsley, and capers to the skillet. Bring to a boil. Whisk in the broth mixture. Reduce the heat and simmer for 2 minutes, whisking constantly until thickened.

CHICKEN AND WAFFLES

PREP TIME: **10 MINUTES** ■ TOTAL TIME: **20 MINUTES**

Makes 4 servings

¼ cup + 2 tablespoons whole wheat pastry flour

2 egg whites, lightly beaten

2 tablespoons 1% milk

1 cup cornflakes, finely crushed

1 tablespoon canola oil

1 pound boneless, skinless chicken breast tenderloins

2 tablespoons unsalted butter

¾ cup low-sodium chicken broth

8 frozen multigrain waffles

1. In a shallow bowl, add ¼ cup flour. In another shallow bowl, whisk together the egg whites and milk. In a third shallow bowl, add the crushed cornflakes.

2. Dredge the chicken tenderloins in the flour to coat. Dip them into the egg mixture to coat, shaking off any excess, and transfer to the cornflakes to coat.

3. In a large nonstick skillet, heat the oil over medium-high heat.

4. In the skillet, cook the chicken for 10 minutes, turning once, or until no longer pink and the juices run clear. Transfer to a serving platter.

5. In the same skillet, melt the butter over medium heat. Whisk in the remaining flour until a smooth paste forms. Slowly whisk in the broth and stir for 5 minutes, or until thickened. Remove from the heat.

6. Prepare the waffles according to package directions.

7. Top the waffles with the chicken and gravy.

SMART START

Switch from cornflakes to bran flakes.

Makeover Magic

BEFORE		AFTER
1,250	CALORIES	456
66 g	FAT	18 g
22 g	SAT FAT	5 g
94 g	CARBS	45 g
6 g	FIBER	9 g
69 g	PROTEIN	32 g
3,950 mg	SODIUM	424 mg

Curb carbs: Using store-bought multigrain waffles is a quick, fiber-full fix that will keep portions of this comfort dish reasonable.

Fill up on fiber: Instead of deep-frying the cutlets, applying whole wheat pastry flour and cornflakes gives crunch and a satisfying fiber boost.

Favor fats: Reduce saturated fat by using boneless, skinless chicken tenderloins and smaller amounts of butter than a traditional version of this dish. For more healthy fats, try this dish with a smear of olive tapenade or avocado instead of the gravy.

Makeover Magic

BEFORE		AFTER
752	CALORIES	368
40 g	FAT	7 g
24 g	SAT FAT	1.5 g
48 g	CARBS	36 g
3 g	FIBER	6 g
45 g	PROTEIN	32 g
842 mg	SODIUM	183 mg

Curb carbs: We used whole wheat egg noodles to accompany this chicken dish instead of regular white pasta and used less of it than you typically would.

Fill up on fiber: Between the whole wheat egg noodles and all of the fresh vegetables added to this classic dish, we really boosted the fiber.

Favor fats: Instead of coating our chicken in a heavy cream sauce, we opted for a savory sauce featuring olive oil.

CHICKEN CACCIATORE

PREP TIME: **10 MINUTES** ■ TOTAL TIME: **50 MINUTES**

Makes 4 servings

4 ounces whole wheat egg noodles

2 teaspoons olive oil

1 pound boneless, skinless chicken breasts (½" thick)

1 package (8 ounces) cremini mushrooms, sliced

1 green bell pepper, sliced

1 red bell pepper, sliced

2 carrots, sliced

1 small onion, sliced

2 cloves garlic, minced

1 can (14.5 ounces) no-salt-added diced tomatoes

1 teaspoon dried oregano

¾ cup dry white wine

1. Prepare the noodles according to package directions. Drain and set aside.

2. In a large nonstick skillet, heat the oil over medium-high heat. Cook the chicken, turning occasionally, for 6 minutes, or until browned on all sides. Transfer to a plate.

3. Add the mushrooms, peppers, carrots, onion, and garlic to the skillet and toss to combine. Reduce the heat to medium, cover, and cook, tossing occasionally, for 3 minutes, or until the mushrooms begin to release liquid. Uncover and cook to evaporate most of the liquid. Add the tomatoes, oregano, wine, and the reserved chicken. Reduce the heat and simmer for 30 minutes, until the mixture has thickened, and a thermometer inserted in the thickest portion of the chicken registers 165°F and the juices run clear.

4. Serve the chicken over the noodles.

CHICKEN-MUSHROOM BAKE

PREP TIME: **10 MINUTES** ■ TOTAL TIME: **45 MINUTES**

Makes 6 servings

8 ounces sprouted whole grain spaghetti

1 tablespoon + 1 teaspoon canola oil

1½ pounds boneless, skinless chicken breast halves cut crosswise into ¼" strips

8 ounces cremini mushrooms, sliced

1¾ cups low-sodium chicken broth, divided

½ cup dry white wine or chicken broth

1 bay leaf

2 tablespoons cornstarch

¼ teaspoon ground black pepper

6 ounces Neufchâtel cheese, softened

½ cup grated Parmesan cheese

1. Preheat the oven to 400°F. Coat an 11" x 8" baking dish with cooking spray.

2. Prepare the pasta according to package directions. Drain well and transfer to a warm, large bowl.

3. In a large nonstick skillet, heat 1 tablespoon of the oil over medium-high heat. Cook the chicken, stirring, for 6 minutes, or until no longer pink and the juices run clear. Transfer to the bowl with the pasta. In the skillet, heat 1 teaspoon of oil. Cook the mushrooms for 5 minutes, or until tender and browned. Remove the mushrooms to the pasta bowl.

4. In the same skillet, bring 1½ cups of the broth, the ½ cup wine or broth, and the bay leaf to a boil.

5. In a cup, combine the cornstarch and the remaining broth. Whisk into the broth mixture and cook for 1 minute, whisking until thickened. Season with the pepper. Remove from the heat. Discard the bay leaf. Add the Neufchâtel cheese and whisk until melted. Pour over the pasta, tossing to mix. Pour into the baking dish. Sprinkle with the Parmesan cheese.

6. Bake on the top rack for 20 minutes, or until light brown and bubbling.

Makeover Magic

BEFORE		AFTER
720	CALORIES	438
40 g	FAT	16 g
21 g	SAT FAT	6 g
58 g	CARBS	32 g
3 g	FIBER	5 g
31 g	PROTEIN	37 g
1,240 mg	SODIUM	358 mg

Curb carbs: Sprouted whole grain pasta is a lower-carb alternative to regular white pasta—it even beats out whole wheat!

Fill up on fiber: Sprouted grain pasta is also high in fiber, and the mushrooms give this recipe the final kick for fiber and nutrients.

Favor fats: With such a creamy dish, instead of full-fat ingredients, we switched to reduced fat when we could. Top this dish with sliced olives to get favored fats.

Makeover Magic

BEFORE		AFTER
1,270	CALORIES	453
84 g	FAT	20 g
41 g	SAT FAT	10 g
54 g	CARBS	35 g
2 g	FIBER	4 g
60 g	PROTEIN	32 g
3,520 mg	SODIUM	523 mg

Curb carbs: Marinara sauce can be a hidden carb bomb. This recipe uses the perfect amount for a moist dish that won't blow up your blood sugar.

Fill up on fiber: Oven-ready whole wheat lasagna noodles and nutrient-dense spinach make this dish hearty and filling.

Favor fats: It wouldn't be lasagna without cheesy goodness, so we made smart picks—part-skim products and hard cheeses like Parmesan decrease the saturated fat but keep our taste buds happy. Using canola oil and olive oil or canola oil–based marinara sauce ensures we incorporate our favored fats.

SMARTSTART

Look for jarred marinara sauce that has olive oil and no added sugar.

QUICK, CREAMY CHICKEN LASAGNA

PREP TIME: **20 MINUTES** ■ TOTAL TIME: **1 HOUR 15 MINUTES**

Makes 8 servings

1 package (9 ounces) oven-ready whole wheat lasagna noodles

4 cups water

1 pound boneless, skinless chicken breasts

1½ teaspoons dried basil

8 ounces Neufchâtel cheese, softened, divided

1 tablespoon canola oil

1½ cups part-skim ricotta cheese

¼ cup grated Parmesan cheese

1½ cups shredded part-skim mozzarella cheese, divided

½ cup low-sodium chicken or vegetable broth

3 cups low-sodium marinara sauce, divided

1 package (10 ounces) frozen chopped spinach, thawed and drained

1. Preheat the oven to 400°F.

2. Place 3 oven-ready noodles in a medium bowl. Cover with warm water for 5 minutes, or until pliable. Reserve.

3. In a large nonstick skillet over medium-high heat, bring the water to a simmer. Cook the chicken for 10 minutes, or until a thermometer inserted in the thickest portion registers 165°F and the juices run clear. Transfer to a cutting board and dice.

4. In a large bowl, combine the chicken, basil, 4 ounces of the Neufchâtel, oil, ricotta, Parmesan, and 1 cup of the mozzarella cheese.

5. In another bowl, whisk together the remaining Neufchâtel and broth until smooth.

6. In a 13" × 9" baking dish, spread ⅓ cup of the sauce. Assemble 3 layers as follows: 4 noodles, ⅔ cup of the sauce, one-third of the chicken mixture, and one-third of the spinach. Top with the softened noodles, the Neufchâtel sauce, the remaining ⅔ cup marinara sauce, and the remaining ½ cup mozzarella. Cover with foil and bake for 30 minutes. Uncover and bake for 15 minutes, or until the cheese melts.

7. Let sit for 10 minutes before serving.

CHICKEN AND SAUSAGE JAMBALAYA

PREP TIME: **10 MINUTES** ■ TOTAL TIME: **55 MINUTES**

Makes 4 servings

3 teaspoons canola oil, divided

½ pound boneless, skinless chicken breasts, cut crosswise into ¼" strips

4 ounces turkey sausage, casing removed, cut into small pieces

1 green bell pepper, chopped

4 scallions, sliced

1 jalapeño chile pepper, seeded and finely chopped (wear plastic gloves when handling)

3 cloves garlic, minced

1 tablespoon salt-free Creole seasoning

1 can (14.5 ounces) no-salt-added diced tomatoes

1 cup no-salt-added canned black beans, drained and rinsed

1½ cups low-sodium chicken broth

½ cup uncooked brown rice

1. In a Dutch oven or large nonstick skillet, heat 1 teaspoon oil over medium-high heat. Cook the chicken for 5 minutes, stirring. Add the sausage and cook for 6 minutes, or until the chicken and sausage are browned, cooked through, and the juices run clear.

2. Add the remaining 2 teaspoons oil, the bell pepper, scallions, jalapeño, garlic, and Creole seasoning. Cook for 3 minutes, stirring, or until the vegetables are browned and softened.

3. Add the tomatoes, beans, chicken broth, and rice and bring to a boil. Reduce the heat to medium low, cover, and cook for 30 minutes or until the rice is tender.

Makeover Magic

BEFORE		AFTER
525	CALORIES	303
22 g	FAT	8 g
8 g	SAT FAT	2 g
47 g	CARBS	32 g
2 g	FIBER	4 g
35 g	PROTEIN	23 g
830 mg	SODIUM	411 mg

Curb carbs: We added brown rice to our jambalaya to make a traditional dish more healthful and cut the amount of rice overall by adding beans, peppers, and more meat.

Fill up on fiber: Beans are the fiber star of this recipe!

Favor fats: We reduced the saturated fat by subbing a mix of lean chicken breast and turkey sausage for the traditional pork sausage. This dish would pair well with an avocado and orange salad, full of healthy fats.

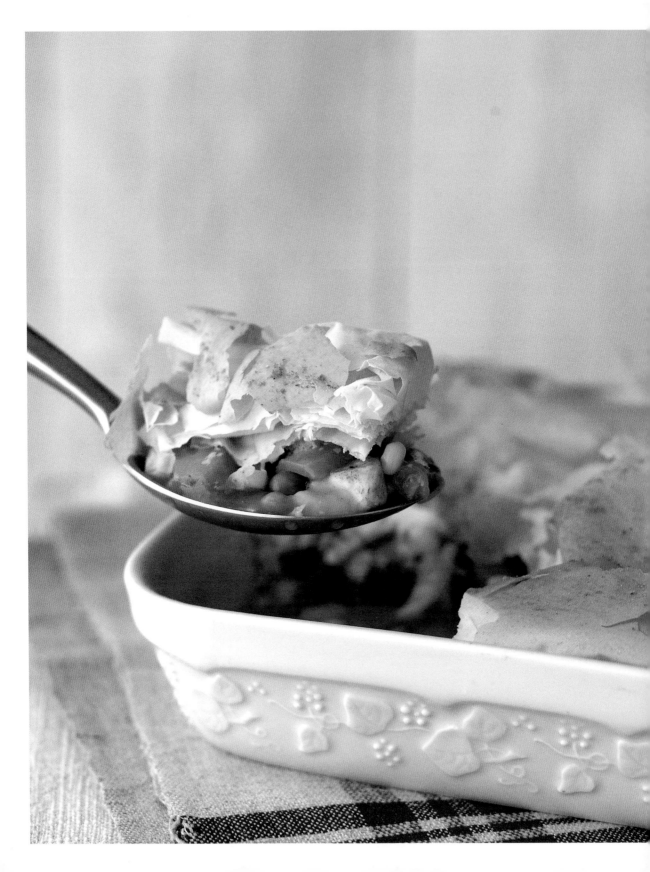

CHICKEN POT PIE

PREP TIME: **5 MINUTES** ■ TOTAL TIME: **45 MINUTES**

Makes 6 servings

2 teaspoons olive oil, divided

1¼ pounds boneless, skinless chicken breasts, cut into ½"–¾" cubes

2 carrots, thinly sliced

2 ribs celery, thinly sliced

1 teaspoon dried rosemary, crushed

2 cups frozen corn, bean, and pea mix, thawed

2 cups low-sodium chicken broth, divided

1 tablespoon cornstarch

8 sheets whole wheat phyllo dough

1. Preheat the oven to 350°F. Coat a 9" × 9" baking dish with cooking spray.

2. In a large nonstick skillet, heat 1 teaspoon of the oil over medium-high heat. Cook the chicken for 8 minutes, stirring, until no longer pink and the juices run clear. Transfer to a bowl and set aside.

3. In the same skillet, in the remaining oil, cook the carrots, celery, and rosemary, stirring, for 5 minutes, or until tender. Stir in the chicken and corn mixture. Transfer to the baking dish. Add 1½ cups broth to the same skillet over medium-low heat and bring to a simmer.

4. In a small bowl, whisk together the remaining ½ cup broth and the cornstarch until smooth. Add the mixture to the broth in the skillet and whisk for 3 minutes, or until thickened. Pour into the chicken and vegetable mixture in the baking dish and stir to combine.

5. Lay 2 phyllo sheets across the top of the dish, tucking the edges into the pan. Lightly coat the sheets with cooking spray. Repeat to make 3 more layers. Bake for 20 minutes, or until golden and bubbling.

Makeover Magic

BEFORE		AFTER
430	CALORIES	222
22 g	FAT	5 g
8 g	SAT FAT	1 g
43 g	CARBS	20 g
1 g	FIBER	3 g
14 g	PROTEIN	24 g
1,020 mg	SODIUM	256 mg

Curb carbs: Substituting whole wheat phyllo dough for store-bought piecrust is a simple trick to curb carbs when baking any kind of pie.

Fill up on fiber: In addition to the whole wheat phyllo dough, tons of vegetables add extra fiber to this classic comfort food.

Favor fats: No store-bought gravy here. We thickened chicken broth with cornstarch to make a homemade, low-fat gravy to coat all of the veggies and chicken!

SMARTSTART

It's okay to have dessert to get your healthy fats. Pair this with Almond Rice Pudding (page 323).

BEFORE		AFTER
721	CALORIES	338
27 g	FAT	9 g
11 g	SAT FAT	3 g
65 g	CARBS	30 g
3 g	FIBER	6 g
50 g	PROTEIN	33 g
1,548 mg	SODIUM	300 mg

Curb carbs: We use half as much flour in this diabetes-friendly dish as the traditional recipe calls for, without sacrificing the flavor.

Fill up on fiber: Whole wheat dumplings help boost the fiber, but more importantly, we added a ton of fresh vegetables to pump up this recipe!

Favor fats: Chicken and dumplings doesn't always have to be a diabetes disaster—we cut out butter and yet still created creamy gravy from light sour cream and broth. For a dose of healthy fats, serve a side salad dressed in flaxseed oil and sunflower seeds.

CHICKEN AND DUMPLINGS

PREP TIME: **10 MINUTES** ■ TOTAL TIME: **50 MINUTES**

Makes 6 servings

1 cup whole wheat pastry flour

1½ teaspoons baking powder

1 large egg, beaten

½ cup buttermilk

1 tablespoon olive oil

1½ pounds boneless, skinless chicken breasts, cut into 1" pieces

1 onion, chopped

3 ribs celery, sliced

2 carrots, sliced

5 cups low-sodium chicken broth, divided

2 tablespoons finely chopped fresh thyme (or 2 teaspoons dried)

1 tablespoon cornstarch or arrowroot

½ cup light sour cream

1½ cups frozen peas, thawed

1. In a bowl, combine the flour and baking powder. Form a well in the center of the mixture.

2. In a liquid measuring glass, whisk together the egg and buttermilk. Pour into the dry ingredients. Stir just until combined. Set aside.

3. In a Dutch oven, heat the oil over medium-high heat. Cook the chicken, stirring often, for 8 minutes, or until no longer pink and the juices run clear.

4. Add the onion, celery, and carrots and cook for 5 minutes, or until browned and softened. Add 4½ cups of the broth and the thyme and bring to a simmer.

5. Reduce the heat to medium low.

6. In a small bowl, whisk together the remaining broth and cornstarch or arrowroot until smooth. Stir into the broth along with the sour cream and peas. Cook for 5 minutes, stirring often, until thickened.

7. Carefully drop spoonfuls of dumpling batter into the thickened sauce and cook for 10 minutes, or until the dumplings are firm on the inside and puffy.

BAKED CHICKEN WITH MUSTARD SAUCE

PREP TIME: **5 MINUTES** ◼ TOTAL TIME: **35 MINUTES**

Makes 4 servings

SAUCE

3 tablespoons honey mustard

3 tablespoons plain 0% Greek yogurt

2 tablespoons orange juice

CHICKEN

2 tablespoons olive oil, divided

1 large egg white

¼ cup honey mustard

½ teaspoon ground black pepper

¼ teaspoon paprika

4 boneless, skinless chicken breasts (6 ounces each, ½" thick)

¾ cup whole wheat panko bread crumbs

1. **To make the sauce:** In a small bowl, whisk the mustard, yogurt, and orange juice together. Place in the refrigerator until the chicken is finished.

2. **To make the chicken:** Preheat the oven to 375°F. Using 1 tablespoon of the oil, coat a rimmed baking sheet.

3. In a large bowl, whisk the egg white until foamy. Whisk in the mustard, pepper, and paprika. Add the chicken and turn to coat well.

4. Place the bread crumbs in a pie plate. One piece at a time, lift the chicken from the mustard mixture and roll in the crumbs, pressing them so they adhere. Place the chicken on the baking sheet. Drizzle the chicken with the remaining 1 tablespoon oil. Bake, turning once, for 25 minutes until crispy and browned, or until a thermometer inserted in the thickest portion registers 165°F and the juices run clear.

Makeover Magic

BEFORE		AFTER
560	CALORIES	347
22 g	FAT	12 g
6 g	SAT FAT	2 g
50 g	CARBS	17 g
0 g	FIBER	2 g
41 g	PROTEIN	40 g
1,280 mg	SODIUM	503 mg

Curb carbs: This dish is often glazed with maple-flavored pancake syrup, which has tons of carbs. Keep it sweet by using a touch of orange juice, which will enhance the mustard's flavor, too!

Fill up on fiber: Whole wheat panko bread crumbs add fiber to this cozy dish.

Favor fats: Olive oil provides healthy fats, but for a bigger boost, pair this dish with the Broccoli-Walnut Farfalle Toss (page 293).

Makeover Magic

BEFORE		AFTER
590	CALORIES	310
33 g	FAT	12 g
11 g	SAT FAT	2 g
40 g	CARBS	23 g
5 g	FIBER	6 g
34 g	PROTEIN	29 g
220 mg	SODIUM	162 mg

Curb carbs: Instead of filling up on traditional roasted potatoes, we mixed in some Brussels sprouts, though you could choose any nonstarchy vegetable side.

Fill up on fiber: The fiber in this surefire favorite comes from keeping the skins on the potatoes and adding delicious Brussels sprouts.

Favor fats: Olive oil and ground flaxseeds provide both MUFAs and ALA fatty acids in this dish.

HERB-ROASTED CHICKEN BREASTS WITH VEGETABLES

PREP TIME: **10 MINUTES** ■ TOTAL TIME: **1 HOUR**

Makes 4 servings

CHICKEN

3 tablespoons lemon juice

2 tablespoons ground flaxseeds

2 cloves garlic, minced

1 tablespoon finely chopped fresh rosemary or 1 teaspoon dried

1 tablespoon olive oil

4 boneless, skinless chicken breasts (4 ounces each)

¼ cup low-sodium chicken broth

VEGETABLES

¾ pound Brussels sprouts, trimmed and halved lengthwise

¾ pound small red potatoes (1¾"–2"), halved

1 tablespoon olive oil

1. Preheat the oven to 400°F. Coat a 13" × 9" baking pan with cooking spray. Coat a rimmed baking sheet with cooking spray.

2. **To make the chicken:** In a small bowl, stir together the lemon juice, flaxseeds, garlic, rosemary, and oil.

3. Place the chicken breasts in the baking pan. Divide the herbed mixture over the chicken breasts and rub on all sides. Bake for 40 minutes, turning once, or until a thermometer inserted in the thickest portion registers 165°F and the juices run clear.

4. **To make the vegetables:** Place the Brussels sprouts and potatoes on the baking sheet. Toss with the oil to coat. Bake for 35 minutes, or until all the vegetables are tender.

ORANGE-SESAME CHICKEN

PREP TIME: **5 MINUTES** ■ TOTAL TIME: **1 HOUR 20 MINUTES**

Makes 4 servings

1½ cups orange juice, divided

6 tablespoons low-sodium soy sauce, divided

1 clove garlic, minced

1 pound boneless, skinless chicken breasts

1¾ cups instant brown rice

2 tablespoons orange zest

1 teaspoon Asian sweet chili sauce (optional)

3 tablespoons water

1 tablespoon cornstarch

2 teaspoons sesame seeds

1. In a resealable plastic bag, combine 1 cup of the orange juice, 2 tablespoons of the soy sauce, and the garlic. Add the chicken, toss, and seal. Place in the refrigerator for 30 minutes, turning once. Remove from the refrigerator and bring to room temperature for 15 minutes.

2. Meanwhile, prepare the rice according to package directions. Remove from the heat and keep covered.

3. Coat a grill rack with cooking spray. Heat the grill over high heat.

4. Remove the chicken from the marinade, discarding the marinade. Grill for 15 minutes, turning once, or until a thermometer inserted in the thickest portion registers 165°F and the juices run clear.

5. Transfer the chicken to a clean cutting board and let it rest for 5 minutes.

6. In a small saucepan over medium-high heat, add the remaining orange juice, remaining soy sauce, orange zest, and chili sauce, if using, and stir. Bring to a simmer.

7. In a small bowl, whisk together the water and cornstarch until a smooth paste forms. Whisk the mixture into the orange sauce and continue to whisk for 3 minutes, or until the orange sauce thickens.

8. Slice the chicken breasts crosswise into ½" pieces. Divide the rice, chicken, sauce, and sesame seeds among 4 plates.

Makeover Magic

BEFORE		AFTER
860	CALORIES	326
41 g	FAT	5 g
7 g	SAT FAT	1 g
66 g	CARBS	39 g
3 g	FIBER	3 g
60 g	PROTEIN	29 g
1,410 mg	SODIUM	552 mg

Curb carbs: Instead of using breading on our chicken, we kept it light with a tangy marinade to curb the carbs so that you can include brown rice in your dish—that's not even accounted for in the take-out version of this recipe.

Fill up on fiber: The brown rice and sesame seeds are the major contributors to fiber in this dish!

Favor fats: We kept this dish low in saturated fats by grilling, not frying. Sesame seeds have some MUFAs, but you can add more by making a side salad dressed with olive oil.

BEFORE		AFTER
400	CALORIES	247
20 g	FAT	12 g
11 g	SAT FAT	4 g
16 g	CARBS	10 g
2 g	FIBER	2 g
37 g	PROTEIN	25 g
230 mg	SODIUM	145 mg

Curb carbs: Our revamped recipe uses less flour. Serve it over a bed of lentils and greens instead of the typical pasta or rice to keep carbs curbed even further.

Fill up on fiber: This protein dish pairs naturally with high-fiber sides like whole wheat pasta or a bed of lentils and greens, like Swiss chard or kale.

Favor fats: Use a small amount of canola oil to lightly fry this dish. Cook your lentils and greens in olive oil for MUFAs with a bit of garlic for more flavor and a slew of other health benefits.

CHICKEN PAPRIKASH

PREP TIME: **5 MINUTES** ■ TOTAL TIME: **45 MINUTES**

Makes 4 servings

1 tablespoon canola oil, divided

1 pound boneless, skinless chicken thighs

1½ tablespoons paprika, divided

1 large onion, sliced lengthwise

1 clove garlic, minced

1 cup low-sodium chicken broth

1 tablespoon no-salt-added tomato paste

½ cup light sour cream

1 tablespoon white whole wheat flour

Chopped parsley for garnish (optional)

1. In a large nonstick skillet, heat 2 teaspoons of oil over medium-high heat.

2. Season the chicken with 1 teaspoon of the paprika. Cook in the skillet for 6 minutes, turning once, or until lightly golden. Transfer to a plate and set aside.

3. Heat the remaining oil in the skillet. Cook the onion and garlic, stirring often, for 6 minutes, or until softened and browned.

4. In a small bowl, whisk together the broth, tomato paste, and remaining paprika until thoroughly combined. Pour into the skillet. Reserve the bowl.

5. Add the chicken pieces back to the skillet. Reduce the heat to low to bring the mixture to a simmer. Cover and cook for 20 minutes, or until a thermometer inserted in the thickest portion registers 165°F and the juices run clear.

6. Transfer the chicken to a plate and keep warm.

7. In the reserved bowl, whisk together the sour cream and flour. Whisk the mixture into the skillet. Cook, stirring constantly, for 4 minutes, or until thickened and bubbling. Serve the chicken topped with the sauce and garnished with the parsley, if using.

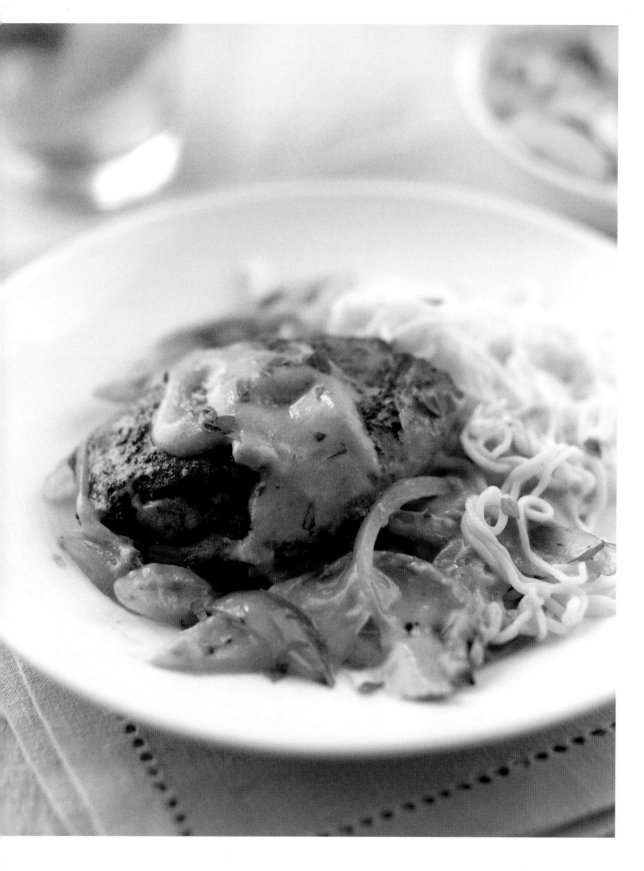

Makeover Magic

BEFORE		AFTER
340	CALORIES	199
14 g	FAT	5 g
6 g	SAT FAT	2 g
26 g	CARBS	9 g
1 g	FIBER	3 g
27 g	PROTEIN	33 g
1,350 mg	SODIUM	247 mg

Curb carbs: Instead of a thick breading, we used a thin, blood sugar–friendly coating of bran flakes, Parmesan cheese, flaxseeds, and spices!

Fill up on fiber: Bran flakes provide some fiber to this dish, but you can add more by serving it with a green salad with sunflower seeds, grated carrots, and baked sweet potato rounds (leave the skins on).

Favor fats: The ground flaxseeds serve up essential omega-3s. Using natural hard cheeses like Parmesan keeps the saturated fats down in this recipe.

PARMESAN CHICKEN FINGERS

PREP TIME: **10 MINUTES** ∎ TOTAL TIME: **25 MINUTES**

Makes 4 servings

1 pound boneless, skinless chicken breast tenderloins	⅓ cup grated Parmesan cheese
¼ teaspoon ground black pepper	2½ tablespoons ground flaxseeds
3 egg whites, lightly beaten	1 teaspoon dried basil
¾ cup bran flakes cereal, finely crushed	½ teaspoon garlic powder

1. Preheat the oven to 450°F. Lightly coat a baking sheet with cooking spray.

2. Season the chicken with the pepper.

3. Whisk the egg whites in a shallow bowl. Combine the crushed bran flakes, cheese, flaxseeds, basil, and garlic powder on a plate.

4. Dip the chicken tenderloins into the egg, shaking off any excess, and toss in the bran flake mixture. Place on the prepared baking sheet. Bake for 12 minutes, or until no longer pink and the juices run clear.

BROCCOLI-STUFFED CHICKEN ROULADE

PREP TIME: **20 MINUTES** ■ TOTAL TIME: **45 MINUTES**

Makes 6 servings

1 shallot, finely chopped

2 cloves garlic, minced, divided

¾ teaspoon crushed red-pepper flakes, divided

2 teaspoons olive oil, divided

2 tablespoons ground flaxseeds

¼ cup grated Parmesan cheese

1 package (10 ounces) frozen chopped broccoli, thawed, drained, and finely chopped

4 chicken breast cutlets (6 ounces each), pounded to ¼" thick

¾ cup low-sodium chicken broth, divided

2 teaspoons cornstarch

1. In a medium nonstick skillet over medium heat, cook the shallot, 1 clove garlic, and ¼ teaspoon pepper flakes in 1 teaspoon of the oil for 3 minutes, or until softened. In a small bowl, combine the shallot mixture, flaxseeds, Parmesan, and broccoli. Lay the chicken on a work surface, smooth side down. Divide the broccoli mixture evenly among the cutlets, spreading it down the center of each.

2. Loosely roll up the sides of the cutlets around the broccoli mixture and secure with wooden picks. Add the remaining 1 teaspoon oil to the skillet set over medium heat. Cook the chicken for 5 minutes, turning occasionally, or until golden brown on all sides. Add ⅔ cup of the broth. Cover and cook over low heat for 10 minutes, or until a thermometer inserted in the thickest portion registers 165°F and the juices run clear. Transfer to a serving platter. Cover to keep warm.

3. Bring the pan juices to a simmer. Add the remaining clove garlic.

4. In a small bowl, whisk together the remaining broth and the cornstarch until smooth. Whisk into the juices in the skillet and cook for 3 minutes, or until the mixture thickens slightly. Stir in the remaining red-pepper flakes. Remove from the heat.

5. Cut the roulades into diagonal slices. Drizzle with the sauce.

Makeover Magic

BEFORE		AFTER
480	CALORIES	204
22 g	FAT	7 g
9 g	SAT FAT	2 g
39 g	CARBS	7 g
1 g	FIBER	2 g
32 g	PROTEIN	27 g
1,190 mg	SODIUM	204 mg

Curb carbs: Instead of breaded and fried chicken, we pan-fried chicken cutlets without breading!

Fill up on fiber: We boosted the fiber in this recipe by adding extra broccoli to fill you up while keeping the overall carb count low.

Favor fats: With such a small amount of oil in this recipe, most of the fat is found in the chicken and naturally lower-saturated-fat Parmesan cheese. The ground flaxseeds provide some omega-3 fatty acids.

Makeover Magic

BEFORE		AFTER
660	CALORIES	314
34 g	FAT	8 g
15 g	SAT FAT	2 g
61 g	CARBS	8 g
1 g	FIBER	3 g
33 g	PROTEIN	55 g
690 mg	SODIUM	579 mg

Curb carbs: We decided not to use a glaze on our chicken, which often contains syrups with many carbs. Instead, we let the jalapeño and bacon speak for themselves. We also used simple grilled chicken without any breading.

Fill up on fiber: Serve this on top of romaine hearts to add not only a good crunch, but fiber too!

Favor fats: Turkey bacon is much leaner than regular bacon, and cooking with olive oil provides MUFAs.

BACON-WRAPPED CHICKEN

PREP TIME: **5 MINUTES** ■ TOTAL TIME: **20 MINUTES**

Makes 4 servings

1 pound boneless, skinless chicken breast tenderloins

1 jalapeño chile pepper, seeded and finely chopped (wear plastic gloves when handling)

8 slices turkey bacon, halved

1 tablespoon olive oil

4 romaine hearts, halved

4 tablespoons reduced-fat blue cheese crumbles

1. Coat a grill rack with cooking spray. Heat the grill over medium-high heat.

2. On a clean cutting board, lay the chicken. Top each tenderloin with a small spoonful of jalapeños. Wrap 1 slice of bacon around the length of each chicken tenderloin. Use a wooden pick to pierce and hold the bacon if needed.

3. Grill for 12 minutes, turning once, or until no longer pink and the juices run clear.

4. Brush the olive oil over the cut side of the romaine hearts. Place the romaine hearts, cut side down, on the grill, sear quickly until there are grill marks, and transfer to a serving platter. Sprinkle with the blue cheese. Serve alongside the chicken tenderloins.

LAYERED CHICKEN AND BEAN ENCHILADAS

PREP TIME: **10 MINUTES** ■ TOTAL TIME: **1 HOUR 5 MINUTES**

Makes 8 servings

1 pound boneless, skinless chicken breast halves cut into bite-size pieces

2 teaspoons olive oil

1 large onion, chopped

1 jalapeño chile pepper, seeded and finely chopped (wear plastic gloves when handling)

1 large green bell pepper, chopped

¾ cup black olives

1 can (10 ounces) + 1 cup medium red enchilada sauce

1 can (15 ounces) no-salt-added black beans, rinsed and drained

10 corn tortillas (6" diameter)

1 cup shredded Cheddar cheese, divided

½ cup light sour cream

1 large tomato, chopped

1. Preheat the oven to 350°F.

2. In a large nonstick skillet coated with cooking spray, cook the chicken over medium heat, stirring, for 5 minutes, or until a thermometer inserted in the thickest portion registers 165°F and the juices run clear. Remove from the heat and set aside.

3. In the same skillet, over medium heat warm the oil. Cook the onion and jalapeño, stirring, for 5 minutes, or until tender. Stir in the bell pepper, olives, and enchilada sauce. Add the chicken. Reduce the heat and simmer for 5 minutes. Stir in the beans.

4. In a 13" × 9" nonstick baking dish, spread half of the chicken mixture evenly. Place the tortillas on top, overlapping them to cover the entire surface. Sprinkle with ½ cup of the cheese. Top with the remaining chicken mixture.

5. Cover with foil and bake for 35 minutes, or until heated through. Uncover. Sprinkle with the remaining cheese mixture. Bake for 5 minutes, or until the cheese is melted.

6. Serve with the sour cream and tomato.

Makeover Magic

BEFORE		AFTER
651	CALORIES	286
38 g	FAT	12 g
18 g	SAT FAT	4 g
37 g	CARBS	24 g
1 g	FIBER	4 g
37 g	PROTEIN	21 g
1,392 mg	SODIUM	563 mg

Curb carbs: Using 6" corn tortillas instead of a larger size helps curb carbs—especially since we use just one tortilla layer instead of two.

Fill up on fiber: We added beans to the traditional chicken enchiladas to boost the fiber in this casserole.

Favor fats: The fat in this recipe comes from the Cheddar cheese and small amounts in the chicken, sour cream, and olive oil. Healthy fats come from the olives.

BEFORE		AFTER
374	CALORIES	292
15 g	FAT	7 g
7 g	SAT FAT	1 g
44 g	CARBS	23 g
5 g	FIBER	7 g
13 g	PROTEIN	30 g
1,117 mg	SODIUM	254 mg

Curb carbs: The majority of carbs in this dish come from the fresh veggies, a hearty substitute for the tortilla chips often used in this type of recipe.

Fill up on fiber: Pinto beans and broccoli work together to bulk up the fiber in this recipe.

Favor fats: Serve with sliced avocado for a creamy topping of healthy fats!

CHICKEN WITH PINTO BEANS SKILLET

PREP TIME: **5 MINUTES** ■ TOTAL TIME: **40 MINUTES**

Makes 4 servings

3 teaspoons canola oil, divided

1 teaspoon ground cumin, divided

1 pound boneless, skinless chicken breasts

1 package (10 ounces) frozen broccoli florets, thawed

1 red or yellow bell pepper, chopped

1 small onion, chopped

3 cloves garlic, finely chopped

1 can (15 ounces) pinto beans, rinsed and drained

1 can (14.5 ounces) no-salt-added diced tomatoes

½ cup low-sodium chicken broth

1. On a plate, combine 1 teaspoon of the oil and ½ teaspoon of the cumin. Add the chicken and rub to coat evenly.

2. In a large nonstick skillet over medium-high heat, cook the chicken for 10 minutes, turning once, or until browned and a thermometer inserted in the thickest portion registers 165°F and the juices run clear. Remove to a cutting surface. Let rest.

3. In the same skillet, heat the remaining 2 teaspoons of oil for 1 minute over medium-high heat. Add the broccoli, pepper, onion, garlic, and the remaining ½ teaspoon cumin. Cover and cook, stirring occasionally, for 5 minutes, or until the vegetables are golden. Add the beans, tomatoes, and broth. Cover and reduce the heat so the mixture simmers. Cook for 10 minutes to flavor the beans.

4. Divide the chicken and bean mixture among 4 plates.

FRIED CHICKEN

PREP TIME: **5 MINUTES** ▪ TOTAL TIME: **4 HOURS 25 MINUTES**

Makes 8 servings

1½ cups buttermilk

3 large cloves garlic, crushed

½ teaspoon ground black pepper, divided

1¼ pounds boneless, skinless chicken breasts (¾" thick)

1¼ pounds boneless, skinless chicken thighs (¾" thick)

¼ cup canola oil

1 cup white whole wheat flour

2 teaspoons paprika

½ teaspoon ground red pepper (optional)

1 tablespoon cornstarch

½ cup 1% milk

1. In a resealable plastic bag combine the buttermilk, garlic, and ¼ teaspoon of the black pepper. Add the chicken pieces and turn to coat. Seal and refrigerate for 4 to 24 hours.

2. In a large, heavy skillet, heat the oil over medium-low heat. Preheat the oven to 250°F. Cover a baking sheet with a double layer of paper towels.

3. In a large, shallow bowl, combine the flour, paprika, and red pepper, if using.

4. Remove the chicken from the marinade and dredge in the flour mixture. Place on a large platter or baking sheet. Discard the marinade.

5. When the oil is hot, add the chicken in batches if necessary and cook for 6 minutes, or until deep brown on the first side. Turn the pieces, cover the skillet loosely with foil, and cook for 5 minutes, or until the chicken is golden, the juices run clear, and a meat thermometer registers 165°F for breasts and thighs. Remove to the lined baking sheet and keep warm in the oven.

6. Using a slotted spoon, remove most of the loose browned bits from the pan. Stir the cornstarch into the oil left in the pan. Cook and stir for 1 minute. Gradually whisk in the milk and cook, stirring, for 3 minutes, or until thickened. Season with the remaining ¼ teaspoon pepper. Serve the gravy with the chicken.

Makeover Magic

BEFORE		AFTER
616	CALORIES	308
35 g	FAT	12 g
9 g	SAT FAT	2 g
24 g	CARBS	15 g
1 g	FIBER	2 g
50 g	PROTEIN	32 g
613 mg	SODIUM	162 mg

Curb carbs: We curbed the carbs by using a smaller amount of flour to bread our chicken pieces.

Fill up on fiber: For just 1 serving of fried chicken, you get 2 grams of fiber, thanks to using white whole wheat flour instead of the traditional white flour.

Favor fats: Instead of submerging the chicken in oil, we used just enough to make the chicken crispy! Canola oil adds heart-healthy MUFAs to this traditionally artery-clogging dish.

SMARTSTART

Serve with a high-fiber side to get your 22 grams of fiber daily.

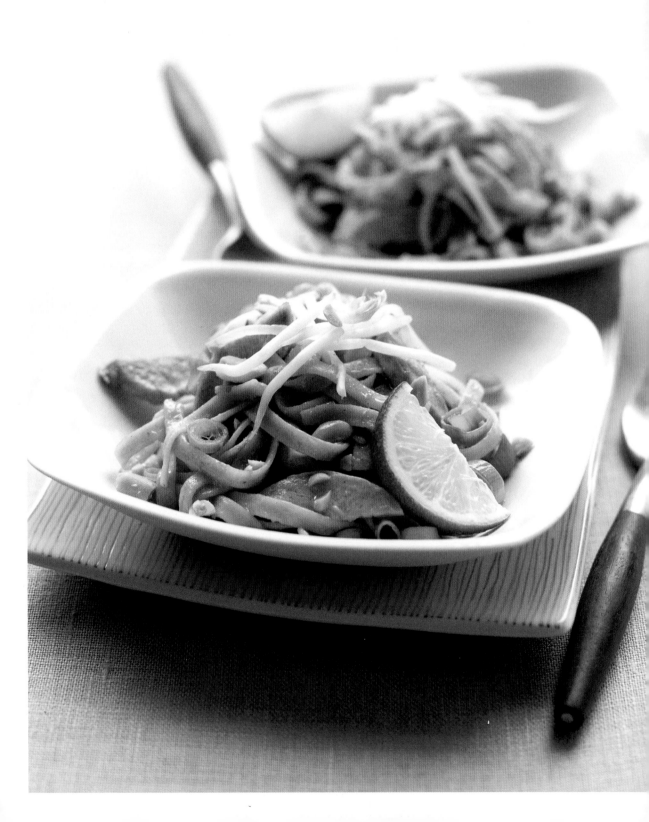

CHICKEN PAD THAI

PREP TIME: **5 MINUTES** ■ TOTAL TIME: **15 MINUTES**

Makes 4 servings

4 ounces flat brown rice noodles

2 tablespoons low-sodium soy sauce

2 tablespoons peanut butter, warmed

1 tablespoon Sriracha sauce

1 teaspoon low-sodium fish sauce

1 tablespoon peanut oil

12 ounces boneless, skinless chicken breast halves, cut into 1½" strips

2 cloves garlic, minced

3 scallions, sliced

1 cup bean sprouts

¼ cup peanuts, chopped

1 lime, quartered, for garnish

1. Prepare the noodles according to package directions.

2. In a small bowl, combine the soy sauce, peanut butter, Sriracha sauce, and fish sauce.

3. In a large nonstick skillet, heat the oil over medium-high heat.

4. Cook the chicken, stirring often, for 5 minutes, or until no longer pink and the juices run clear. Add the garlic and cook for 30 seconds. Stir in the noodles and cook for 1 minute, or until hot. Add the soy sauce mixture and cook, tossing, for 1 minute. Stir in the scallions and remove from the heat.

5. Divide among 4 plates, garnishing each with ¼ cup of the bean sprouts and sprinkling with the peanuts. Serve with the lime wedges.

Makeover Magic

BEFORE		AFTER
650	CALORIES	355
19 g	FAT	15 g
2 g	SAT FAT	3 g
83 g	CARBS	32 g
5 g	FIBER	5 g
38	PROTEIN	26 g
2,280 mg	SODIUM	560 mg

Curb carbs: With so many great toss-ins, we don't need to use such a large portion of noodles.

Fill up on fiber: Using brown rice noodles instead of white boosts the fiber, as does a generous serving of bean sprouts!

Favor fats: Peanut butter, peanut oil, and chopped peanuts are all great sources of healthy MUFAs!

BEFORE		AFTER
526	CALORIES	267
17 g	FAT	11 g
8 g	SAT FAT	4 g
51 g	CARBS	19 g
4 g	FIBER	3 g
39 g	PROTEIN	23 g
845 mg	SODIUM	246 mg

Curb carbs: We swapped out pasta and added wild rice, which has 10 grams fewer carbs than even healthy brown rice!

Fill up on fiber: Broccoli, onions, and whole grains all boost the fiber.

Favor fats: We used ground flaxseeds to boost healthy fats and reduced saturated fat by thickening our sauce with milk and sour cream instead of using a canned cream soup.

BROCCOLI-CHICKEN CASSEROLE

PREP TIME: **10 MINUTES** ■ TOTAL TIME: **1 HOUR**

Makes 6 servings

1½ cups wild rice

1 tablespoon canola oil

¾ pound boneless, skinless chicken breasts

1 package (10 ounces) frozen chopped broccoli, thawed

1 small onion, chopped

2 cloves garlic, minced

1¼ cups 1% milk, divided

¾ cup light sour cream

¾ cup reduced-fat shredded Cheddar cheese

2 tablespoons whole wheat panko bread crumbs

2 tablespoons ground flaxseeds

1. Preheat the oven to 350°F. Lightly coat an 8" × 8" baking dish with cooking spray.

2. In a saucepan, prepare the rice according to package directions. Remove from the heat and set aside.

3. In a large nonstick skillet, heat the oil over medium-high heat. Cook the chicken for 10 minutes, turning once, or until browned and a thermometer inserted in the thickest portion registers 165°F and the juices run clear. Transfer to a clean cutting board and let rest for 5 minutes. Using a fork, shred the chicken into small pieces.

4. In the same skillet, cook the broccoli, onion, and garlic for 5 minutes, or until the onion softens. Stir into the rice.

5. Add ¾ cup of the milk to the skillet and bring to a simmer over medium-low heat.

6. Whisk the remaining milk, sour cream, and cheese into the skillet and stir for 5 minutes, or until thickened. Pour the mixture into the baking dish. Add the reserved rice mixture and chicken. Stir until all ingredients are combined. In a bowl, combine the bread crumbs and flaxseeds. Sprinkle this mixture over the rice mixture. Place the baking dish in the oven and bake for 20 minutes, or until the cheese is melted and the mixture is thickened.

SWEET POTATO AND TURKEY SHEPHERD'S PIE

PREP TIME: 10 MINUTES ■ **TOTAL TIME: 50 MINUTES**

Makes 6 servings

2 sweet potatoes (8 ounces), peeled and cut into ½" pieces

1 tablespoon olive oil

1 onion, chopped

2 teaspoons dried thyme

12 ounces 99% fat-free, lean ground turkey

1 cup low-sodium chicken broth

3 tablespoons whole wheat flour

3 carrots, chopped

1 cup frozen peas, thawed

1 cup frozen corn, thawed

1 cup frozen cut green beans, thawed

¼ cup dried cranberries

1. Preheat the oven to 350°F. Coat an 8" × 8" baking dish with cooking spray.

2. Fill a large saucepan halfway with water and bring to a boil over high heat. Cook the sweet potatoes for 15 minutes, or until tender. Remove from the heat. Drain. Place the potatoes back in the saucepan and drizzle with the oil. Using a potato masher, mash the potatoes until smooth. Set aside.

3. Coat a nonstick skillet with cooking spray and heat over medium-high heat. Cook the onion and thyme, stirring occasionally, for 4 minutes, or until starting to soften. Add the turkey and cook for 5 minutes or until no longer pink.

4. Combine the broth and flour and pour into the skillet. Bring the mixture to a boil, stirring constantly. Reduce the heat to medium low and simmer for 5 minutes, or until thickened. Stir in the carrots, peas, corn, beans, and cranberries. Pour the filling into the baking dish.

5. Spread the mashed sweet potatoes over the top of the mixture. Bake for 20 minutes, or until the top is browned and the filling is hot and bubbly.

Makeover Magic

BEFORE		AFTER
460	CALORIES	228
23 g	FAT	6 g
10 g	SAT FAT	2 g
37 g	CARBS	29 g
2 g	FIBER	5 g
25 g	PROTEIN	15 g
980 mg	SODIUM	119 mg

Curb carbs: We turned a bread-based casserole into one filled with meat and vegetables with a sweet potato "crust."

Fill up on fiber: The veggies, dried fruit, and whole wheat flour help this nostalgic recipe to not only feel like Thanksgiving, but also give you a 5-gram dose of fiber.

Favor fats: Olive oil adds MUFAs to this dinner.

BEFORE		AFTER
440	CALORIES	235
15 g	FAT	10 g
2 g	SAT FAT	1 g
38 g	CARBS	9 g
2 g	FIBER	3 g
37 g	PROTEIN	31 g
710 mg	SODIUM	87 mg

Curb carbs: Instead of using a ready-made stuffing mix, we created our own with apples, onions, and pecans—no bread needed!

Fill up on fiber: Leave the skins on the apples for added fiber.

Favor fats: Ground flaxseeds provide omega-3s, and pecans are a delicious source of MUFAs.

STUFFED TURKEY TENDERLOIN

PREP TIME: **10 MINUTES** ■ TOTAL TIME: **40 MINUTES**

Makes 4 servings

1 tablespoon canola oil, divided

½ small onion, finely chopped

1 Granny Smith apple, cored and chopped

3 tablespoons finely chopped pecans

2 tablespoons ground flaxseeds

2 cloves garlic, minced

1 pound turkey breast tenderloins (2 tenderloins)

1 cup low-sodium chicken broth

2 tablespoons plain 0% Greek yogurt

2 teaspoons finely chopped fresh thyme or ⅔ teaspoon dried

1. In a large nonstick skillet, heat ½ tablespoon of the oil over medium heat. Cook the onion for 5 minutes, or until softened. Add the apple, pecans, flaxseeds, and garlic and cook for 2 minutes, or until the garlic is fragrant and the apples are slightly softened. Transfer the mixture to a bowl.

2. On a clean cutting board, pat the tenderloins dry with a paper towel. Cut a slit, or a pocket, in the tenderloins lengthwise across the side of the tenderloin three-quarters of the way through, to make a deep enough pocket.

3. Stuff each pocket with the reserved mixture.

4. In the same skillet, heat the remaining oil over medium heat. Cook the turkey for 4 minutes, turning once, until browned. Add the broth. Cover, reduce the heat, and simmer for 15 minutes, or until a thermometer inserted in the thickest portion registers 165°F and the juices run clear.

5. Transfer the turkey to a plate and keep warm. Increase the heat and cook the broth for 3 minutes, or until reduced by half. Whisk in the yogurt and thyme.

TURKEY MEAT LOAF WITH CRANBERRY CHUTNEY

PREP TIME: **10 MINUTES** ■ TOTAL TIME: **1 HOUR 35 MINUTES**

Makes 8 servings

½ tablespoon olive oil

1 shallot, finely chopped

2 cups cranberries

½ cup quinoa

1 cup water

1 tablespoon olive oil

1 onion, chopped

2 cloves garlic, minced

3 pounds 99% fat-free, lean ground turkey

¼ cup ketchup

2 egg whites, lightly beaten

2 tablespoons ground flaxseeds

1. Preheat the oven to 350°F.

2. In a saucepan, heat the oil over medium-high heat. Cook the shallot for 5 minutes. Add the cranberries and cook for 10 minutes.

3. Meanwhile, in a saucepan, bring the quinoa and water to a boil. Reduce the heat to low, cover, and cook for 15 minutes. Remove from the heat, transfer to a bowl, and set aside.

4. In a skillet, heat the oil over medium heat. Cook the onion and garlic for 5 minutes, or until lightly browned. Transfer to a bowl.

5. Add the turkey, prepared quinoa, ketchup, egg whites, and flaxseeds to the bowl with the onion mixture. Stir to combine.

6. Transfer the meat loaf into a baking dish and loosely form into a rectangular log. Cover with half of the chutney. Bake the meat loaf for 60 minutes, or until a thermometer inserted in the center registers 165°F and the meat is no longer pink. Serve the meat loaf with the remaining chutney.

Makeover Magic

BEFORE		AFTER
515	CALORIES	288
26 g	FAT	6 g
10 g	SAT FAT	0.5 g
29 g	CARBS	16 g
1 g	FIBER	3 g
39 g	PROTEIN	46 g
948 mg	SODIUM	198 mg

Curb carbs: Many meat loaves are high in carbohydrates because of the thick sauces in and on top of them. We went with a basic meat loaf base with the addition of quinoa to add texture and healthy carbs.

Fill up on fiber: The cranberries and quinoa give this meat loaf a kick of fiber!

Favor fats: Instead of the traditional, and more fatty, ground beef, we used lean ground turkey with only a small amount of fat. The olive oil and flaxseeds provide the healthy fats!

Makeover Magic

Curb carbs: We used an average-size whole wheat hamburger bun instead of an oversize white bun, which helped us to maintain proper portion sizes.

Fill up on fiber: A whole wheat bun loaded with mushrooms, pepper, and onion—we made sure you got a good amount of fiber from this burger!

Favor fats: Add a thin slice of avocado for a creamy burger topping that's full of MUFAs. Or pair with a salad drizzled in olive oil.

TURKEY CHEESEBURGERS

PREP TIME: **5 MINUTES** ■ TOTAL TIME: **20 MINUTES**

Makes 4 servings

1 pound 99% fat-free, lean ground turkey

2 egg whites

1½ tablespoons reduced-sodium Worcestershire sauce

8 ounces mushrooms, trimmed and sliced

2 teaspoons olive oil

4 slices onion (¼" thick)

1 green bell pepper, sliced

4 whole wheat hamburger buns

2 ounces reduced-fat Cheddar cheese

4 tablespoons barbecue sauce

1. In a large bowl, combine the turkey, egg whites, and Worcestershire sauce. Gently form into 4 burgers, pressing down to create a shallow well in the center of each.

2. Coat a grill rack with cooking spray. Preheat the grill for medium heat. Toss the mushrooms with the oil and cook in a grill basket (or cast-iron skillet) for 6 minutes, stirring, until golden brown. Remove from the heat and keep warm.

3. Coat the onion and bell pepper with olive oil spray. Grill the onion, turning, for 4 minutes, or until tender. Grill the buns cut side down for 2 minutes, or until marked. Grill the burgers for 8 minutes, turning once, or until a thermometer inserted in the center registers 165°F and the meat is no longer pink. Top with cheese and grill, covered, for 30 seconds, or until melted.

4. Serve the burgers on buns and top with the onion, pepper, mushrooms, and barbecue sauce.

TURKEY AND ORZO STUFFED PEPPERS

PREP TIME: **5 MINUTES** ■ TOTAL TIME: **40 MINUTES**

Makes 4 servings

⅓ cup whole wheat orzo

4 quarts water

4 large red bell peppers

2 teaspoons canola oil

1 pound 99% fat-free, lean ground turkey

1 small onion, chopped

2 cloves garlic, minced

1 tablespoon finely chopped fresh thyme

1 pound baby kale

½ cup frozen peas, thawed

1 can (14.5 ounces) no-salt-added tomato sauce

1. Preheat the oven to 350°F. Prepare the orzo according to package directions.

2. In a large pot, bring the water to a boil over high heat. Cut off and discard the stems of the 4 large bell peppers. Seed the peppers, being careful not to puncture them. Cook the whole peppers in the boiling water for 2 minutes, or until slightly softened. Drain the peppers on paper towels. In an 8" × 8" baking dish, stand the peppers upright. Set aside.

3. In a large nonstick skillet, heat the oil over medium-high heat until hot but not smoking. Cook the turkey, stirring, for 3 minutes, breaking up any clumps with a spoon. Add the onion, garlic, and thyme. Cook for 3 minutes, or until the onions are softened. Add the kale and peas. Cover and cook for 3 minutes, or until the kale is wilted. Remove the pan from the heat.

4. Add the reserved orzo to the kale mixture and stir to combine. Spoon the mixture into the bell peppers. Pour the tomato sauce into the baking dish in and around the peppers. Bake for 15 minutes, or until the peppers and filling are hot.

Makeover Magic

BEFORE		AFTER
560	CALORIES	353
28 g	FAT	6 g
14 g	SAT FAT	0.5 g
42 g	CARBS	40 g
6 g	FIBER	11 g
34 g	PROTEIN	37 g
990 mg	SODIUM	215 mg

Curb carbs: This dish's carbs come primarily from the vegetables and orzo. But our makeover dish is so high in fiber that the magic carbs come out to just 29 grams!

Fill up on fiber: Kale and whole wheat orzo are great sources of fiber that set this recipe apart from more traditional stuffed peppers.

Favor fats: Add olives and pine nuts for flavor and some favored fats.

BEFORE		AFTER
520	CALORIES	307
28 g	FAT	11 g
12 g	SAT FAT	4 g
41 g	CARBS	31 g
4 g	FIBER	17 g
27 g	PROTEIN	34 g
1,210 mg	SODIUM	445 mg

Curb carbs: Use a sprouted grain wrap when trying to find ways to decrease carbs and increase fiber. Ezekiel brand has a delicious sprouted wrap.

Fill up on fiber: The sprouted grain wrap, vegetables, and beans we added set this quesadilla apart from the rest because it is a superstar in fiber! This recipe has a whopping 17 grams of fiber, which you can subtract from the total carbs to count this dish as just 14 grams of carbs.

Favor fats: Using 50% reduced-fat cheese allowed us to make these quesadillas very cheesy, with only 5 grams of fat from the cheese. The avocado is the heart-healthy fat of choice in this recipe.

TURKEY AND BEAN QUESADILLAS

PREP TIME: **5 MINUTES** ■ TOTAL TIME: **30 MINUTES**

Makes 8 servings

1 pound turkey breast cutlets

1 teaspoon canola oil

1 green bell pepper, finely chopped

1 small onion, finely chopped

½ cup frozen corn kernels, thawed

1 jalapeño chile pepper, seeded and finely chopped (wear plastic gloves when handling)

1 can (15 ounces) black beans, rinsed and drained

16 sprouted whole wheat tortillas (7" diameter)

8 ounces 50% reduced-fat Cheddar cheese, shredded

1 cup salsa

½ avocado, pitted and chopped

1. Coat a grill rack with cooking spray. Preheat the grill to medium.

2. On the grill, cook the turkey cutlets for 10 minutes, turning once, or until no longer pink. Transfer to a cutting board and use a fork to shred the meat.

3. In a nonstick skillet, heat the oil over medium-high heat. Cook the bell pepper and onion for 5 minutes, or until tender. Add the corn, jalapeño, black beans, and turkey and cook for 5 minutes, or until heated through. Remove from the heat.

4. On a clean work surface, lay out 8 tortillas. Sprinkle half of the cheese on the 8 tortillas and top them with the vegetable mixture. Sprinkle the remaining cheese on top of the vegetable mixture and top with the remaining tortillas.

5. Place the tortillas on the grill, working in batches if necessary, and cook for 6 minutes, turning once, or until the cheese is melted and the tortillas are golden brown. Adjust the heat if necessary to prevent burning. Transfer the quesadillas to serving plates. Top with salsa and avocado.

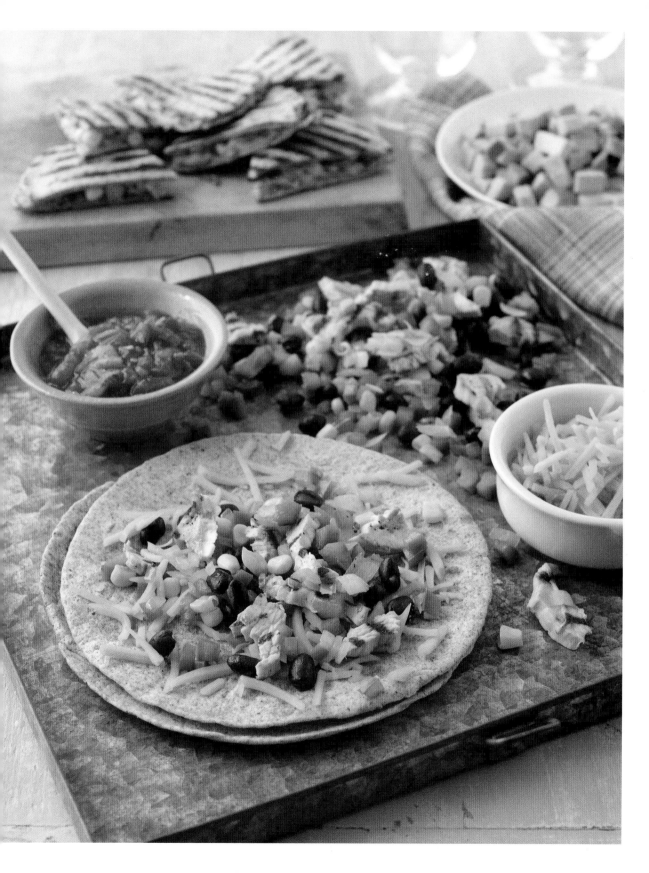

Makeover Magic

BEFORE		AFTER
510	CALORIES	298
22 g	FAT	9 g
9 g	SAT FAT	1 g
42 g	CARBS	21 g
5 g	FIBER	7 g
38 g	PROTEIN	36 g
1,552 mg	SODIUM	467 mg

Curb carbs: We replaced traditional linguine with succulent strands of zucchini for a dramatic cut in carbs.

Fill up on fiber: Zucchini is the main source of fiber in this recipe.

Favor fats: Flaxseeds create a great foundation of healthy fats. Add olives and pine nuts for flavor and even more good fats.

TURKEY MEATBALLS AND ZUCCHINI PASTA

PREP TIME: **5 MINUTES** ■ TOTAL TIME: **35 MINUTES**

Makes 4 servings

1 pound 99% fat-free, lean ground turkey

3 cloves garlic, minced, divided

1 egg white

¼ cup ground flaxseeds

1 tablespoon canola oil

1 onion, chopped

2 teaspoons Italian seasoning

1 can (28 ounces) whole peeled tomatoes, chopped, juice reserved

1 tablespoon no-salt-added tomato paste

3 large zucchini, cut into matchsticks

1. Preheat the oven to 400°F. Coat a baking sheet with cooking spray.

2. In a bowl, combine the turkey, 1 clove of the garlic, the egg white, and the ground flaxseeds. With slightly damp hands, form the mixture into sixteen 1½" balls and set them 1" apart on the prepared baking sheet. Bake, turning once, for 25 minutes, or until a thermometer inserted in the center registers 165°F and the meat is no longer pink.

3. In a large saucepan, heat the oil over medium-high heat. Cook the remaining 2 cloves of garlic, onion, and Italian seasoning, stirring occasionally, for 3 minutes, or until the onion begins to soften. Stir in the tomatoes and their juice, and the tomato paste. Bring to a boil. Reduce the heat to medium low and simmer, partially covered, for 15 minutes, or until the sauce starts to thicken. Stir in the meatballs and simmer for 5 minutes, or until the sauce has thickened and the meatballs are hot.

4. Place the zucchini in a large microwave-safe bowl and cook in the microwave oven on high for 1 minute, or until slightly softened.

5. Divide the zucchini among 4 shallow bowls and top each with 4 meatballs and sauce.

BAKED SPAGHETTI WITH TURKEY MEAT SAUCE

PREP TIME: **5 MINUTES** ■ TOTAL TIME: **1 HOUR 15 MINUTES**

Makes 8 servings

8 ounces whole wheat spaghetti, broken into 2" pieces

⅓ cup grated Parmesan cheese

2 egg whites

1 tablespoon canola oil

1 pound 99% fat-free, lean ground turkey

2 cups low-sodium, olive oil–based pasta sauce

½ teaspoon dried oregano

1 clove garlic, minced

1 cup 2% cottage cheese

4 ounces part-skim mozzarella cheese, shredded

1. Prepare the spaghetti according to package directions. Drain. Preheat the oven to 350°F.

2. Place the spaghetti in a 13" × 9" baking dish. Stir in the Parmesan cheese and egg whites until thoroughly combined. Spread the mixture evenly in the pan.

3. In a large skillet, heat the oil over medium-high heat. Cook the turkey for 5 minutes, or until the meat is brown. Drain. Stir in the pasta sauce, oregano, and garlic.

4. Spread the cottage cheese over the spaghetti layer and top with the meat mixture.

5. Bake for 30 minutes. Sprinkle the mozzarella cheese over the top and bake an additional 10 minutes, or until the cheese is melted and just begins to brown. Let stand for 15 minutes before cutting.

Makeover Magic

BEFORE		AFTER
434	CALORIES	312
17 g	FAT	9 g
8 g	SAT FAT	4 g
43 g	CARBS	32 g
3 g	FIBER	5 g
26 g	PROTEIN	28 g
732 mg	SODIUM	330 mg

Curb carbs: Our dish uses whole wheat spaghetti instead of regular pasta—and less of it than a traditional baked spaghetti.

Fill up on fiber: The pasta is a great sources of fiber. Pair this dish with a side salad to boost the fiber even more!

Favor fats: We swapped out ground beef and went with 99% lean ground turkey, which is less fatty but just as tasty. Top with olives for added healthy fats.

Makeover Magic

BEFORE		AFTER
630	CALORIES	407
30 g	FAT	11 g
15 g	SAT FAT	4 g
45 g	CARBS	43 g
3 g	FIBER	7 g
45 g	PROTEIN	34 g
878 mg	SODIUM	573 mg

Curb carbs: The carbohydrates in our recipe are similar to our comparison, but by upping the fiber, we're able to use magic carbs to bring the recipe down to 36 grams.

Fill up on fiber: Kale and our whole wheat penne raise the fiber!

Favor fats: For a dose of healthy fats, add a side salad drizzled with olive oil, canola oil, or even flaxseed oil.

BAKED ZITI WITH TURKEY

PREP TIME: **10 MINUTES** ▨ TOTAL TIME: **55 MINUTES**

Makes 4 servings

1½ cups (5 ounces) whole wheat penne pasta

6 ounces lean Italian-style turkey sausage (sweet or mild), cut into 4" pieces

8 ounces 99% fat-free, lean ground turkey

1 large green bell pepper, chopped

1 small onion, chopped

4 ounces button mushrooms, chopped

3 cloves garlic, minced

2 teaspoons Italian seasoning

2 cups low-sodium pasta sauce

½ pound baby kale

¾ cup (3 ounces) shredded part-skim mozzarella cheese

1. Preheat the oven to 375°F. Coat a shallow 3-quart baking dish with cooking spray and set aside.

2. Cook the pasta according to package directions. Drain and set aside.

3. Heat a large nonstick skillet over medium heat. Cook the sausage and ground turkey for 10 minutes, or until browned and no longer pink inside. Transfer the sausage to a clean plate and allow to cool while preparing the rest of the sauce.

4. In the same skillet, cook the bell pepper, onion, mushrooms, garlic, and Italian seasoning, stirring occasionally, for 7 minutes, or until the onion is almost soft. Stir in the pasta sauce and kale.

5. Cut the sausage into ¼" slices and place in the prepared baking dish along with the sauce and pasta. Toss to combine. Sprinkle with the cheese. Bake for 25 minutes, or until heated through and the cheese is melted and slightly browned.

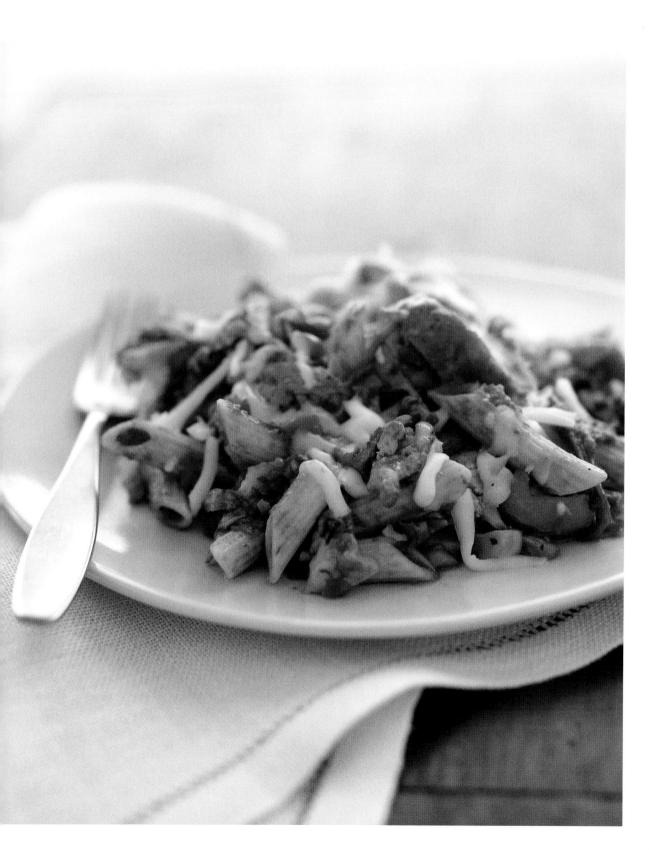

BEFORE		AFTER
710	CALORIES	260
42 g	FAT	11 g
20 g	SAT FAT	3 g
45 g	CARBS	8 g
2 g	FIBER	3 g
35 g	PROTEIN	34 g
1,580 mg	SODIUM	147 mg

Curb carbs: Instead of using bread crumbs, we opted for ground flaxseeds, which dramatically cut the carbohydrates.

Fill up on fiber: This dish is typically low fiber, so be sure to serve it along with a whole grain or other fiber superstar.

Favor fats: We love lean ground turkey because it really cuts the saturated fat compared to most Swedish meatball recipes. Serve with toasted almonds and pine nuts over a spinach salad for a delicious serving of healthy fats.

TURKEY SWEDISH MEATBALLS

PREP TIME: **5 MINUTES** ■ TOTAL TIME: **25 MINUTES**

Makes 4 servings

1 pound 99% fat-free, lean ground turkey

1 small onion, finely chopped

1 large egg

¼ cup ground flaxseeds

¼ teaspoon ground allspice

¾ cup low-sodium chicken broth

2 teaspoons cornstarch

2 teaspoons Worcestershire sauce

2 teaspoons canola oil

½ cup light sour cream

1. In a large bowl, combine the turkey, onion, egg, flaxseeds, and allspice. Mix until well combined and form into 24 (1") meatballs.

2. In a small bowl, combine the broth, cornstarch, and Worcestershire sauce and set aside.

3. In a large nonstick skillet, heat the oil over medium heat. Cook the meatballs for 14 minutes, turning occasionally, until browned and cooked through. Transfer the meatballs to paper towels to drain.

4. Increase the heat to medium high and add the broth mixture to the skillet. Bring to a boil, shaking the pan often, and cook for 2 minutes to thicken. Remove from the heat and stir in the sour cream until well blended.

5. Return the meatballs to the pan and gently turn to coat with the sauce.

SLOPPY JOES

PREP TIME: **10 MINUTES** ■ TOTAL TIME: **25 MINUTES**

Makes 4 servings

1 onion, chopped

1 green bell pepper, chopped

1 rib celery, chopped

2 cloves garlic, chopped

1 pound 99% fat-free, lean ground turkey

1½ cups no-salt-added crushed tomatoes

2 tablespoons maple syrup

1 tablespoon cider vinegar

2 teaspoons Worcestershire sauce

4 whole wheat sandwich buns

1. Heat a large nonstick skillet coated with cooking spray to medium. Cook the onion, bell pepper, celery, and garlic for 7 minutes, or until soft.

2. Add the turkey. Cook for 5 minutes, breaking the meat up with a spoon, or until no longer pink. Add the crushed tomatoes, maple syrup, vinegar, and Worcestershire sauce. Cook, stirring occasionally, for 5 minutes, or until hot and bubbly. Spoon into the buns.

Makeover Magic

BEFORE		AFTER
439	CALORIES	315
16 g	FAT	4 g
6 g	SAT FAT	0.5 g
46 g	CARBS	40 g
2 g	FIBER	6 g
27 g	PROTEIN	34 g
1,360 mg	SODIUM	324 mg

Curb carbs: We chose a whole wheat bun over the average white bun. Instead of fries, serve with a nonstarchy side like asparagus to keep carbs curbed.

Fill up on fiber: We added pepper, onion, and celery to give this classic sandwich an extra kick of fiber!

Favor fats: Serve this classic dish with grilled asparagus coated in olive oil and slivered almonds for favored fats.

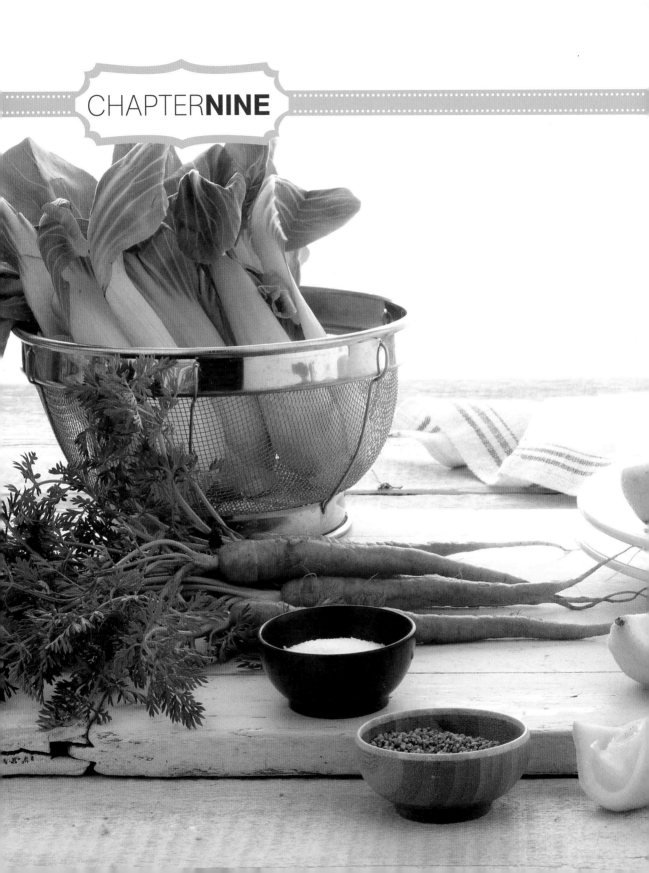

CHAPTER**NINE**

Seafood

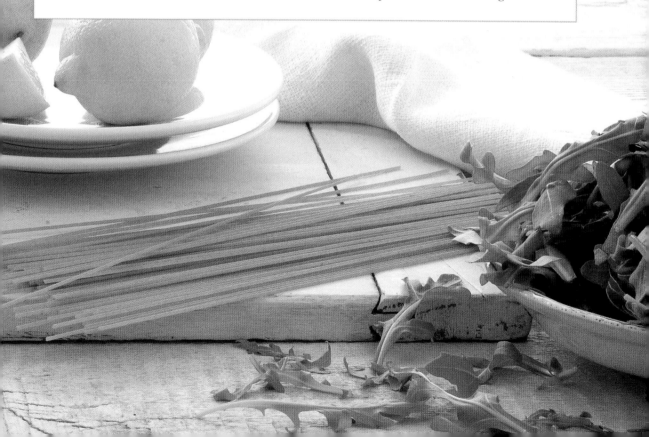

Makeover Magic

BEFORE		AFTER
1,041	CALORIES	347
55 g	FAT	6 g
8 g	SAT FAT	1 g
82 g	CARBS	43 g
10 g	FIBER	8 g
56 g	PROTEIN	33 g
2,562 mg	SODIUM	405 mg

Curb carbs: Most po' boys are breaded and fried, adding carbs, fat, and calories. This seasoned version is a fresh, flavorful take on the comfort food favorite.

Fill up on fiber: Adding coleslaw to this dish boosts the fiber while adding tanginess.

Favor fats: Baking the fish instead of frying it greatly reduces the trans fats. Cod is a great source of the omega-3 fatty acids EPA and DHA.

FISH PO' BOY WITH CAJUN SLAW

PREP TIME: **20 MINUTES** ■ TOTAL TIME: **35 MINUTES**

Makes 4 servings

3 tablespoons plain 0% Greek yogurt

2 tablespoons olive oil mayonnaise

2 tablespoons agave nectar or honey

1 tablespoon cider vinegar

¼ teaspoon hot-pepper sauce (optional)

1 bag (14 ounces) preshredded coleslaw mix

1 red bell pepper, cut into 1" strips, each halved

½ small onion, grated

2 teaspoons blackening seasoning

4 thick cod fillets (5 ounces each)

1 cup mixed greens

1 large tomato, thinly sliced

1 whole wheat baguette (12 ounces), sliced lengthwise in half and cut crosswise into 4 pieces

1. Preheat the oven to 350°F. Coat a baking sheet with cooking spray.

2. In a large bowl, whisk together the yogurt, mayonnaise, nectar or honey, vinegar, and hot-pepper sauce (if using). Add the coleslaw mix, bell pepper, and onion. Toss to coat well. Chill until ready to serve.

3. Rub the seasoning over the fish. Place the fish on the baking sheet and bake, turning once, for 15 minutes, or until the fish flakes easily.

4. Divide the greens and tomato on the baguettes. Top each with a fish fillet, folding the fish to fit, if necessary. Serve with the coleslaw.

FISH AND CHIPS

PREP TIME: **20 MINUTES** ▥ TOTAL TIME: **1 HOUR**

Makes 4 servings

2 medium sweet potatoes, peeled and cut into large wedges

1 tablespoon canola oil

1 teaspoon salt, divided

1 teaspoon ground black pepper, divided

2 egg whites

1 tablespoon Dijon mustard

1 cup whole wheat panko bread crumbs

½ teaspoon dried thyme

4 wild halibut fillets (6 ounces each), skinned

Malt vinegar

1. Preheat the oven to 425°F. On a large baking sheet, place the potatoes and drizzle with the oil and ½ teaspoon each of the salt and pepper. Toss to coat. Bake for 30 minutes.

2. Meanwhile, in a shallow bowl, whisk together the egg whites, mustard, and the remaining ½ teaspoon each of salt and pepper. In another shallow bowl, combine the bread crumbs and thyme. Dip the fish into the egg whites and then into the crumbs.

3. After the fries have baked for 15 minutes, add the fish to the same baking sheet and return to the oven. Bake for 15 minutes, or until the fish flakes easily. Serve with the vinegar.

Makeover Magic

BEFORE		AFTER
579	CALORIES	350
33 g	FAT	8 g
4 g	SAT FAT	1 g
53 g	CARBS	26 g
3 g	FIBER	4 g
14 g	PROTEIN	41 g
759 mg	SODIUM	413 mg

Curb carbs: Each serving of "chips" equals just half a potato, a plentiful amount alongside the fish fillets.

Fill up on fiber: Both the panko breading and the sweet potatoes contribute fiber to this pub favorite.

Favor fats: Halibut is full of marine omega-3s. By baking the fillets, we avoid frying in saturated fats.

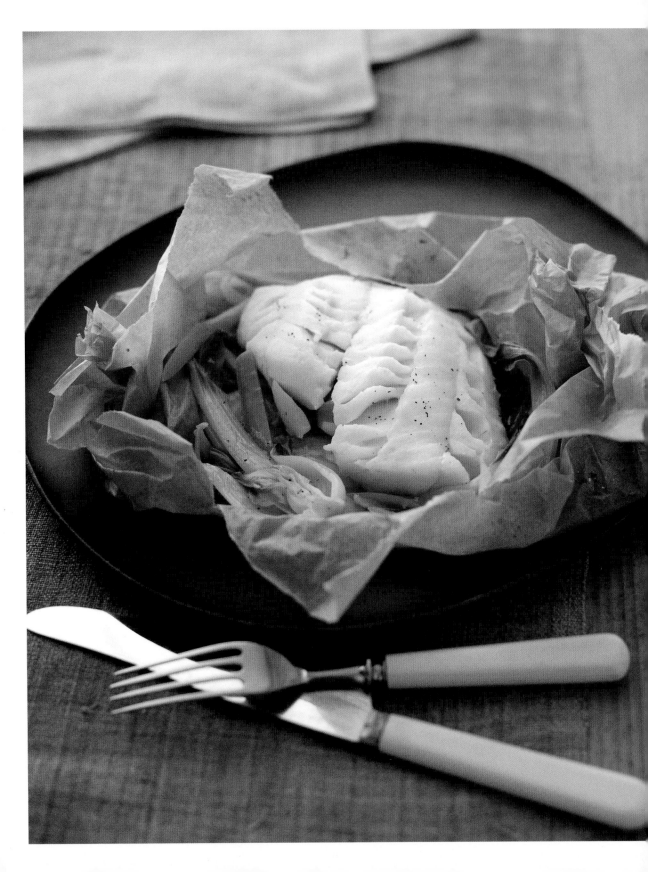

ASIAN FISH PACKETS

PREP TIME: **15 MINUTES** ■ TOTAL TIME: **25 MINUTES**

Makes 4 servings

4 baby bok choy

2 carrots, cut into matchsticks

1 onion, cut into thin wedges

4 wild halibut fillets (6 ounces each)

2 teaspoons low-sodium soy sauce, divided

1 teaspoon rice wine vinegar, divided

2 teaspoons freshly grated ginger, divided

1. Preheat the oven to 450°F. Coat one side of four 20" × 12" sheets of parchment with cooking spray.

2. Divide the bok choy, carrots, and onion among the packets. Drizzle each with ½ teaspoon soy sauce, ¼ teaspoon vinegar, and ½ teaspoon ginger. Add the fillets.

3. Fold the other half of each sheet over the filling and fold the edges to make a tight seal.

4. Arrange the packets on a large baking sheet. Bake for 10 minutes, or until the packets are puffed. Transfer each packet to a serving plate. Carefully slit the top of each to allow the steam to escape. After a minute, peel back the paper. Check to make sure the fish flakes easily.

Makeover Magic

BEFORE		AFTER
830	CALORIES	233
60 g	FAT	4 g
9 g	SAT FAT	0.5 g
16 g	CARBS	10 g
5 g	FIBER	4 g
58 g	PROTEIN	39 g
810 mg	SODIUM	280 mg

Curb carbs: Instead of a sweet, sugary sauce, these fish packets are flavored with fresh ginger and a touch of rice wine vinegar.

Fill up on fiber: Bok choy offers not just fiber, but also a lovely, sweet flavor.

Favor fats: Halibut is our source of EPA and DHA omega-3 fatty acids.

Makeover Magic

BEFORE		AFTER
764	CALORIES	426
42 g	FAT	18 g
7 g	SAT FAT	3 g
46 g	CARBS	40 g
4 g	FIBER	5 g
47 g	PROTEIN	29 g
1,369 mg	SODIUM	115 mg

Curb carbs: Nothing says southern comfort like catfish! This dish is typically fried and dredged in flour and cornmeal, adding unnecessary carbs. Our version cuts straight to the cornmeal, using smaller amounts of the blood sugar–busting ingredients overall.

Fill up on fiber: Topping the fish with corn and black beans adds classic flavor—and lots of fiber.

Favor fats: Catfish contains our heart-healthy omega-3 fatty acids. Plus, using our simple skillet sauté method takes saturated fats from deep-frying out of the equation.

CORNMEAL CATFISH WITH BLACK-EYED PEAS

PREP TIME: **15 MINUTES** ■ TOTAL TIME: **30 MINUTES**

Makes 4 servings

4 teaspoons canola oil, divided

1 cup fresh or frozen and thawed corn kernels

1 clove garlic, minced

½ teaspoon dried thyme

1 can (15 ounces) black-eyed peas, rinsed and drained

1 roasted red pepper, patted dry and chopped

1 cup yellow cornmeal

¼ teaspoon salt

4 catfish fillets (6 ounces each)

1. In a medium saucepan, heat 1 teaspoon of the oil over medium-high heat. Cook the corn kernels, garlic, and thyme for 5 minutes, stirring occasionally, until lightly browned. Add the peas and red pepper and cook for 1 minute, or until heated through. Keep warm.

2. On a large plate, combine the cornmeal and salt. Dredge the fillets in the cornmeal, pressing to adhere.

3. In a large nonstick skillet, heat the remaining 3 teaspoons of oil over medium heat. Cook the catfish for 8 minutes, turning once, or until golden and the fish flakes easily. Serve the fish topped with the black-eyed pea mixture.

TROUT PAELLA

PREP TIME: 15 MINUTES ■ **TOTAL TIME: 35 MINUTES**

Makes 4 servings

1   teaspoon canola oil

1   small onion, chopped

1   red bell pepper, chopped

3   cloves garlic, finely chopped

1   teaspoon paprika

½   teaspoon ground turmeric

¼   teaspoon dried thyme

1   cup no-salt-added canned chickpeas, rinsed and drained

2   cups fat-free, reduced-sodium chicken broth

½   cup quinoa, rinsed well

3   cups chopped kale or collards

1   pound wild rainbow trout, cut into 2" chunks

1. In a large saucepot, heat the oil over medium-high heat. Cook the onion, bell pepper, garlic, paprika, turmeric, and thyme, stirring occasionally, for 5 minutes, or until lightly browned. Stir in the chickpeas, broth, and quinoa. Cover and simmer for 10 minutes, or until most of the broth is absorbed.

2. Stir in the kale or collards. Cook for 1 minute, or until partially wilted. Stir in the trout. Cover and simmer for 5 minutes, or until the trout flakes easily.

Makeover Magic

BEFORE		AFTER
540	CALORIES	350
23 g	FAT	8 g
9 g	SAT FAT	1 g
56 g	CARBS	36 g
2 g	FIBER	10 g
28 g	PROTEIN	33 g
1,420 mg	SODIUM	304 mg

Curb carbs: We use ½ cup of quinoa in this dish instead of a cup or more of white rice.

Fill up on fiber: Quinoa and kale both pack fiber—enough to use the magic carbs effect!

Favor fats: Trout is an under-appreciated fish when it comes to dining, but just as great a source of healthy fats as the more common salmon and tuna.

Makeover Magic

BEFORE		AFTER
650	CALORIES	371
31 g	FAT	12 g
17 g	SAT FAT	2 g
46 g	CARBS	42 g
2 g	FIBER	12 g
43 g	PROTEIN	26 g
440 mg	SODIUM	500 mg

Curb carbs: Going with a moderate amount of whole grain pasta (6 ounces in this case) is an easy way to curb carbs.

Fill up on fiber: While whole grain pasta is naturally higher in fiber, the real stars of this recipe are the spinach and artichokes, which add a whopping 5 grams!

Favor fats: Typically a dish like this is laden with heavy cream and butter. Here, we substituted MUFA-rich canola oil mayonnaise and replaced the high-carb bread crumbs with golden flaxseeds to keep the crunch but add more MUFAs and ALA omega-3s. Plus, salmon is naturally plentiful in the EPA and DHA forms of omega-3s, which you should aim to get into your diet through marine sources twice per week.

SALMON PASTA CASSEROLE

PREP TIME: **10 MINUTES** ■ TOTAL TIME: **50 MINUTES**

Makes 4 servings

6 ounces whole grain farfalle pasta (bow ties)

2 pouches (5 ounces each) wild pink salmon, drained

1 package (10 ounces) frozen artichoke hearts, thawed and chopped

1 package (10 ounces) frozen chopped spinach, thawed and drained

¼ cup canola oil mayonnaise

¼ cup grated Parmesan cheese, divided

1 tablespoon lemon juice

¼ cup ground golden flaxseeds

1. Preheat the oven to 350°F. Coat an 8" × 8" baking dish with cooking spray.

2. Prepare the pasta according to package directions. Drain and set aside.

3. Meanwhile, in a large bowl, combine the salmon, artichokes, spinach, mayonnaise, 2 tablespoons of the cheese, and the lemon juice. Toss gently until blended. Stir in the pasta and spread in the baking dish. Top with the flaxseeds and remaining 2 tablespoons cheese.

4. Bake for 30 minutes, or until heated through.

SMARTSTART

You can add a lower-carb dessert or a cup of berries to this dinner dish if you are craving sweets.

SALMON WITH AVOCADO SALSA

PREP TIME: **15 MINUTES** ■ TOTAL TIME: **30 MINUTES + STANDING TIME**

Makes 4 servings

1 avocado, pared, pitted, and chopped

1 red bell pepper, chopped

1 small red onion, chopped

3 tablespoons freshly squeezed lime juice

¼ cup chopped fresh cilantro

1 clove garlic, minced

¼ teaspoon salt

1 tablespoon canola oil

2 wild salmon fillets (6 ounces each)

1. In a small bowl, combine the avocado, pepper, onion, lime juice, cilantro, garlic, and salt. Cover and let stand for at least 30 minutes to blend the flavors.

2. In a large nonstick skillet, heat the oil over medium-high heat. Sear the fillets for 10 minutes, turning once, or until opaque. Divide the salmon among 4 plates. Serve with the salsa.

Makeover Magic

BEFORE		AFTER
830	CALORIES	375
45 g	FAT	22 g
10 g	SAT FAT	3 g
61 g	CARBS	10 g
7 g	FIBER	4 g
44 g	PROTEIN	35 g
1,920 mg	SODIUM	372 mg

Curb carbs: Ditch the taco shell and pair this naturally low-carb dish with a higher-carb side like Baked Risotto (page 292) or Scalloped Red Potatoes (page 284).

Fill up on fiber: Avocado is a great source of fiber, and the bell pepper adds fiber as well.

Favor fats: While this dish seems high in fat, most of that represents good fats from both the salmon and the avocado.

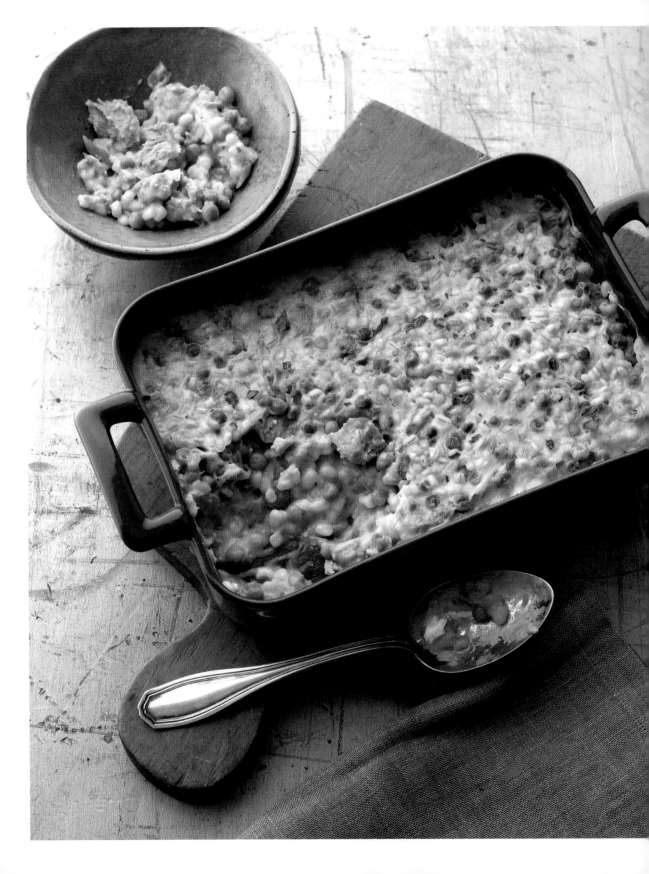

SALMON-BARLEY BAKE

PREP TIME: **15 MINUTES** ■ TOTAL TIME: **45 MINUTES**

Makes 4 servings

1 cup water

½ cup quick-cooking barley

¾ cup reduced-sodium, fat-free chicken broth

3 medium carrots, sliced diagonally

1 onion, finely chopped

1½ cups 1% milk

¼ teaspoon ground black pepper

1 tablespoon arrowroot, dissolved in 2 tablespoons cold water

1 can (14.7 ounces) wild red salmon, drained, with skin and bones removed

1 package (9 ounces) frozen peas, thawed

2 tablespoons chopped fresh tarragon or 2 teaspoons dried

1. Preheat the oven to 400°F. Coat a shallow 1½-quart baking dish with cooking spray. In a small saucepan, bring the water to a boil over medium-high heat. Stir in the barley, reduce the heat to medium low, cover, and cook for 10 minutes, or just until tender. Remove from the heat.

2. Meanwhile, in a large skillet over medium heat, bring the broth to a boil. Add the carrots and onion, cover, and cook, stirring often, for 3 minutes, or until crisp-tender. Transfer to the prepared baking dish with a slotted spoon.

3. Add the milk and pepper to the broth in the skillet and bring to a boil. Stir the arrowroot mixture and add it to the milk mixture. Cook, stirring constantly, until thickened. Reduce the heat to medium and stir in the salmon, barley, peas, and tarragon. Bring to a simmer and pour into the prepared baking dish.

4. Bake for 15 minutes, or until bubbly.

Makeover Magic

BEFORE		AFTER
480	CALORIES	329
22 g	FAT	6 g
13 g	SAT FAT	2 g
53 g	CARBS	40 g
2 g	FIBER	8 g
20 g	PROTEIN	31 g
560 mg	SODIUM	464 mg

Curb carbs: Barley is a delicious whole grain. Using just ½ cup in this recipe gives the casserole body without affecting blood sugar.

Fill up on fiber: Barley and peas are the main sources of fiber in this dish.

Favor fats: Wild canned salmon is an excellent source of healthy fats—choose the darker-color variety for more omega-3s.

TUNA TETRAZZINI

PREP TIME: **15 MINUTES** ■ TOTAL TIME: **1 HOUR**

Makes 4 servings

8 ounces multigrain spaghetti

4 cups broccoli florets

¼ pound mushrooms, sliced

1 onion, chopped

¼ cup water

1 jar (2 ounces) diced pimientos, drained

1½ teaspoons Italian seasoning

⅓ cup whole grain pastry flour

2½ cups 1% milk

⅓ cup (1½ ounces) grated Parmesan cheese

2 cans (5 ounces each) light tuna packed in water, drained

1. Preheat the oven to 350°F. Coat a medium baking dish with cooking spray. Prepare the pasta according to package directions and drain.

2. In a large saucepan coated with cooking spray over medium-high heat, cook the broccoli, mushrooms, onion, and water, stirring occasionally, for 5 minutes, or until the broccoli is tender-crisp. Stir in the pimientos and Italian seasoning. Place in a bowl.

3. In the same saucepan, add the flour. Gradually add the milk, whisking constantly, until smooth. Cook, whisking constantly, over medium heat for 6 minutes, or until slightly thickened and bubbling.

4. Remove from the heat. Stir in the Parmesan until smooth. Stir in the tuna, the reserved broccoli mixture, and the spaghetti. Toss to mix. Pour into the prepared baking dish.

5. Cover and bake for 20 minutes. Uncover and bake for 10 minutes, or until bubbly. Remove from the oven and let stand for 5 minutes before serving.

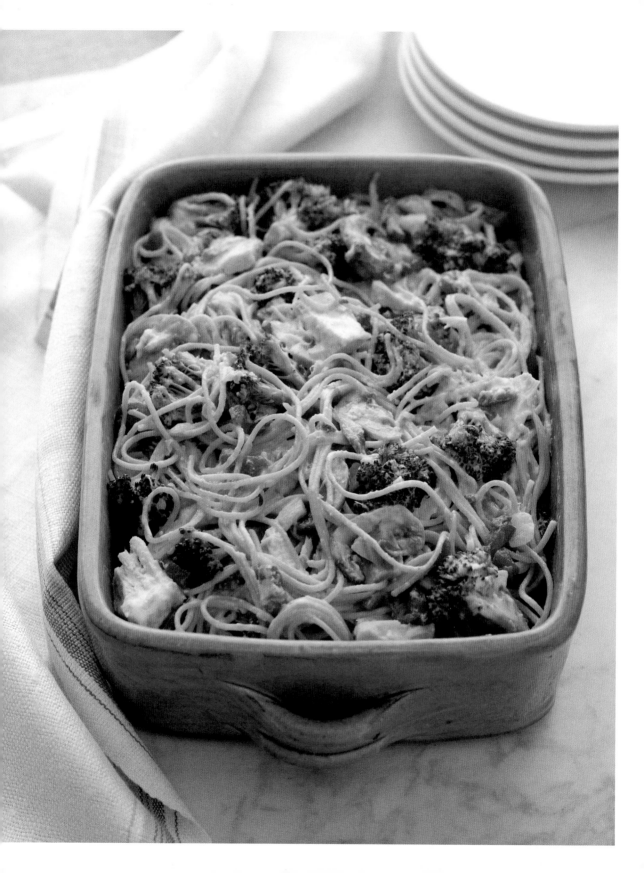

BEFORE		AFTER
460	CALORIES	327
12 g	FAT	20 g
6 g	SAT FAT	2 g
45 g	CARBS	8 g
7 g	FIBER	5 g
42 g	PROTEIN	19 g
780 mg	SODIUM	296 mg

Curb carbs: No need to serve these steaks on a roll—the flavor is so strong and delicious that a bed of greens makes a perfect platter. Plus, at only 8 grams of carbs, you've got room to add a higher-carb side dish or enjoy a slice of cake for dessert!

Fill up on fiber: Our fiber comes from the mixed greens, cucumber, and avocado. The roll in the comparison recipe adds fiber—but also lots of carbs.

Favor fats: This dish is full of amazing fats! Tuna is a nice source of omega-3 fatty acids, while canola oil mayonnaise and avocado are both full of MUFAs.

TUNA STEAKS ON GREENS

PREP TIME: **5 MINUTES** ■ TOTAL TIME: **15 MINUTES**

Makes 4 servings

¼ cup canola oil mayonnaise

2 scallions, thinly sliced

1 tablespoon lime juice

1 small clove garlic, minced

½ teaspoon ground cumin

4 yellowfin tuna steaks (4 ounces each)

2 teaspoons canola oil

¼ teaspoon salt

4 cups mixed greens

1 small cucumber, sliced

1 avocado, thinly sliced

2 tablespoons chopped fresh cilantro (optional)

1. Coat a grill rack or broiler pan with cooking spray. Preheat the grill or broiler to medium-high heat.

2. In a medium bowl, stir together the mayonnaise, scallions, lime juice, garlic, and cumin until well blended. Refrigerate until serving.

3. Brush the tuna steaks with the oil and sprinkle with the salt. Set on the grill rack or broiler pan. Grill or broil for 4 minutes, turning once, or until well marked and opaque.

4. Divide the greens, cucumber, and avocado among 4 plates. Top each with 1 tuna steak and a dollop of the mayonnaise mixture. Sprinkle with the cilantro, if using.

SWEET AND SOUR SHRIMP

PREP TIME: **5 MINUTES** ■ TOTAL TIME: **10 MINUTES**

Makes 2 servings

- 2 teaspoons canola oil
- 2 cups (half of a 16-ounce package) frozen bell pepper strips
- ⅓ cup apricot all-fruit jam
- 2 teaspoons red wine vinegar
- 6 ounces cooked, peeled, and deveined shrimp
- 4 cups steamed broccoli

In a large nonstick skillet, heat the oil over medium-high heat. Cook the peppers for 3 minutes, stirring, until lightly browned. Stir in the jam, vinegar, and shrimp. Cook for 2 minutes, or until bubbly. Serve with the broccoli.

Makeover Magic

BEFORE		AFTER
483	CALORIES	283
29 g	FAT	6 g
4 g	SAT FAT	1 g
46 g	CARBS	31 g
1 g	FIBER	3 g
13 g	PROTEIN	27 g
1,928 mg	SODIUM	283 mg

Curb carbs: Instead of using a sugary prepackaged sauce, we've used all-fruit jam that adds natural sweetness.

Fill up on fiber: The steamed broccoli in this dish is the main source of fiber, but the bell pepper strips also contribute.

Favor fats: Instead of deep-frying the shrimp, we cut out saturated fat by cooking the shrimp right in the pan with the veggies and jam. For added healthy fats (and to give this recipe some extra crunch), toss in sliced almonds.

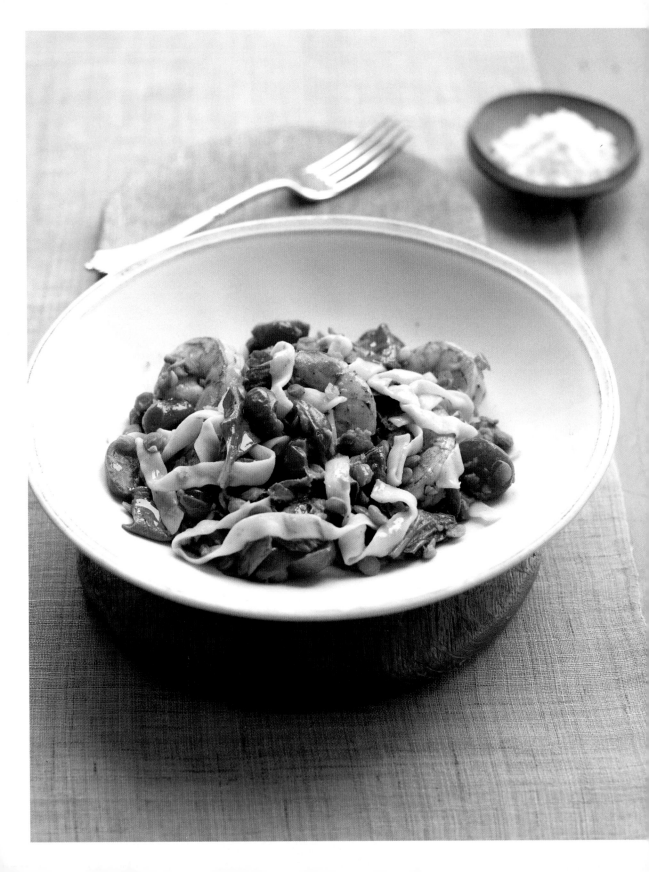

SHRIMP SCAMPI LINGUINE

PREP TIME: **10 MINUTES** ■ TOTAL TIME: **20 MINUTES**

Makes 4 servings

1 package (8 ounces) shirataki fettuccine

2 tablespoons canola oil

1 pound medium shrimp, peeled and deveined

4 cloves garlic, minced

½ teaspoon red-pepper flakes

1 pint cherry tomatoes, halved

½ cup dry white wine

Juice of 1 lemon

4 cups packed baby spinach leaves

1 can (15 ounces) lentils, rinsed and drained

½ cup grated Parmesan cheese

1. Prepare the fettuccine according to package directions.

2. Meanwhile, in a large skillet, heat the oil over medium heat. Cook the shrimp, garlic, and red-pepper flakes for 2 minutes, stirring, or until the shrimp start to turn pink.

3. Add the tomatoes, wine, and lemon juice. Cook for 2 minutes, or until the tomatoes start to soften. Add the spinach and lentils and cook, stirring, for 1 minute, or until the spinach wilts. Stir in the drained fettuccine and toss to coat well. Divide among 4 plates and sprinkle each with 2 tablespoons of the cheese.

Makeover Magic

BEFORE		AFTER
587	CALORIES	336
28 g	FAT	12 g
10 g	SAT FAT	3 g
45 g	CARBS	19 g
7 g	FIBER	7 g
34 g	PROTEIN	33 g
554 mg	SODIUM	446 mg

Curb carbs: Using shirataki noodles in place of wheat-based linguine cuts the carbs dramatically while still serving up satisfying, slurpable noodles.

Fill up on fiber: Adding lentils and spinach to this classic dish pumps up the fiber, as well as other important nutrients, like iron.

Favor fats: Shrimp is very low in saturated fats and high in omega-3s. As for the topping, no need to bathe this dish in lots of butter. Instead, we flavor the sauce with wine, lemon, and fresh tomatoes.

Makeover Magic

BEFORE		AFTER
400	CALORIES	320
10 g	FAT	12 g
2 g	SAT FAT	2 g
56 g	CARBS	27 g
4 g	FIBER	6 g
22 g	PROTEIN	27 g
560 mg	SODIUM	484 mg

Curb carbs: The best way to make a taco healthy and satisfying is to select 6" corn tortillas over the larger white flour ones. This move cuts the carbs while adding some fiber.

Fill up on fiber: The fiber in this dish comes not just from the tortillas, but also the avocado.

Favor fats: Shrimp and avocado team up in this recipe to bring you both omega-3 fatty acids and essential MUFAs.

SHRIMP TACOS

PREP TIME: **10 MINUTES** ■ TOTAL TIME: **15 MINUTES**

Makes 4 servings

1 Hass avocado, cubed

3 tablespoons finely chopped red onion

2 tablespoons chopped fresh cilantro or 2 teaspoons dried

½ jalapeño chile pepper, seeded and finely chopped (wear plastic gloves when handling)

1 tablespoon fresh lime juice

½ teaspoon salt, divided

1 pound peeled and deveined medium shrimp

1½ teaspoons chili powder

1 tablespoon olive oil

8 corn tortillas (6" diameter)

1 cup shredded romaine

1. In a small bowl, toss together the avocado, onion, cilantro, pepper, lime juice, and ¼ teaspoon of the salt. Set aside.

2. In a medium bowl, combine the shrimp, chili powder, and remaining ¼ teaspoon salt.

3. In a large nonstick skillet, heat the oil over medium-high heat. Cook the shrimp, stirring, for 5 minutes, or until opaque. Transfer to a plate and keep warm.

4. Heat the tortillas in a dry skillet over medium-high heat for 1 minute, turning once, or until hot and lightly toasted. Place 2 tortillas on 4 plates. Divide the romaine, shrimp, and avocado mixture among the tortillas.

SCALLOPS WITH BEANS AND ARUGULA

PREP TIME: **5 MINUTES** ▪ TOTAL TIME: **20 MINUTES**

Makes 4 servings

2 tablespoons canola oil, divided

1 red onion, finely chopped

1 clove garlic, minced

1½ cans white beans (14.5 ounces each), rinsed and drained

4 cups baby arugula

1 pound large sea scallops

Pinch of salt

Pinch of ground black pepper

1. In a large skillet, heat 1 tablespoon of the oil over medium heat. Cook the onion and garlic for 3 minutes, or until the onion is softened. Add the beans and arugula and cook, stirring, for 3 minutes, or until the beans are hot and the arugula is wilted. Place on a serving plate. Cover and keep warm.

2. In the same skillet, heat the remaining 1 tablespoon of the oil over medium-high heat. Blot the scallops dry with a paper towel and sprinkle with salt and pepper. Cook the scallops for 5 minutes, turning once, or until browned and opaque.

3. Place over the bean mixture.

Makeover Magic

BEFORE		AFTER
386	CALORIES	298
19 g	FAT	12 g
5 g	SAT FAT	3 g
36 g	CARBS	22 g
0 g	FIBER	6 g
16 g	PROTEIN	28 g
919 mg	SODIUM	267 mg

Curb carbs: The scallops are so flavorful, there's no need for extra breading. Enjoy them au naturel with the beans and arugula for company.

Fill up on fiber: Adding beans to any dish pumps up the fiber.

Favor fats: There's no need to fry scallops—searing them in healthy canola oil adds good fats and nice flavor.

CHAPTER**TEN**

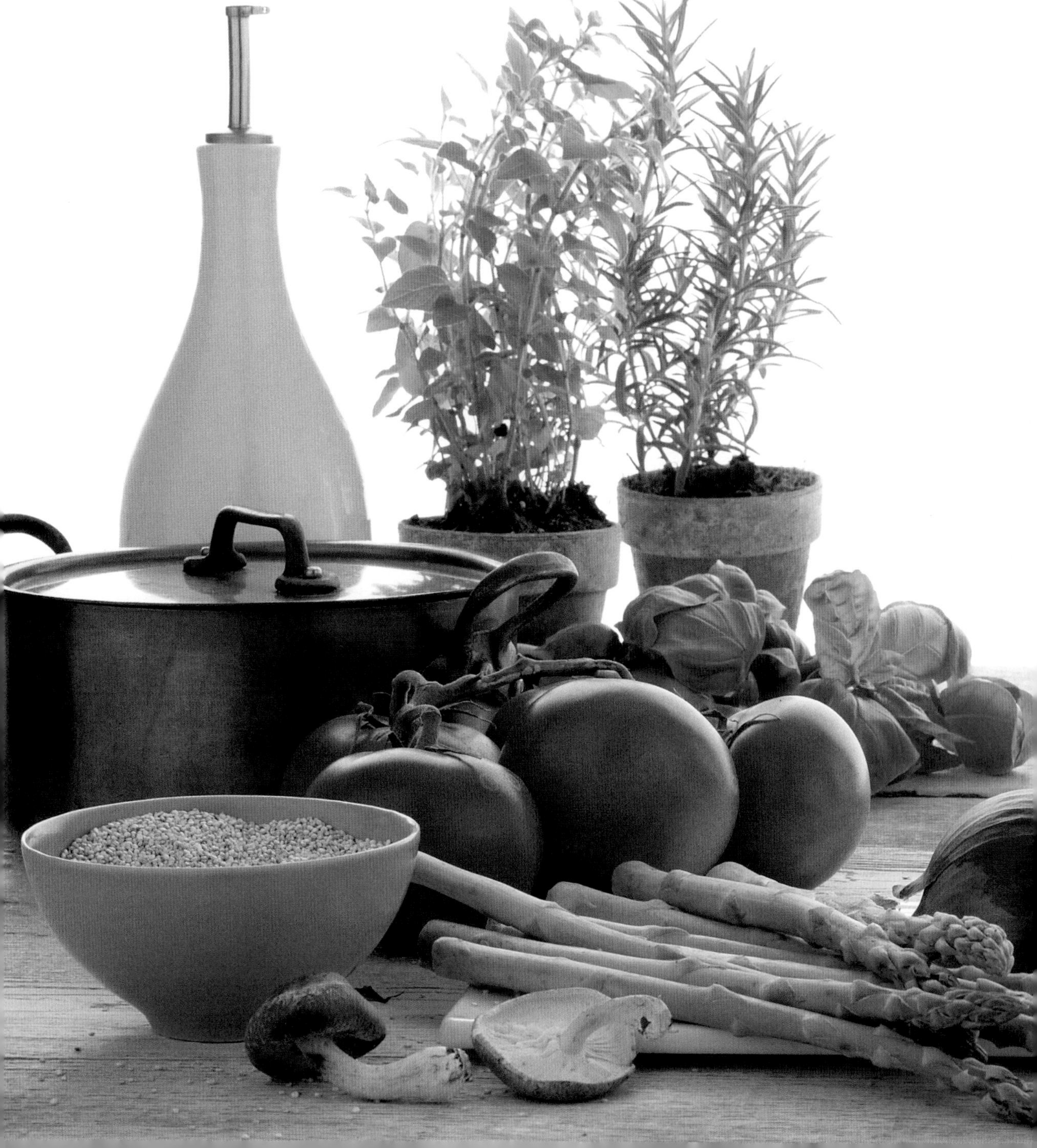

Vegetarian

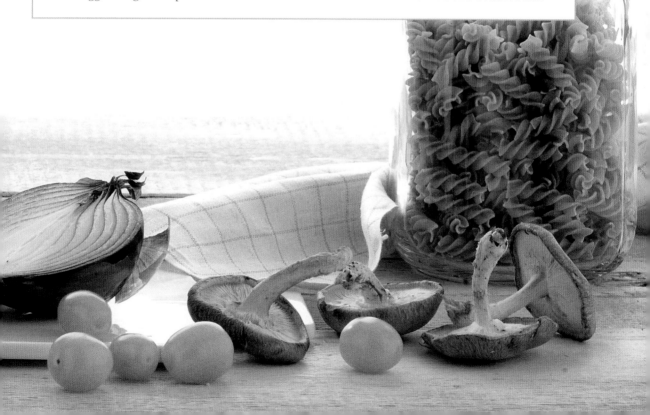

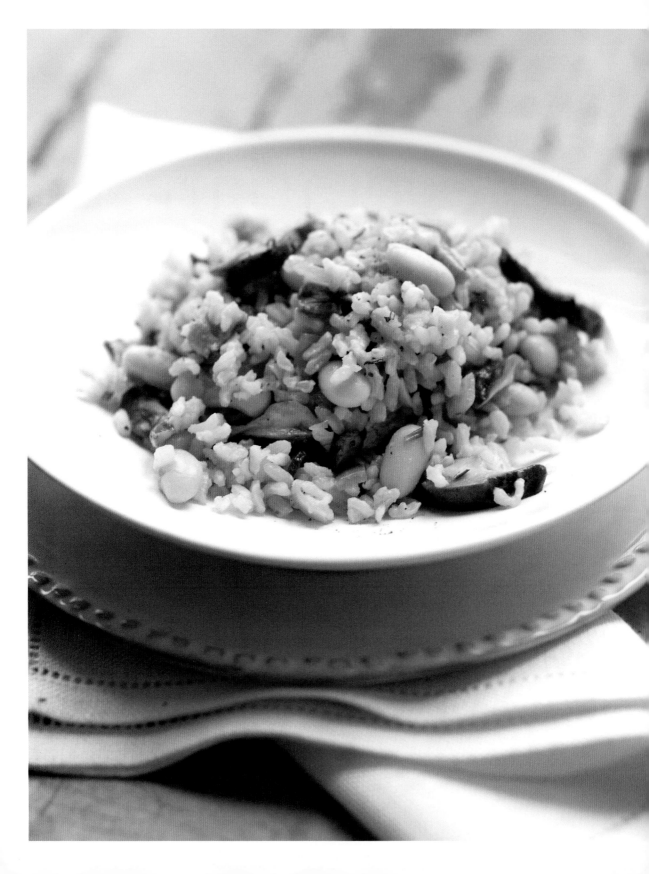

WILD MUSHROOM AND WHITE BEAN RISOTTO

PREP TIME: **10 MINUTES** ■ TOTAL TIME: **40 MINUTES**

Makes 4 servings

1 cup brown rice

½ ounce dried porcini mushrooms

¾ cup boiling water

2 tablespoons olive oil

1 onion, chopped

½ pound shiitake mushrooms, stems discarded, caps thinly sliced

2 cloves garlic, minced

1 teaspoon chopped fresh rosemary or ⅓ teaspoon dried

¼ teaspoon salt

¼ cup dry white wine

1 can (14–19 ounces) low-sodium cannellini beans, rinsed and drained

2 tablespoons grated Parmesan cheese

1. Prepare the rice according to package directions.

2. Meanwhile, in a small bowl, combine the dried mushrooms and boiling water. Let the mushrooms stand for 10 minutes, or until softened. With a slotted spoon, remove the mushrooms to a sieve. Rinse and coarsely chop. Reserve the mushroom soaking liquid.

3. In a large nonstick skillet, heat the oil over medium-high heat. Cook the onion for 6 minutes, stirring, or until softened. Add the chopped mushrooms, shiitake mushrooms, garlic, rosemary, and salt. Cook for 6 minutes, stirring occasionally, or until tender.

4. Add the wine and bring to a boil. Boil for 30 seconds, scraping any browned bits from the bottom of the pan, or until the wine is almost evaporated. Carefully pour in the reserved soaking liquid, leaving any grit in the bottom of the bowl. Bring to a boil. Reduce the heat and simmer for 5 minutes, or until the liquid is reduced by half. Stir in the beans and the rice and cook for 2 minutes, or until hot. Sprinkle with the Parmesan.

Makeover Magic

BEFORE		AFTER
590	CALORIES	273
22 g	FAT	7 g
10 g	SAT FAT	2 g
83 g	CARBS	35 g
2 g	FIBER	4 g
14 g	PROTEIN	8 g
1,140 mg	SODIUM	352 mg

Curb carbs: By "beefing up" this vegetarian classic with porcinis, shiitakes, and cannellini beans, we were able to use less rice.

Fill up on fiber: Brown rice and cannellini beans work together to pack fiber into this savory dish.

Favor fats: Olive oil provides some MUFAs, but for more healthy fats, try adding a side salad drizzled with flaxseed oil or a salad Niçoise.

BEFORE		AFTER
450	CALORIES	315
20 g	FAT	13 g
4 g	SAT FAT	2 g
60 g	CARBS	44 g
2 g	FIBER	11 g
7 g	PROTEIN	9 g
700 mg	SODIUM	379 mg

Curb carbs: Quinoa has fewer carbs and more fiber and protein than white rice.

Fill up on fiber: Don't forget asparagus when selecting vegetables—it offers 5 grams of fiber per serving.

Favor fats: Avocado not only adds MUFAs but is also a good source of fiber.

VEGETABLE SAUTÉ WITH QUINOA

PREP TIME: **20 MINUTES** ■ TOTAL TIME: **50 MINUTES**

Makes 4 servings

1½ cups water

¾ cup quinoa, rinsed

¼ teaspoon salt

1 tablespoon canola oil

1 onion, cut into wedges

1 pound asparagus, trimmed and cut in half

1 bunch radishes, trimmed and halved

2 cloves garlic, minced

¼ cup fat-free, low-sodium vegetable broth

2 tablespoons apricot all-fruit spread

1 tablespoon balsamic vinegar

8 ounces baby spinach

1 avocado, cubed

1. In a large skillet, bring the water to a boil over high heat. Stir in the quinoa and salt and return to a boil. Reduce the heat to low, cover, and simmer for 20 minutes, or until all of the water is absorbed and the quinoa is tender.

2. Meanwhile, in a large nonstick skillet, heat the oil over medium-high heat. Cook the onion, stirring, for 3 minutes, or until tender. Stir in the asparagus, radishes, and garlic and cook for 2 minutes. Add the broth, apricot spread, and vinegar and stir for 1 minute to deglaze the pan. Add the spinach, cover, and cook for 3 minutes, or until wilted.

3. Divide the quinoa and vegetables among 4 plates. Sprinkle with the avocado.

PASTA WITH SUMMER VEGETABLES

PREP TIME: **15 MINUTES** ■ TOTAL TIME: **35 MINUTES**

Makes 4 servings

8 ounces whole grain shell pasta with added protein and omega-3s

1 tablespoon olive oil

1 small red onion, thinly sliced

2 cloves garlic, sliced

1 medium zucchini, cut into 1" chunks

1 yellow squash, cut into 1" chunks

1 cup cherry tomatoes, halved

1 cup small fresh mozzarella balls (ciliegini), halved

¼ cup chopped fresh basil or 8 teaspoons dried

1. Prepare the pasta according to package directions.

2. Meanwhile, in a large nonstick skillet, heat the oil over medium-high heat. Cook the onion and garlic for 2 minutes, stirring occasionally, or until softened. Stir in the zucchini and squash and cook for 8 minutes, stirring occasionally, or until the vegetables are tender-crisp. Stir in the tomatoes and cook for 3 minutes, or just until the tomatoes begin to burst.

3. Stir in the pasta and mozzarella. Cook for 2 minutes, stirring, or until the pasta is hot and the mozzarella just begins to melt. Remove the skillet from the heat and stir in the basil.

Makeover Magic

BEFORE		AFTER
670	CALORIES	390
27 g	FAT	7 g
9 g	SAT FAT	1 g
91 g	CARBS	49 g
5 g	FIBER	8 g
17 g	PROTEIN	34 g
100 mg	SODIUM	490 mg

Curb carbs: Cutting the pasta with veggies helps to bring down the carbs.

Fill up on fiber: By using whole wheat pasta and high-fiber veggies, there's enough fiber in this dish to bring the magic carbs down to 41 grams per serving!

Favor fats: Sneak in some extra healthy fats by using omega-3–enriched pasta! Reduce saturated fat by using fresh mozzarella balls instead of a thick cheese sauce.

BEFORE		AFTER
630	CALORIES	346
34 g	FAT	13 g
21 g	SAT FAT	7 g
55 g	CARBS	42 g
2 g	FIBER	6 g
27 g	PROTEIN	22 g
850 mg	SODIUM	470 mg

Curb carbs: Halve the typical amount of pasta and toss in cauliflower, onion, and bell pepper.

Fill up on fiber: Whole grain pasta and vegetables add fiber, not to mention a satisfying, sophisticated flavor, to a childhood favorite!

Favor fats: We use reduced-fat dairy to minimize the saturated fat and rely on canola oil for a helping of MUFAs. Add more by tossing in some toasted pine nuts.

ROASTED VEGETABLE MAC AND CHEESE

PREP TIME: **20 MINUTES** ■ TOTAL TIME: **1 HOUR 15 MINUTES**

Makes 6 servings

1 head cauliflower, cut into large florets

1 large onion, cut into wedges

1 yellow or red bell pepper, cut into eighths

2 teaspoons canola oil

8 ounces whole grain elbow pasta

2 cups 1% milk

2 tablespoons whole wheat flour

½ teaspoon dried mustard

¼ teaspoon salt

1½ cups shredded reduced-fat sharp Cheddar cheese

2 tablespoons grated Romano cheese

1. Preheat the oven to 350°F. Coat an 11" × 7" baking dish with cooking spray.

2. On a rimmed baking sheet, roast the cauliflower, onion, bell pepper, and oil for 30 minutes, stirring once, or until the cauliflower is golden brown. Remove from the oven to a cutting board and chop the roasted vegetables coarsely. Add to the prepared dish.

3. Meanwhile, prepare the pasta according to package directions. Drain and place in the dish with the roasted vegetables.

4. In a medium saucepan, whisk together the milk, flour, mustard, and salt. Cook for 4 minutes, whisking, or until the mixture begins to thicken. Stir in the Cheddar and Romano and cook for 2 minutes, or until melted. Pour over the pasta and vegetables, tossing to coat. Bake for 20 minutes, or until bubbling.

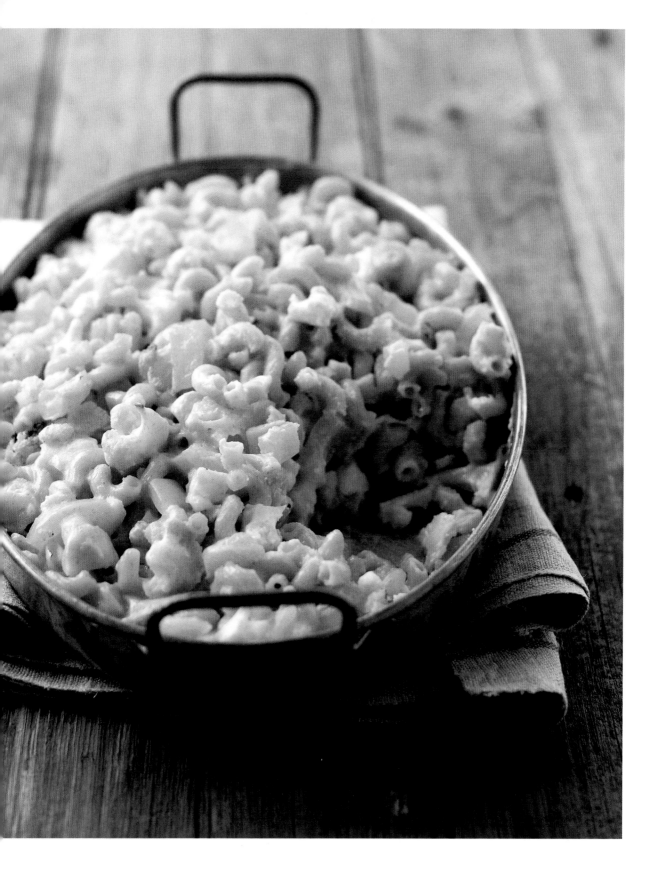

BEFORE		AFTER
800	CALORIES	341
48 g	FAT	15 g
30 g	SAT FAT	5 g
69 g	CARBS	34 g
4 g	FIBER	5 g
24 g	PROTEIN	20 g
810 mg	SODIUM	228 mg

Curb carbs: This dish uses half the pasta thanks to added broccoli and tomatoes.

Fill up on fiber: We used multigrain pasta for a fiber boost, and broccoli adds both fiber and flavor.

Favor fats: Pesto sauce, full of healthy MUFAs, is a great substitute for saturated fat–laden Alfredo sauce. And the multigrain pasta adds some omega-3 fatty acids to the dish, too.

BROCCOLI PENNE

PREP TIME: **15 MINUTES** ■ TOTAL TIME: **25 MINUTES**

Makes 4 servings

6 ounces multigrain penne pasta

2 cups fresh broccoli florets

1 cup grape tomatoes, halved

6 ounces fresh mozzarella cheese, cubed

¼ cup pesto sauce

1 tablespoon lemon juice

1. Prepare the pasta according to package directions. Add the broccoli to the pot for the last 2 minutes of cooking. Drain, reserving ½ cup of the pasta water.

2. In a large bowl, place the pasta, broccoli, tomatoes, cheese, pesto, and lemon juice. Add the reserved water, 1 tablespoon at a time, stirring gently, until smooth.

BAKED PASTA AND VEGETABLES

PREP TIME: **10 MINUTES** ■ TOTAL TIME: **45 MINUTES**

Makes 4 servings

4 ounces whole grain spaghetti

1 pound asparagus, trimmed and cut into 3" pieces

2 carrots, sliced

2 tablespoons canola oil

1 red onion, cut into thin wedges

½ teaspoon dried basil

2 tablespoons whole grain pastry flour

1 cup 1% milk

2 ounces reduced-fat cream cheese, cut into cubes

¼ cup grated Parmesan cheese

¼ cup ground golden flaxseeds

1. Preheat the oven to 450°F. Coat an 8" × 8" baking dish with cooking spray. Prepare the pasta according to package directions, adding the asparagus and carrots during the last 3 minutes of cooking. Drain.

2. Meanwhile, in a large skillet, heat the oil over medium heat. Cook the onion and basil, stirring, for 5 minutes, or until soft. Add the flour and cook, stirring constantly with a wooden spoon, for 2 minutes, or until lightly browned. Gradually whisk in the milk.

3. Cook, whisking, for 5 minutes, or until thickened. Remove from the heat and stir in the cream cheese until blended. Add the pasta mixture and toss to coat well. Pour into the prepared dish. Sprinkle with the cheese and flaxseeds. Bake for 15 minutes, or until lightly browned.

Makeover Magic

BEFORE		AFTER
550	CALORIES	257
20 g	FAT	6 g
11 g	SAT FAT	2 g
69 g	CARBS	38 g
4 g	FIBER	8 g
23 g	PROTEIN	6 g
960 mg	SODIUM	243 mg

Curb carbs: This creamy dish is lower in carbs because we substitute vegetables for half of the pasta.

Fill up on fiber: Aside from the whole grain pasta, the main sources of fiber in this recipe are asparagus, carrots, and red onion.

Favor fats: Canola oil and flaxseeds are our sources of favored fats. We used reduced-fat cream cheese to keep this dish heart healthy.

BEFORE		AFTER
490	CALORIES	292
6 g	FAT	6 g
0.5 g	SAT FAT	0.5 g
94 g	CARBS	49 g
6 g	FIBER	11 g
19 g	PROTEIN	11 g
2,870 mg	SODIUM	458 mg

Curb carbs: Cutting the vegetables into matchstick-thin pieces allows them to replace some of the pasta without losing any of the flavor.

Fill up on fiber: In addition to using whole wheat spaghetti instead of white lo mein noodles, we use lots of fibrous vegetables for a dish bursting with flavor.

Favor fats: Canola oil and sesame oil both have healthy fats. For additional MUFAs, sprinkle on a few tablespoons of sesame seeds.

VEGETABLE LO MEIN

PREP TIME: **15 MINUTES** ■ TOTAL TIME: **20 MINUTES**

Makes 4 servings

8 ounces whole wheat spaghetti

1 tablespoon canola oil

1 red onion, thinly sliced

3 baby bok choy, thinly sliced

2 carrots, thinly sliced

½ cup low-sodium vegetable broth

2 cloves garlic, minced

3 tablespoons low-sodium soy sauce

2 tablespoons rice wine vinegar

2 teaspoons cornstarch

1 teaspoon toasted sesame oil

4 ounces snow peas, sliced lengthwise

1. Prepare the pasta according to package directions.

2. Meanwhile, in a large skillet, heat the canola oil over medium-high heat. Cook the onion, bok choy, and carrots for 3 minutes, or until tender-crisp.

3. In a small bowl, whisk together the broth, garlic, soy sauce, vinegar, cornstarch, and sesame oil and add it to the skillet. Add the snow peas and cook, stirring constantly, for 3 minutes, or until the sauce is thickened. Add the pasta and toss to combine.

VEGGIE BURGER WRAPS

PREP TIME: **5 MINUTES** ■ TOTAL TIME: **15 MINUTES**

Makes 2 servings

2 frozen vegetarian garden burgers, thawed

2 whole wheat tortillas (6" diameter)

1 cup fresh baby spinach leaves

1 plum tomato, sliced

1 scallion, thinly sliced

2 tablespoons unsalted stone-ground mustard

½ avocado, sliced

1. In a nonstick skillet over medium-high heat, cook the burgers for 6 minutes, turning once, until browned and heated through.

2. Cut the burgers in half and place 2 halves in each tortilla. Top with the spinach, tomato, scallion, mustard, and avocado slices.

Makeover Magic

BEFORE		AFTER
420	CALORIES	238
20 g	FAT	11 g
4 g	SAT FAT	1 g
28 g	CARBS	25 g
4 g	FIBER	13 g
30 g	PROTEIN	18 g
1,310 mg	SODIUM	377 mg

Curb carbs: Who said a burger has to be on a bun? Cut the burger in half and it fits perfectly into a wrap!

Fill up on fiber: Between the tortilla, veggie burger, and fresh toppings, this meal comes in at an awesome 13 grams of fiber!

Favor fats: The avocado in this dish provides MUFAs as well as a creamy, flavorful condiment for this veggie burger wrap.

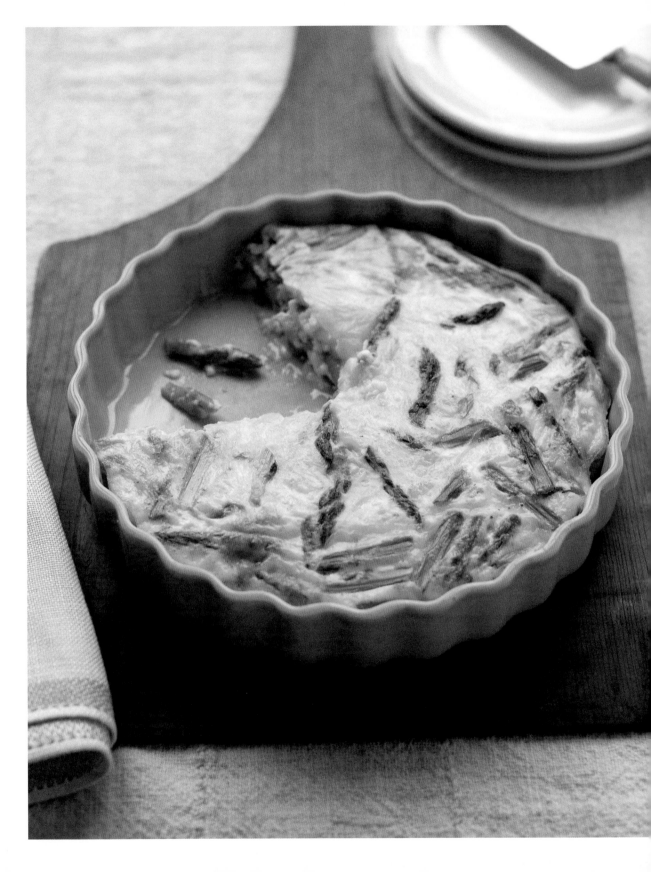

ASPARAGUS SWISS QUICHE

PREP TIME: **10 MINUTES** ■ TOTAL TIME: **1 HOUR 5 MINUTES**

Makes 4 servings

3 tablespoons ground golden flaxseeds

1 tablespoon water

1 pound asparagus, trimmed and cut into 1½" pieces

4 scallions, thinly sliced

1½ cups 1% milk

1 cup shredded reduced-fat Swiss cheese

4 egg whites

2 omega-3–enriched eggs

2 teaspoons Dijon mustard

¼ teaspoon ground black pepper

⅛ teaspoon salt

2 tablespoons grated Parmesan cheese

1. Preheat the oven to 350°F. Coat a 9" quiche or pie plate with cooking spray. Sprinkle with the flaxseeds.

2. In a nonstick skillet, heat the water over medium-high heat. Cook the asparagus and scallions, stirring, for 5 minutes, or until tender-crisp.

3. Meanwhile, in a large bowl, whisk together the milk, Swiss cheese, egg whites, eggs, mustard, pepper, and salt. Stir in the asparagus mixture. Pour into the pie pan and sprinkle with the Parmesan.

4. Bake for 40 minutes, or until a knife inserted in the center comes out clean. Let stand for 10 minutes before serving.

Makeover Magic

BEFORE		AFTER
620	CALORIES	217
52 g	FAT	8 g
25 g	SAT FAT	3 g
20 g	CARBS	15 g
0 g	FIBER	4 g
17 g	PROTEIN	23 g
580 mg	SODIUM	387 mg

Curb carbs: Eliminating the crust typical of quiche reduces both carbs and fat in this recipe, without losing the gooey goodness.

Fill up on fiber: Asparagus adds some fiber to the dish. Serve it with a green salad with apple wedges and a sprinkle of walnuts for more fiber and nutrients.

Favor fats: Dusting the quiche pan with flaxseeds creates a slight crust while adding good fats. We also boost healthy fats by using omega-3–rich eggs.

Makeover Magic

BEFORE		AFTER
450	CALORIES	345
25 g	FAT	16 g
14 g	SAT FAT	5 g
35 g	CARBS	24 g
2 g	FIBER	4 g
21 g	PROTEIN	30 g
780 mg	SODIUM	570 mg

Curb carbs: We use less bread in this strata and fill in the rest with savory vegetables.

Fill up on fiber: Multigrain bread is chock-full of fiber.

Favor fats: Kalamata olives provide healthy fats in this dish.

BROCCOLI-CHEDDAR STRATA

PREP TIME: **10 MINUTES** ■ TOTAL TIME: **50 MINUTES**

Makes 4 servings

5 slices low-carb multigrain bread, toasted and broken into 2" pieces

2 cups 1% milk

4 large eggs

3 large egg whites

2 tablespoons flour

½ teaspoon ground black pepper

2 cups frozen broccoli florets

½ cup frozen chopped onion

2 tablespoons chopped kalamata olives

1½ cups shredded reduced-fat, low-sodium Cheddar cheese

1. Preheat the oven to 350°F. Coat an 11" × 7" baking dish with cooking spray. Place the bread in the pan.

2. In a large bowl, whisk together the milk, eggs, egg whites, flour, and pepper. Stir in the broccoli, onion, and olives. Pour over the bread. Top with the cheese. Let stand at room temperature for 10 minutes.

3. Bake for 35 minutes, or until a knife inserted in the center comes out clean.

AFRICAN STEW

PREP TIME: **15 MINUTES** ■ TOTAL TIME: **50 MINUTES**

Makes 4 servings

1 large onion, chopped

1 Japanese eggplant, chopped

1 small zucchini, chopped

1 clove garlic, minced

1 teaspoon ground ginger

1 teaspoon dried thyme

4 cups fat-free, low-sodium vegetable or chicken broth

1 can (14.5 ounces) diced tomatoes, drained

1 large sweet potato, peeled and cut into ½" pieces

⅓ cup omega-3–enriched peanut butter

1 can (14.5 ounces) white beans, rinsed and drained

½ cup unsalted peanuts, coarsely chopped

1. In a large saucepan coated with cooking spray over medium-high heat, cook the onion, eggplant, zucchini, garlic, ginger, and thyme for 5 minutes, stirring, or until the vegetables are lightly browned.

2. Stir in the broth, tomatoes, and sweet potato and bring to a boil. Reduce the heat to low, cover, and simmer for 15 minutes, or until the potatoes are just tender.

3. Place the peanut butter in a small bowl. Remove 1 cup of the simmering broth and whisk into the peanut butter. Return to the pan with the beans and cook for 10 minutes, or until the flavors are blended.

4. Divide the stew among 4 bowls and sprinkle with the peanuts.

Makeover Magic

BEFORE		AFTER
639	CALORIES	355
23 g	FAT	17 g
5 g	SAT FAT	3 g
55 g	CARBS	41 g
7 g	FIBER	10 g
53 g	PROTEIN	13 g
866 mg	SODIUM	283 mg

Curb carbs: By mixing 1 sweet potato with other lower-carb veggies, we're able to curb carbs in this dish while boosting fiber.

Fill up on fiber: This hearty stew is full of fiber-toting veggies, including white beans, sweet potato, eggplant, and zucchini.

Favor fats: The omega-3–enriched peanut butter and chopped nuts add healthful MUFAs and omega-3 fats.

Makeover Magic

Curb carbs: All the carbs in this hearty dish come from high-fiber legumes and veggies.

Fill up on fiber: Beans, corn, and tomatoes pump up the fiber in this dish. Serve with ½ cup brown rice or quinoa for added flavor and fiber.

Favor fats: Choosing this vegetarian chili over a meaty version cuts out saturated fat. Canola oil provides some healthy fats, but you could top with sliced avocado in addition to the yogurt to get even more MUFAs.

FIRE-ROASTED CHILI

PREP TIME: **15 MINUTES** ■ TOTAL TIME: **50 MINUTES**

Makes 4 servings

2 tablespoons canola oil

1 large onion, chopped

1 green bell pepper, chopped

3 cloves garlic, minced

1 can (14.5 ounces) fire-roasted diced tomatoes with green chiles

1 can (14.5 ounces) no-salt-added diced tomatoes

1 can (14–19 ounces) no-salt-added red kidney beans, rinsed and drained

1 cup frozen shelled edamame

1 cup fresh or thawed frozen corn kernels

1 can (4 ounces) chopped mild green chiles, drained

2 tablespoons chili powder

1 teaspoon ground cumin

¼ cup chopped fresh cilantro

¼ cup plain 0% Greek yogurt

1. In a Dutch oven or large saucepot, heat the oil over medium-high heat. Cook the onion, bell pepper, and garlic for 8 minutes, stirring occasionally, or until tender. Stir in the tomatoes (with juice), beans, edamame, corn, chiles, chili powder, and cumin.

2. Bring to a boil. Reduce the heat to low, cover, and simmer, stirring occasionally, for 25 minutes, or until the flavors are blended. Stir in the cilantro. Serve with the yogurt.

BEAN ENCHILADAS

PREP TIME: **15 MINUTES** ■ TOTAL TIME: **1 HOUR 5 MINUTES**

Makes 4 servings

2 teaspoons canola oil

1 onion, chopped

2 cloves garlic, finely chopped

½ teaspoon ground cumin

3 cups chopped fresh kale

1 can (15 ounces) no-salt-added black beans, rinsed and drained

2 tablespoons ground flaxseeds

1 can (15 ounces) no-salt-added diced tomatoes, drained

½ cup loosely packed chopped fresh cilantro

8 corn tortillas (6" diameter)

4 slices reduced-sodium pepper Jack cheese, halved

½ avocado, thinly sliced into 8 pieces

1. Preheat the oven to 350°F. Coat a 13" × 9" baking dish with cooking spray.

2. In a large nonstick skillet, heat the oil over medium heat. Cook the onion, garlic, and cumin, stirring occasionally, for 3 minutes, or until softened. Add the kale and cook for 5 minutes, stirring, or until wilted. Stir in the beans and flaxseeds. Cook for 5 minutes, or until simmering. Smash some of the beans with the back of a spoon to thicken the mixture.

3. In a medium bowl, stir together the tomatoes and cilantro. Set aside.

4. Wrap the tortillas in paper towels and microwave for 1 minute, or until softened. Remove to a work surface. Evenly divide the bean mixture down the center of each tortilla. Roll each into a tube. Place seam side down in the baking dish. Spoon the tomato mixture over the enchiladas. Cover tightly with foil.

5. Bake for 20 minutes. Carefully remove the foil and place 1 piece of the cheese over each enchilada. Bake for 10 minutes, or until the cheese melts. Remove from the oven and allow the enchiladas to sit for 5 minutes before serving.

6. Place 2 enchiladas on 4 plates, along with 2 slices of avocado.

Makeover Magic

BEFORE		AFTER
505	CALORIES	366
27 g	FAT	16 g
14 g	SAT FAT	4 g
35 g	CARBS	45 g
3 g	FIBER	10 g
30 g	PROTEIN	14 g
760 mg	SODIUM	243 mg

Curb carbs: Choose smaller 6" corn tortillas over the huge flour ones to cut the carbs while adding nice flavor.

Fill up on fiber: Black beans and kale work together in this dish for a great source of fiber.

Favor fats: Ground flaxseeds and avocado are the favored fats in this recipe. Serve with mixed greens drizzled with olive oil, vinegar, and pepitas.

SMARTSTART

To make this meal complete, serve with a seafood seviche to start. Not only will you meet your protein needs, but you will get your omega-3s.

Makeover Magic

Curb carbs: Using sandwich thins instead of white burger buns not only lowers carbs, but ensures each bite is full of juicy burger instead of mostly bread.

Fill up on fiber: The beans and whole wheat sandwich thins mean the magic carbs in this dish come out to just 33—still allowing room for a starchy vegetable side like an ear of corn, if desired.

Favor fats: Going meatless cuts saturated fat, as does using reduced-fat cheese; add healthy fats by spreading some olive tapenade or guacamole onto your burger.

BLACK BEAN BURGERS

PREP TIME: **15 MINUTES** ■ TOTAL TIME: **25 MINUTES**

Makes 4 servings

6 ounces mushrooms, quartered

½ red onion, quartered

½ cup chopped fresh cilantro

¼ cup ground flaxseeds

2 cloves garlic

1 egg white

1 teaspoon salt

1 can (15 ounces) no-salt-added black beans, rinsed and drained

1 tablespoon canola oil

4 slices reduced-fat pepper Jack cheese

4 whole grain sandwich thins, split

4 lettuce leaves

1 small tomato, sliced

1. In a food processor, process the mushrooms, onion, cilantro, flaxseeds, garlic, egg white, and salt until finely chopped. Add the beans and pulse 15 times, or until coarsely chopped. Evenly divide the mixture into 4 burgers.

2. In a large skillet, heat the oil over medium heat. Cook the burgers for 6 minutes, turning once. Top each burger with a slice of cheese. Cover the skillet and cook for 3 minutes, or until the cheese melts.

3. Place on the sandwich thins and top with the lettuce and tomato.

VEGETABLE PIZZA

PREP TIME: **20 MINUTES** ■ TOTAL TIME: **1 HOUR 20 MINUTES**

Makes 8 servings

⅔ cup warm water (105°–115°F)

1 envelope (¼ ounce) active dry yeast (2¼ teaspoons)

2 teaspoons olive oil

2 cups whole wheat pastry or white whole wheat flour, divided

¼ teaspoon salt

1 tablespoon olive oil

1½ cups frozen mixed bell peppers, thawed

1 package (10 ounces) frozen chopped spinach, thawed and drained well

1 clove garlic, minced

1 can (14.5 ounces) diced tomatoes, well drained

4 ounces fresh mozzarella cheese, shredded

1. Coat a large bowl with cooking spray. Set aside.

2. In a glass measuring cup, mix the water and the yeast to dissolve. Stir in the oil.

3. In a food processor, pulse 1¾ cups of the flour and the salt to mix. With the machine running, add the yeast water through the feed tube. Process for 2 minutes, or until the mixture forms a moist ball. Transfer the dough to a work surface lightly floured with some of the remaining ¼ cup flour. Knead for 1 minute, or until the dough is smooth. Place the dough in the prepared bowl. Coat lightly with cooking spray. Cover with plastic wrap. Set aside to rise for about 30 minutes, or until doubled in size.

4. Coat a 14" round pizza pan with cooking spray. Punch down the dough. Transfer to a lightly floured surface. Let stand for 5 minutes. With floured hands or a rolling pin, pat or roll into a 14" circle. Transfer to the prepared pan. Pinch the edges to make a border. Cover with plastic wrap and let stand for 15 minutes. Preheat the oven to 375°F.

5. In a large skillet, heat the oil over medium-high heat. Cook the peppers for 3 minutes or until lightly browned. Stir in the spinach and garlic and cook, stirring, for 3 minutes. Add the tomatoes and cook, stirring, for 3 minutes, or until any liquid evaporates.

6. Spread the tomato mixture over the crust. Sprinkle with the cheese. Bake for 15 minutes, or until golden and bubbly. Cut into 8 slices.

Makeover Magic

BEFORE		AFTER
330	CALORIES	243
11 g	FAT	8 g
6 g	SAT FAT	3 g
39 g	CARBS	27 g
3 g	FIBER	5 g
14 g	PROTEIN	14 g
890 mg	SODIUM	452 mg

Curb carbs: Making this delicious, doughy whole wheat pizza crust from scratch eliminates extra sugars and processed ingredients that can drive the carb count way up and wreak havoc on your health.

Fill up on fiber: Whole grain pizza dough contributes the bulk of fiber in this recipe—add on your own homemade sauce and you have a great, fresh, fiber-full pizza.

Favor fats: Olive oil provides plenty of MUFAs, but for more healthy fats, you can always top with sliced olives.

BEFORE		AFTER
548	CALORIES	240
19 g	FAT	8 g
10 g	SAT FAT	4 g
69 g	CARBS	35 g
3 g	FIBER	8 g
22 g	PROTEIN	10 g
1,022 mg	SODIUM	315 mg

Curb carbs: A thin 11" pizza crust makes a delicious and crunchy low-carb pizza.

Fill up on fiber: We chose a whole wheat crust, and using beans as a pizza sauce pumps up both the fiber and protein in this dish.

Favor fats: We use olive oil in this delicious slice of the Mediterranean; for a bigger boost of healthy fats, top the pizza with sliced kalamata olives.

CARAMELIZED ONION AND FENNEL PIZZA

PREP TIME: **10 MINUTES** ■ TOTAL TIME: **45 MINUTES**

Makes 6 servings

1 large red onion, cut into 8 wedges

1 small fennel bulb, thinly sliced

2 plum tomatoes, chopped

3 cloves garlic, thinly sliced

1 tablespoon olive oil

1 tablespoon chopped fresh rosemary or 1 teaspoon dried

¼ teaspoon red-pepper flakes

1 cup no-salt-added cannellini beans, rinsed and drained

1 thin whole wheat pizza crust (11" diameter)

2 ounces reduced-fat goat cheese, crumbled

1. Preheat the oven to 450°F. On a baking sheet or roasting pan, combine the onion, fennel, tomatoes, and garlic. Add the oil, rosemary, and red-pepper flakes. Toss to coat well.

2. Roast for 25 minutes, stirring occasionally, or until the vegetables are tender and lightly browned.

3. In a medium bowl, mash the beans until coarsely mashed. Spread evenly over the pizza crust, leaving a ½" border all around. Scatter the vegetables over the top. Sprinkle with the cheese. Bake for 10 minutes, or until the topping is hot and the crust is crisp. Let stand for 5 minutes before cutting into 6 slices.

Vegetarian

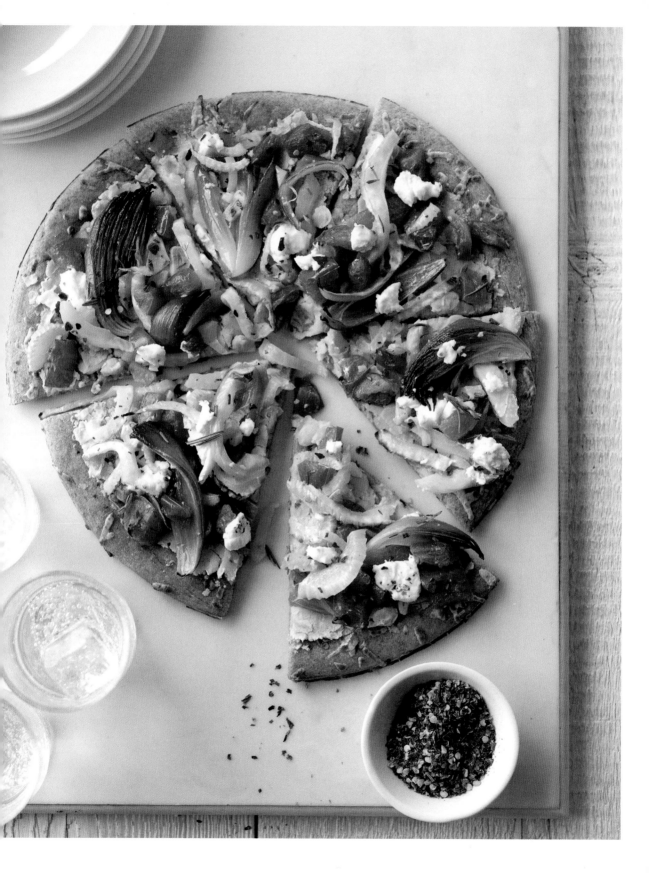

CHAPTER**ELEVEN**

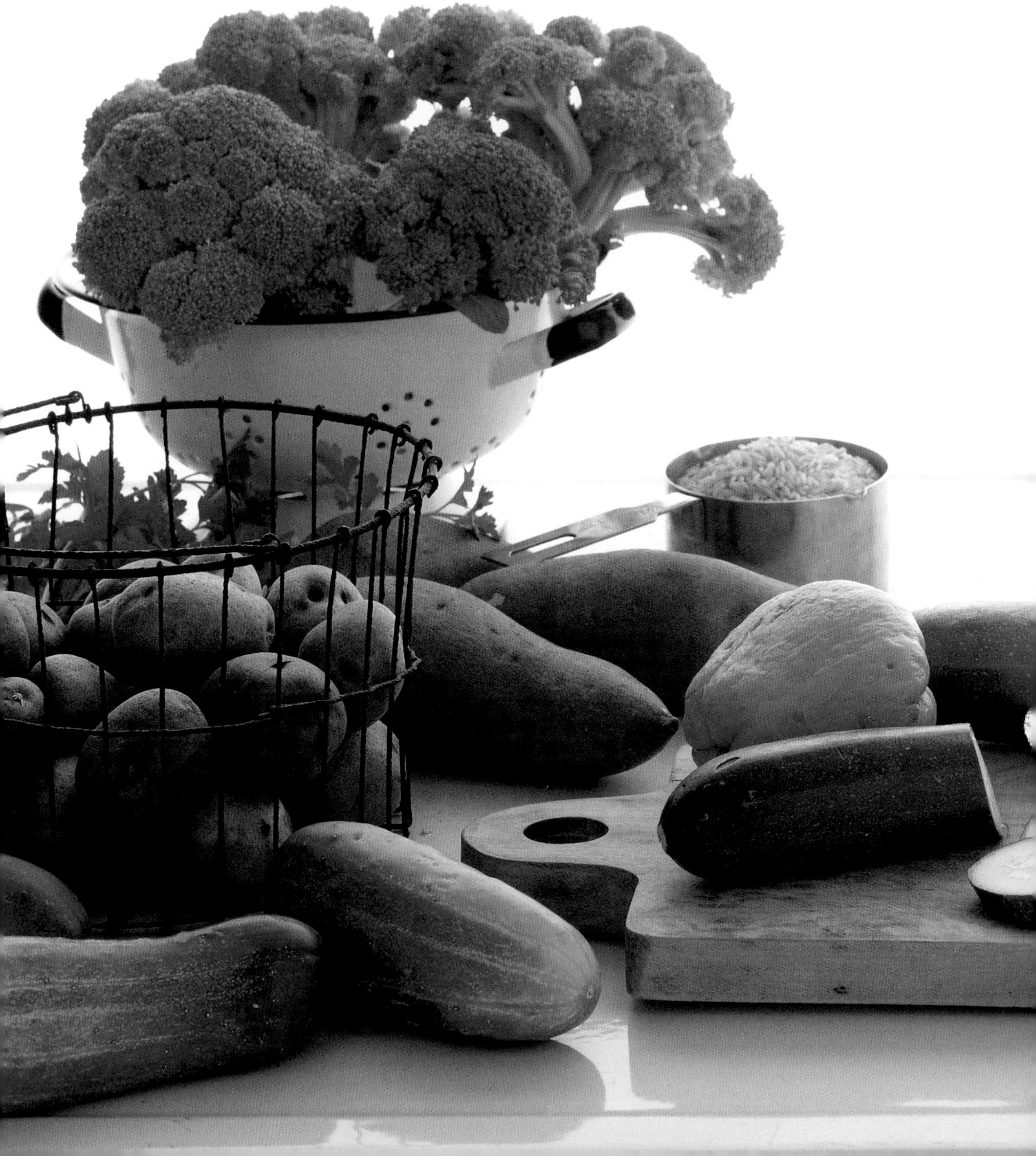

Sides

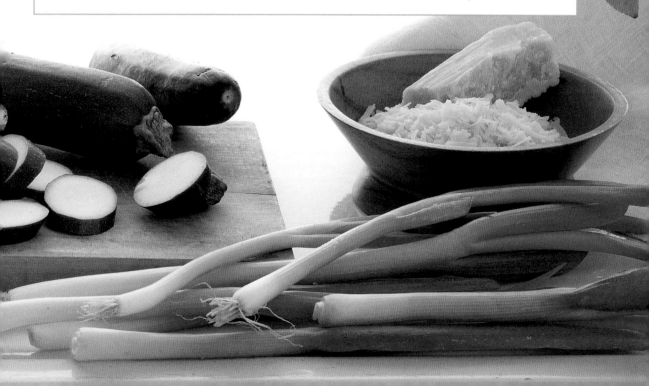

BEFORE		AFTER
175	CALORIES	86
7 g	FAT	4 g
1 g	SAT FAT	0.5 g
16 g	CARBS	11 g
4 g	FIBER	5 g
3 g	PROTEIN	4 g
550 mg	SODIUM	135 mg

Curb carbs: This naturally low-carb dish was made over to raise the fiber and get healthy fats into your meal. It would pair well with Tuna Tetrazzini (page 244) or Chicken Pad Thai (page 217).

Fill up on fiber: Asparagus contributes the bulk of the fiber in this dish at nearly 4 grams.

Favor fats: Sesame seeds, sesame oil, and canola oil are all full of diabetes-friendly fats, making this a great side to pair with low-in-fat main course recipes.

STIR-FRIED ASPARAGUS WITH GINGER, SESAME, AND SOY

PREP TIME: **15 MINUTES** ■ TOTAL TIME: **25 MINUTES**

Makes 4 servings

1½ pounds thin asparagus, trimmed and cut into 2" pieces

2 teaspoons canola oil

1 red bell pepper, seeded and cut into strips

1 tablespoon chopped fresh ginger or 1 teaspoon ground

1 tablespoon reduced-sodium soy sauce

1 teaspoon toasted sesame oil

1 teaspoon sesame seeds

1. In a large nonstick skillet, bring ¼" of water to a boil over high heat. Add the asparagus and return to a boil. Reduce the heat to low, cover, and simmer for 5 minutes, or until tender-crisp. Drain and cool briefly under cold running water. Wipe the skillet dry with a paper towel.

2. Heat the canola oil in the same skillet over high heat. Cook the pepper, stirring constantly, for 3 minutes, or until tender-crisp. Add the asparagus, ginger, and soy sauce and cook for 2 minutes, or until heated through. Remove from the heat and stir in the sesame oil and sesame seeds.

GREEN BEAN CASSEROLE

PREP TIME: **15 MINUTES** ■ TOTAL TIME: **1 HOUR 5 MINUTES**

Makes 8 servings

½ cup buttermilk

½ cup whole wheat panko bread crumbs

1 onion, cut crosswise into ¼"-thick slices and separated into rings

½ pound mushrooms, sliced

1 small onion, chopped

½ teaspoon dried thyme

¼ teaspoon salt

¼ cup whole wheat pastry flour

3 cups 1% milk

1 bag (16 ounces) frozen French-cut green beans, thawed and drained

¼ cup almonds, sliced

1. Preheat the oven to 500°F. Coat a medium baking dish with cooking spray. Coat a baking sheet with cooking spray.

2. In a shallow bowl, place the buttermilk. In another shallow bowl, place the bread crumbs. Dip the onion rings into the buttermilk, dredge in the bread crumbs, and place on the baking sheet. Coat lightly with cooking spray. Bake for 20 minutes, or until tender and golden brown.

3. Meanwhile, coat a large saucepan with cooking spray. Set over medium heat. Add the mushrooms, chopped onion, thyme, and salt. Coat with cooking spray. Cook, stirring occasionally, for 5 minutes, or until the mushrooms give off liquid. Sprinkle with the flour. Cook, stirring, for 1 minute. Add the milk. Cook, stirring constantly, for 4 minutes, or until thickened. Add the green beans and almonds. Stir to mix.

4. Reduce the oven temperature to 400°F. Pour the bean mixture into the prepared baking dish. Scatter the onion rings over the top. Bake for 30 minutes, or until hot and bubbly.

Makeover Magic

BEFORE		AFTER
315	CALORIES	115
22 g	FAT	2 g
11 g	SAT FAT	0.5 g
23 g	CARBS	20 g
4 g	FIBER	4 g
11 g	PROTEIN	7 g
711 mg	SODIUM	146 mg

Curb carbs: For an autumnal feel, pair this naturally low-carb dish with a turkey-centered main, like Sweet Potato and Turkey Shepherd's Pie (page 219).

Fill up on fiber: The green beans are a fiber boss! Using homemade onion rings with panko breading instead of the prepackaged kind also adds fiber.

Favor fats: Almonds are a great source of healthy MUFAs for this holiday favorite!

BEFORE		AFTER
190	CALORIES	120
13 g	FAT	6 g
8 g	SAT FAT	2 g
13 g	CARBS	15 g
2 g	FIBER	7 g
6 g	PROTEIN	4 g
660 mg	SODIUM	216 mg

Curb carbs: While this dish is typically not high in carbs, we've still worked our magic on it by eliminating flour from the sauce and instead using cream cheese to thicken it. While our carbs are slightly higher than typical creamed spinach, we make up for it with a huge boost in the fiber content!

Fill up on fiber: Spinach is already a great source of fiber. Toss in artichokes and you'll be surprised how high the fiber count rises in this classic dish.

Favor fats: Sautéing in healthy olive oil instead of butter adds MUFAs to this dish. Be sure to serve this with a main dish high in healthy fats to get enough to reap the benefits on your blood sugar.

CREAMED SPINACH AND ARTICHOKES

PREP TIME: **10 MINUTES** ■ TOTAL TIME: **20 MINUTES**

Makes 4 servings

1 tablespoon olive oil

1 onion, chopped

1 clove garlic, minced

¼ cup vegetable broth

1 pound baby spinach

1 box (9 ounces) frozen artichokes, thawed and chopped

3 ounces reduced-fat cream cheese, cubed

⅛ teaspoon ground black pepper

⅛ teaspoon ground nutmeg

1. In a large nonstick skillet, heat the oil over medium-high heat. Cook the onion and garlic for 5 minutes, stirring occasionally, or until softened. Add the broth and bring to a simmer. Cook the spinach for 4 minutes, tossing frequently, or just until wilted.

2. Stir in the artichokes, cream cheese, pepper, and nutmeg and cook for 1 minute, or until the cream cheese melts and is well blended.

CREAMED SWEET CORN

PREP TIME: 5 MINUTES ■ **TOTAL TIME: 25 MINUTES**

Makes 4 servings

1 tablespoon olive oil

1 small onion, diced

1 red bell pepper, diced

2 ribs celery, diced

2 cups fresh or frozen
  corn kernels

1 clove garlic, minced

¾ teaspoon salt

½ cup 2% evaporated milk

1 tablespoon ground
  flaxseeds

1. Heat the oil in a medium saucepan over medium heat. Cook the onion, pepper, and celery for 4 minutes, stirring often, or until soft. Add the corn, garlic, and salt and cook for 10 minutes, stirring often.

2. Pour in the milk and the ground flaxseeds. Cook over low heat for 2 minutes, or until the mixture is creamy.

Makeover Magic

BEFORE		AFTER
378	CALORIES	150
26 g	FAT	6 g
16 g	SAT FAT	1 g
34 g	CARBS	22 g
4 g	FIBER	3 g
8 g	PROTEIN	6 g
439 mg	SODIUM	492 mg

Curb carbs: We use less corn than a typical creamed corn recipe and fill the remainder with fresh bell pepper, onion, and celery.

Fill up on fiber: The fiber in this recipe comes from a riot of veggies tossed together here. The comparison only has more fiber because it contains twice the amount of corn.

Favor fats: Ground flaxseeds add ALA omega-3s to this dish. Using evaporated milk means there's no need for added butter and sugar.

BEFORE		AFTER
520	CALORIES	226
27 g	FAT	14 g
14 g	SAT FAT	4 g
59 g	CARBS	13 g
2 g	FIBER	4 g
12 g	PROTEIN	15 g
350 mg	SODIUM	353 mg

Curb carbs: This clever spaghetti squash swap means fewer carbs *and* way more nutrients than basic spaghetti has to offer.

Fill up on fiber: Flaxseeds, kale, and squash all work together to bring fiber to this side dish.

Favor fats: Keeping saturated fat low is easy when you choose reduced-fat cheese or simply use less of the full-fat variety. For MUFAs, almonds and canola oil go a long way!

CHEESE AND VEGETABLE BAKE

PREP TIME: **15 MINUTES** ■ TOTAL TIME: **1 HOUR 25 MINUTES**

Makes 6 servings

1 spaghetti squash, halved and seeded

2 tablespoons canola oil

4 cups chopped kale

2 plum tomatoes, chopped

2 cloves garlic, chopped

1 cup 1% cottage cheese

½ cup shredded low-fat mozzarella cheese

¼ teaspoon salt

¼ cup grated Parmesan cheese

3 tablespoons ground flaxseeds

¼ cup finely chopped almonds

1. Preheat the oven to 400°F. Coat a 13" × 9" baking dish and a baking sheet with cooking spray. On the prepared baking sheet, place the squash, cut side down. Bake for 30 minutes, or until tender. With a fork, scrape the squash strands into a large bowl.

2. Meanwhile, heat the oil in a medium skillet over medium heat. Cook the kale for 10 minutes, stirring, or until tender. Add the tomatoes and garlic and cook for 3 minutes.

3. Add the cottage cheese, mozzarella, salt, and the tomato mixture to the bowl with the squash. Toss to coat. Place in the prepared baking dish. Sprinkle the Parmesan, flaxseeds, and almonds over the top.

4. Bake for 30 minutes, or until hot and bubbly.

GARLIC OVEN FRIES

PREP TIME: **5 MINUTES** ■ TOTAL TIME: **40 MINUTES**

Makes 4 servings

1 pound russet (baking) potatoes, cut into 3½" × ½" sticks

3 carrots, quartered lengthwise and cut into 3⅓" sticks

2 tablespoons canola oil

¼ teaspoon garlic salt

¼ teaspoon ground black pepper

1. Preheat the oven to 450°F. Coat 2 large baking sheets with cooking spray.

2. In a large bowl, combine the potatoes, carrots, oil, garlic salt, and pepper, tossing to coat well. On the baking sheets, arrange the potatoes and carrots in a single layer. Bake for 30 minutes, turning once, or until golden and crisp.

Makeover Magic

BEFORE		AFTER
500	CALORIES	221
25 g	FAT	4 g
4 g	SAT FAT	2 g
63 g	CARBS	27 g
6 g	FIBER	2 g
6 g	PROTEIN	3 g
350 mg	SODIUM	97 mg

Curb carbs: Carrots may seem an unlikely choice for fries, but this root vegetable is a delicious low-carb choice that fits in great with the russet potatoes.

Fill up on fiber: The potatoes take the lead when it comes to fiber—just remember to include the skins! The comparison has higher fiber only because it solely uses potatoes instead of including carrots.

Favor fats: Instead of deep frying, use a small amount of canola oil, our favored fat in this recipe.

Makeover Magic

BEFORE		AFTER
570	CALORIES	303
30 g	FAT	9 g
11 g	SAT FAT	2 g
58 g	CARBS	48 g
8 g	FIBER	5 g
18 g	PROTEIN	8 g
1,200 mg	SODIUM	77 mg

Curb carbs: The homemade version of this fast-food favorite is still high in carbs, so be sure to pair it with a low-carb, high-fiber main dish such as the Cobb Salad–Style Buffalo Dogs (page 176).

Fill up on fiber: The best way to keep fiber in a potato-based dish is to keep the skin on the potatoes.

Favor fats: Instead of using real chili on these fries, get the same flavor without all the saturated fat by using chili powder and Cheddar cheese instead. Using olive oil to cook the fries adds MUFA power!

CHILI CHEESE FRIES

PREP TIME: **10 MINUTES** ■ TOTAL TIME: **40 MINUTES**

Makes 4 servings

2 tablespoons olive oil

2 teaspoons chili powder

½ teaspoon ground cumin

2 medium russet potatoes, each cut into 16 wedges

¼ cup shredded reduced-fat Cheddar cheese

1. Preheat the oven to 450°F. Coat 2 large-rimmed baking sheets with cooking spray.

2. In a large bowl, combine the oil, chili powder, and cumin until blended. Add the potatoes and toss to coat well. Arrange the potatoes in a single layer on the baking sheets.

3. Bake for 30 minutes, turning once, or until golden brown and crisp. Sprinkle with the cheese and bake for 1 minute, or until the cheese is melted.

CREAMY MASHED POTATOES

PREP TIME: **10 MINUTES** ■ TOTAL TIME: **30 MINUTES**

Makes 6 servings

1 pound russet (baking) potatoes, peeled and halved

1 small head cauliflower, cut into florets

⅓ cup vegetable broth

2 tablespoons olive oil

½ cup plain 0% Greek yogurt

1. In a large pot, combine the potatoes and cauliflower and cover with water. Over high heat, bring to a boil. Reduce the heat to medium and simmer for 20 minutes, or until the potatoes and cauliflower are easily pierced with a fork. Drain.

2. In a large bowl, place the drained potatoes, cauliflower, broth, and oil. With an electric mixer on medium speed, beat until creamy. Add the yogurt and beat just until blended.

Makeover Magic

BEFORE		AFTER
250	CALORIES	132
8 g	FAT	5 g
5 g	SAT FAT	1 g
39 g	CARBS	19 g
2 g	FIBER	3 g
5 g	PROTEIN	5 g
370 mg	SODIUM	347 mg

Curb carbs: This is the ultimate in sneaky substitutions—by cutting half of the potatoes by substituting cauliflower, we also cut the carbs in half, while adding a rich, creamy flavor.

Fill up on fiber: Just one little cauliflower head contributes twice as much fiber to this dish as a whole pound of potatoes. To up the fiber more, try leaving the potato peels intact and going for "smashed" potatoes instead.

Favor fats: Typically, mashed potatoes are full of butter. Adding olive oil for healthy fat and Greek yogurt for creaminess is a healthier alternative.

Makeover Magic

BEFORE		AFTER
740	CALORIES	256
46 g	FAT	5 g
28 g	SAT FAT	3 g
54 g	CARBS	42 g
11 g	FIBER	5 g
3 g	PROTEIN	12 g
1,260 mg	SODIUM	181 mg

Curb carbs: We reduced the flour in this dish and added chia seeds to help thicken the milk.

Fill up on fiber: Chia seeds are an excellent source of fiber, but of course the potatoes here provide the most fiber of all!

Favor fats: By using a smaller amount of cheese, we reduced the saturated fat, while adding chia seeds offers up ALA omega-3 fatty acids.

SCALLOPED RED POTATOES

PREP TIME: **20 MINUTES** ■ TOTAL TIME: **1 HOUR 5 MINUTES**

Makes 4 servings

3 tablespoons whole wheat flour

2 tablespoons white chia seeds

¼ teaspoon ground nutmeg

6 medium red potatoes, scrubbed and cut into ½" slices

6 scallions, chopped

1 cup shredded 4-cheese Italian blend, divided

1 cup 1% milk

1. Preheat the oven to 400°F. Coat an 11" × 7" baking dish with cooking spray. In a small bowl, stir together the flour, chia seeds, and nutmeg.

2. Arrange one-third of the potatoes in the dish. Sprinkle with one-third of the flour mixture, one-third of the scallions, and one-third of the cheese. Repeat the layers twice. Pour the milk over the top. Cover and bake for 25 minutes.

3. Uncover and bake for 20 minutes, or until the potatoes are tender and browned.

SMARTSTART

Serve with wild salmon or grilled chicken.

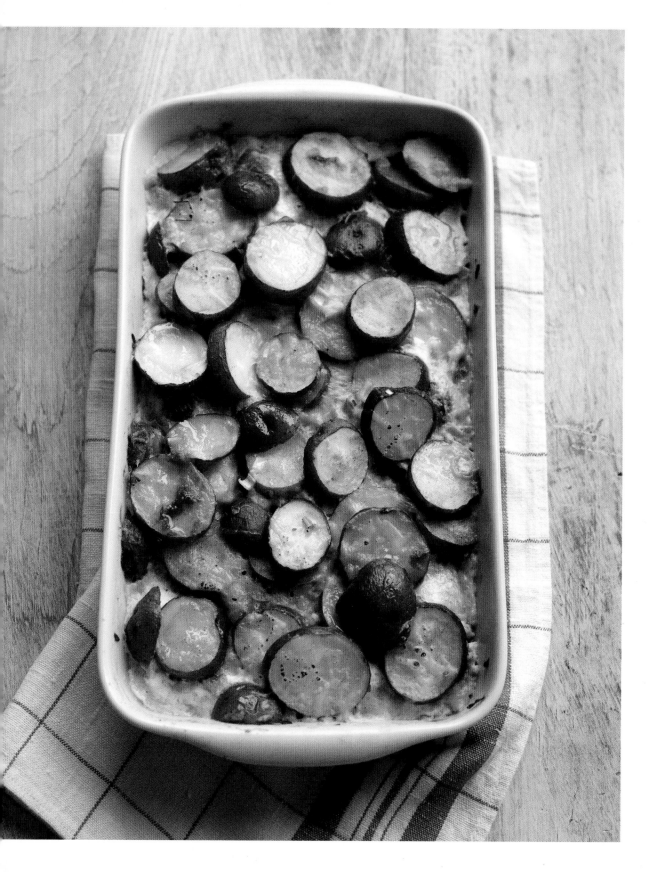

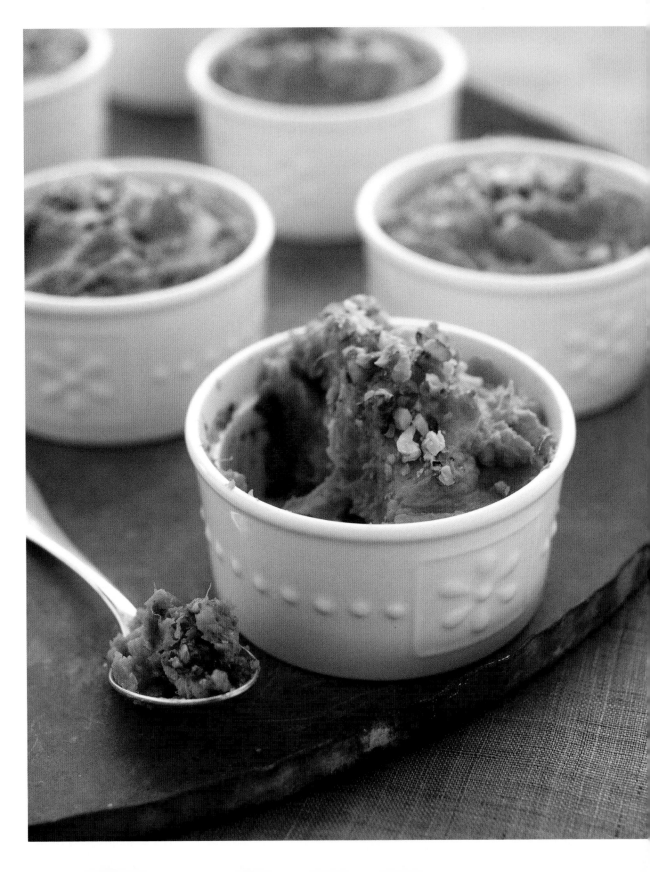

WHIPPED SWEET POTATO CASSEROLES

PREP TIME: **10 MINUTES** ▪ TOTAL TIME: **35 MINUTES**

Makes 6 servings

8 tablespoons walnuts, finely chopped, divided

2 tablespoons ground flaxseeds

2½ tablespoons canola oil, divided

1½ pounds sweet potatoes, peeled and cut into ½" cubes

⅓ cup orange juice

2 tablespoons fat-free half-and-half

½ teaspoon pumpkin pie spice

⅛ teaspoon salt

⅛ teaspoon ground black pepper

1. Preheat the oven to 400°F. Coat six 4-ounce ramekins with cooking spray. Place on a baking sheet.

2. In a small bowl, combine 6 tablespoons of the walnuts, the flaxseeds, and 1½ tablespoons of the oil until blended. Divide the mixture among the ramekins and press with a fork to cover the bottoms of the ramekins.

3. In a large saucepan with a steamer basket inserted, bring 2" of water to a boil over high heat. Add the sweet potatoes, cover, and cook over medium heat for 15 minutes, or until very tender.

4. In a medium bowl, place the potatoes. Add the orange juice, half-and-half, pumpkin pie spice, salt, pepper, and the remaining 1 tablespoon oil. With an electric mixer, beat the mixture until smooth. Divide among the ramekins. Sprinkle with the remaining 2 tablespoons walnuts.

5. Bake for 10 minutes, or until golden brown.

Makeover Magic

BEFORE		AFTER
480	CALORIES	222
22 g	FAT	13 g
10 g	SAT FAT	1 g
69 g	CARBS	24 g
4 g	FIBER	5 g
5 g	PROTEIN	4 g
190 mg	SODIUM	112 mg

Curb carbs: There's no need to sweeten this side with sugar—pumpkin pie spice adds nice flavor to these already-sweet potatoes.

Fill up on fiber: Walnuts are our main source of fiber in this dish.

Favor fats: This dish is full of beneficial fats. MUFAs come from the canola oil and walnuts, while ALA omega-3 fatty acids come from the ground flaxseeds.

Makeover Magic

BEFORE		AFTER
310	CALORIES	196
11 g	FAT	4 g
6 g	SAT FAT	1 g
46 g	CARBS	35 g
3 g	FIBER	7 g
6 g	PROTEIN	7 g
500 mg	SODIUM	238 mg

Curb carbs: Turn this dish into a blood sugar buster by switching from a base of bread (usually low-fiber white) to barley. Thanks to the rule of magic carbs, this makes a great side dish to just about any main course recipe.

Fill up on fiber: Barley and mushrooms both lead to a high fiber count.

Favor fats: Canola oil and chia seeds provide delicious healthy fats.

MUSHROOM-BARLEY STUFFING

PREP TIME: **15 MINUTES** ■ TOTAL TIME: **1 HOUR 20 MINUTES**

Makes 8 servings

1 ounce dried porcini mushrooms

2 cups hot water

2 tablespoons canola oil

1 package (8 ounces) sliced mushrooms

2 ribs celery, chopped

1 large red onion, chopped

2 cloves garlic, minced

½ teaspoon dried rosemary

½ teaspoon dried thyme

2 cups pearl barley

3 cups reduced-sodium chicken broth

¼ cup chia seeds

2 tablespoons grated Romano cheese

¼ teaspoon salt

¼ teaspoon ground black pepper

1. Preheat the oven to 400°F. Coat a 3-quart baking dish with cooking spray.

2. In a small bowl, combine the porcini mushrooms and water and let stand for 20 minutes, or until the mushrooms are soft. Using a slotted spoon, remove the mushrooms. Chop and set aside. Strain the liquid into a small bowl through a fine sieve lined with cheesecloth or a coffee filter. Set aside.

3. In a medium saucepan, heat the oil over medium-high heat. Cook the sliced mushrooms, celery, onion, garlic, rosemary, and thyme, stirring, for 10 minutes, or until the mushroom liquid has evaporated.

4. Add the reserved porcini mushrooms and the barley. Cook, stirring, for 4 minutes. Add the reserved mushroom liquid and the broth and bring to a boil. Remove from the heat. Stir in the chia seeds, cheese, salt, and pepper.

5. Place in the prepared dish. Cover and bake for 40 minutes, or until the barley is tender.

BARLEY PILAF WITH ARTICHOKES AND KALE

PREP TIME: **15 MINUTES** ■ TOTAL TIME: **1 HOUR 5 MINUTES**

Makes 6 servings

1 tablespoon canola oil

1 onion, chopped

1 carrot, chopped

1 rib celery, chopped

½ cup barley

1 clove garlic, minced

2½ cups reduced-sodium vegetable or chicken broth

½ cup water

¼ cup bulgur wheat

4 cups chopped kale

1 package (9 ounces) frozen artichoke hearts

½ teaspoon lemon zest

1. In a medium saucepan, heat the oil over medium-high heat. Cook the onion, carrot, and celery for 5 minutes, stirring, or until softened. Add the barley and garlic and cook, stirring, for 3 minutes.

2. Stir in the broth and water and bring to a boil over high heat. Reduce the heat to low, cover, and simmer for 25 minutes. Stir in the bulgur and kale and cook for 5 minutes. Stir in the artichokes and lemon zest and cook for 10 minutes, or until all of the broth is absorbed and the barley is al dente.

Makeover Magic

BEFORE		AFTER
260	CALORIES	162
7 g	FAT	4 g
3 g	SAT FAT	0.5 g
42 g	CARBS	30 g
0 g	FIBER	8 g
7 g	PROTEIN	6 g
700 mg	SODIUM	262 mg

Curb carbs: Barley is much more nutritious than white rice. To reduce carbs, reduce the amount of grain and bulk the dish up with vegetables.

Fill up on fiber: Artichokes, kale, and barley work together to give this dish 8 grams of fiber! Using the magic carbs rule makes this a perfect accompaniment to a low-carb main dish recipe.

Favor fats: Artichokes and canola oil are the healthy fat stars in this pilaf.

Makeover Magic

BEFORE		AFTER
470	CALORIES	235
18 g	FAT	12 g
8 g	SAT FAT	1 g
71 g	CARBS	26 g
3 g	FIBER	9 g
11 g	PROTEIN	7 g
440 mg	SODIUM	295 mg

Curb carbs: Quinoa has fewer carbs per serving than rice and is always a smart pick for blood sugar control.

Fill up on fiber: Quinoa is also high in fiber, bringing this meal over the "magic carbs" number all on its own at more than 7 grams per serving.

Favor fats: Pistachios are a great source of MUFAs. Meanwhile, olive oil is a smart pick over vegetable oil to keep saturated fat low and healthy fats abundant.

QUINOA PILAF WITH PISTACHIOS

PREP TIME: **10 MINUTES** ■ TOTAL TIME: **35 MINUTES**

Makes 6 servings

2 tablespoons olive oil
1 cup quinoa, rinsed
4 scallions, chopped
1 clove garlic, minced
1½ cups water

1 cup vegetable broth
¼ teaspoon ground cardamom
½ cup pistachios, chopped

1. In a medium saucepan, heat the oil over medium heat. Cook the quinoa, scallions, and garlic for 3 minutes, stirring, or until the vegetables are softened.

2. Add the water, broth, and cardamom and bring to a boil. Reduce the heat to low, cover, and simmer for 20 minutes, or until the quinoa is tender. Remove from the heat and set aside for 5 minutes. Stir in the pistachios.

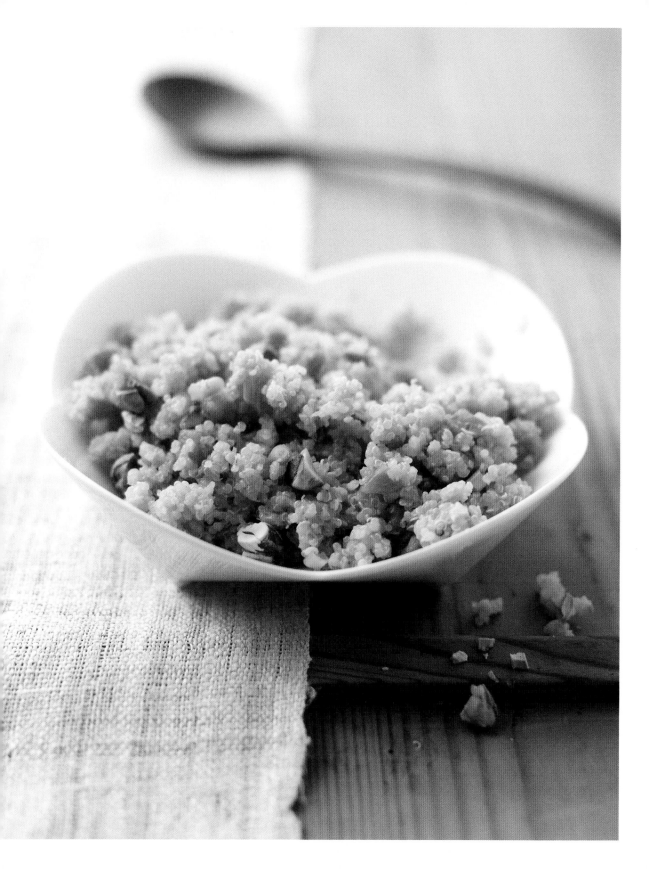

Makeover Magic

BEFORE		AFTER
470	CALORIES	236
23 g	FAT	8 g
12 g	SAT FAT	2 g
50 g	CARBS	32 g
2 g	FIBER	3 g
18 g	PROTEIN	8 g
970 mg	SODIUM	383 mg

Curb carbs: Using half wild rice, half brown rice cuts down on the carbs while adding variety to the flavor and texture of this risotto.

Fill up on fiber: Rice and peas are both packed with fiber.

Favor fats: Typically this dish would be cooked in lots of butter, but using canola oil cuts down on saturated fat while boosting your dose of good fats.

BAKED RISOTTO

PREP TIME: **10 MINUTES** ■ TOTAL TIME: **1 HOUR 10 MINUTES**

Makes 4 servings

2 tablespoons canola oil

1 onion, chopped

1 medium red bell pepper, chopped

½ cup brown rice, preferably short or medium grain

½ cup wild rice

1 clove garlic, minced

3 cups vegetable broth

1 cup frozen peas, thawed

⅓ cup grated Romano cheese

1. Preheat the oven to 425°F. In a large ovenproof saucepan or Dutch oven, heat the oil over medium heat. Cook the onion and pepper for 3 minutes. Add the brown rice, wild rice, and garlic and cook, stirring, for 2 minutes, or until the rice is coated.

2. Add the broth and bring to a boil. Cover and place in the oven. Bake for 55 minutes, or until the broth is absorbed and the rice is just tender. Remove from the oven and stir in the peas and cheese. Cover and let stand for 5 minutes.

BROCCOLI-WALNUT FARFALLE TOSS

PREP TIME: **10 MINUTES** ■ TOTAL TIME: **25 MINUTES**

Makes 4 servings

4   ounces whole grain farfalle (bow-tie) pasta

1   bunch broccoli, cut into florets

2   tablespoons canola oil

1   small red onion, thinly sliced

¼   teaspoon salt

⅛   teaspoon ground black pepper

1½ ounces crumbled goat cheese

⅓   cup walnuts, toasted and coarsely chopped

1. Prepare the pasta according to package directions, adding the broccoli during the last 4 minutes of cooking time. Drain, reserving ¼ cup of the cooking water. Transfer the pasta and broccoli to a bowl.

2. In the same pot, heat the oil over medium heat. Cook the onion for 5 minutes, stirring occasionally, or until softened.

3. Stir in the drained pasta and broccoli, reserved pasta cooking water, salt, and pepper. Cook for 1 minute, stirring, or until heated through. Remove from the heat and stir in the goat cheese. Sprinkle with the walnuts.

Makeover Magic

BEFORE		AFTER
680	CALORIES	307
39 g	FAT	16 g
6 g	SAT FAT	3 g
63 g	CARBS	32 g
5 g	FIBER	7 g
19 g	PROTEIN	13 g
830 mg	SODIUM	249 mg

Curb carbs: We reduced the pasta in this recipe by half and tossed in broccoli, which—while also high in carbs—packs more fiber.

Fill up on fiber: Using whole grain varieties is an easy way to up the fiber in any pasta recipe. Toss in high-fiber veggies like broccoli and you're all set!

Favor fats: Walnuts and canola oil bring the MUFAs and omega-3 fatty acids to this dish. Goat cheese is a delicious gourmet dairy item that's also relatively low in saturated fat.

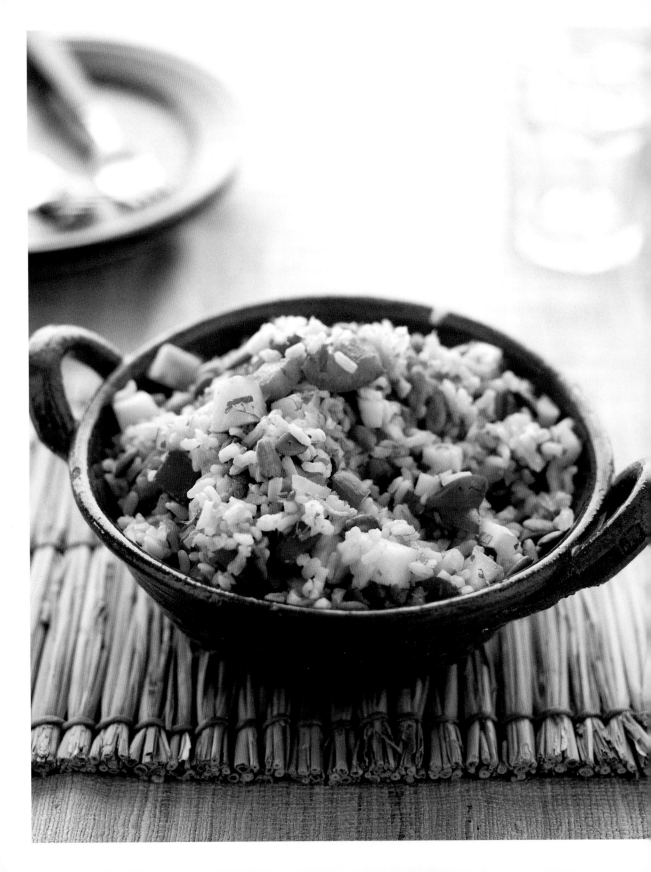

MEXICAN FRIED RICE

PREP TIME: **15 MINUTES** ▪ TOTAL TIME: **25 MINUTES**

Makes 8 servings

1 tablespoon olive oil

1 onion, chopped

1 medium zucchini, chopped

1 chayote squash, peeled, seeded, and chopped

1 red bell pepper, chopped

1 teaspoon ground cumin

1½ cups cooked brown rice, chilled

1 cup pumpkin seeds, toasted

½ teaspoon salt

2 tablespoons chopped fresh cilantro

1 teaspoon freshly grated lime zest

1. In a large nonstick skillet, heat the oil over medium-high heat. Cook the onion, zucchini, squash, pepper, and cumin, stirring, for 5 minutes, or until tender-crisp.

2. Add the rice and cook, stirring often, for 2 minutes, or until lightly toasted.

3. Stir in the pumpkin seeds and salt and cook for 1 minute. Remove from the heat and stir in the cilantro and lime zest.

Makeover Magic

BEFORE		AFTER
260	CALORIES	118
8 g	FAT	6 g
2 g	SAT FAT	1 g
33 g	CARBS	14 g
2 g	FIBER	3 g
14 g	PROTEIN	6 g
700 mg	SODIUM	106 mg

Curb carbs: We can use less rice in this side because of the large amount of vegetables tossed in.

Fill up on fiber: Brown rice is higher in fiber than the white rice typically used in this type of recipe. The chopped veggies also add fiber.

Favor fats: Pumpkin seeds are a delicious source of diabetes-friendly fats that add unexpected flavor to fried rice.

BEFORE		AFTER
730	CALORIES	219
43 g	FAT	18 g
21 g	SAT FAT	3 g
63 g	CARBS	8 g
3 g	FIBER	3 g
22 g	PROTEIN	7 g
370 mg	SODIUM	154 mg

Curb carbs: Shirataki noodles are naturally low in carbs and make a great swap for traditional wheat pasta.

Fill up on fiber: Spinach adds fiber and flavor to this blood-sugar–friendly pasta dish.

Favor fats: Walnuts, rich in ALAs, are the base of this sauce that's so rich and delicious you'd swear it was loaded with heavy cream.

FETTUCCINE WITH BASIL-WALNUT SAUCE

PREP TIME: **20 MINUTES** ■ TOTAL TIME: **20 MINUTES**

Makes 4 servings

1 package (8 ounces) shirataki fettuccine

½ cup walnuts, toasted and coarsely chopped

¼ cup fresh basil or 8 teaspoons dried

2 cloves garlic

2 tablespoons olive oil

3 cups baby spinach

½ cup plain 1% Greek yogurt

¼ cup grated Romano cheese

1. In a medium saucepan, prepare the fettuccine according to package directions. Drain and return to the saucepan.

2. Meanwhile, in a food processor or blender, process the walnuts, basil, and garlic until blended. Add the oil and pulse until well blended.

3. Add the pesto and spinach to the pan with the fettuccine. Over low heat, cook for 3 minutes, stirring, or until the spinach wilts. Remove from the heat and stir in the yogurt and cheese.

Sides

TEX-MEX PASTA AND BEANS

PREP TIME: **10 MINUTES** ■ TOTAL TIME: **25 MINUTES**

Makes 4 servings

1 cup whole wheat rotelle pasta

1 red onion, chopped

1 green bell pepper, chopped

½ teaspoon ground cumin

1 cup canned black beans, rinsed and drained

¾ cup salsa

2 tablespoons chopped fresh cilantro

½ avocado, peeled, seeded, and chopped

1. Prepare the pasta according to package directions.

2. Meanwhile, in a large nonstick skillet coated with cooking spray over medium-high heat, cook the onion and pepper for 5 minutes, stirring occasionally, or until softened. Add the cumin and cook for 1 minute, stirring, or until fragrant.

3. Stir in the pasta, beans, salsa, and cilantro. Cook for 1 minute, or until hot. Top with the avocado.

Makeover Magic

BEFORE		AFTER
460	CALORIES	230
17 g	FAT	5 g
9 g	SAT FAT	0.5 g
60 g	CARBS	41 g
4 g	FIBER	8 g
17 g	PROTEIN	8 g
940 mg	SODIUM	275 mg

Curb carbs: We use half the amount of pasta called for in typical dishes of this type and pump up the volume with vegetables like pepper and onion.

Fill up on fiber: Adding beans increases the fiber, as does switching from white pasta to whole wheat.

Favor fats: Not all pasta has to be bathed in rich, saturated fat–laden cheese sauce. Here, avocado adds favored fats and creaminess to this dish.

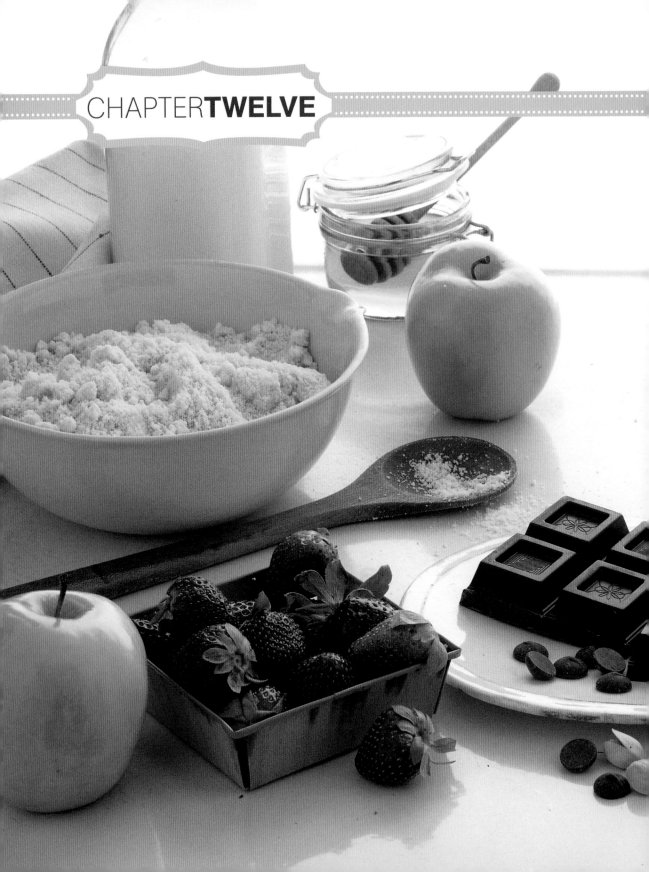

CHAPTER**TWELVE**

Desserts

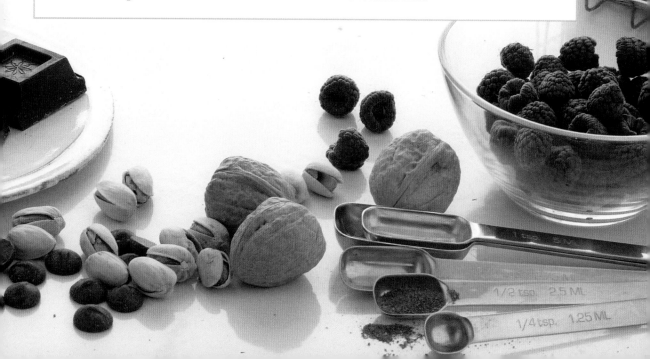

Makeover Magic

BEFORE		AFTER
499	CALORIES	151
27 g	FAT	8 g
4 g	SAT FAT	1 g
60 g	CARBS	18 g
2 g	FIBER	2 g
5 g	PROTEIN	3 g
407 mg	SODIUM	61 mg

Curb carbs: The average coffee cake recipe uses over a cup of sugar! Get delicious results with just 4 tablespoons of honey instead.

Fill up on fiber: Adding nuts and whole wheat flour boosts the fiber.

Favor fats: Pecans and canola oil are high in MUFAs. We cut the standard amount of butter from this recipe too, which decreases saturated fat.

ORANGE-PECAN TEA BREAD

PREP TIME: **15 MINUTES** ■ TOTAL TIME: **50 MINUTES**

Makes 9 servings

1 cup whole grain pastry flour

½ cup finely chopped pecans

2 tablespoons ground flaxseeds

1 teaspoon baking powder

½ teaspoon grated orange zest

¼ teaspoon ground cardamom

½ cup 1% milk

1 egg, lightly beaten

2 tablespoons canola oil

4 tablespoons honey, divided

1 tablespoon orange juice

1. Preheat the oven to 350°F. Coat a 9" × 5" loaf pan with cooking spray.

2. In a medium bowl, whisk together the flour, pecans, flaxseeds, baking powder, orange zest, and cardamom.

3. In a small bowl, whisk together the milk, egg, oil, and 2 tablespoons of the honey. Stir into the flour mixture just until combined.

4. In the prepared pan, spread the batter. Bake for 30 minutes, or until a wooden pick inserted in the center comes out clean. Cool in the pan on a rack for 10 minutes.

5. In a small saucepan, heat the remaining 2 tablespoons of honey and the orange juice until warm.

6. Using the tines of a fork, poke holes over the surface of the cake. Spoon on the honey mixture. Remove the cake from the pan and cut into 9 slices.

SMARTSTART

Serve with a cup of green or black tea for added antioxidants.

CHOCOLATE-ALMOND CAKE

PREP TIME: **15 MINUTES** ■ TOTAL TIME: **45 MINUTES**

Makes 12 servings

3 ounces bittersweet (60–75%) chocolate, coarsely chopped

½ cup blanched almonds

8 tablespoons sugar, divided

½ cup reduced-fat sour cream

¼ cup ground flaxseeds

3 omega-3–enriched egg yolks

2 tablespoons canola oil

1 teaspoon vanilla extract

½ teaspoon almond extract

3 tablespoons unsweetened cocoa powder

5 omega-3–enriched egg whites, at room temperature

¼ teaspoon salt

1. Preheat the oven to 350°F. Coat an 8" or 9" springform pan with cooking spray.

2. In a glass bowl, microwave the chocolate on high for 2 minutes, stirring every 30 seconds, or until smooth.

3. In a food processor, finely grind the almonds with 1 tablespoon of the sugar.

4. In a large bowl, stir together the melted chocolate, sour cream, flaxseeds, egg yolks, oil, vanilla, almond extract, 5 tablespoons of the remaining sugar, and the cocoa powder until well blended.

5. In another large bowl, with an electric mixer on high speed, beat the egg whites and salt until foamy. Gradually add the remaining 2 tablespoons of sugar, beating, until stiff peaks are formed.

6. Stir one-quarter of the beaten whites into the chocolate mixture. Gently fold in the remaining whites. Spoon into the pan. Smooth the top.

7. Bake for 30 minutes, or until the cake is dry on the top, and a wooden pick inserted in the center comes out with a few moist crumbs. Cool in the pan on a rack. The cake will fall dramatically. Loosen the edges of the cake with a knife and remove the pan sides.

Makeover Magic

BEFORE		AFTER
490	CALORIES	184
33 g	FAT	12 g
14 g	SAT FAT	3 g
47 g	CARBS	18 g
3 g	FIBER	3 g
6 g	PROTEIN	5 g
292 mg	SODIUM	80 mg

Curb carbs: Choose this cake over a frosted chocolate cake, which is loaded with carbs. By eliminating the flour and using nuts instead, not only did we curb the carbs, but we added healthy fats and pumped up the vitamins and minerals.

Fill up on fiber: The combination of chocolate with strawberries is delicious and also adds fiber.

Favor fats: Canola oil offers up both omega-3 fatty acids and MUFAs, and almonds add MUFAs, too.

Makeover Magic

BEFORE		AFTER
636	CALORIES	229
43 g	FAT	5 g
26 g	SAT FAT	1 g
52 g	CARBS	38 g
1 g	FIBER	6 g
9 g	PROTEIN	11 g
387 mg	SODIUM	214 mg

Curb carbs: Cut carbs by using a small amount of honey instead of sugar. Replacing cream cheese with cottage cheese adds protein, which is ideal for blood sugar control.

Fill up on fiber: Oat bran gives the crust a boost in fiber.

Favor fats: Ground flaxseeds serve up favored fats.

LEMON-RASPBERRY CHEESECAKE

PREP TIME: **15 MINUTES** ▪ TOTAL TIME: **55 MINUTES +
STANDING AND CHILLING TIMES**

Makes 8 servings

¼ cup oat bran

¼ cup ground golden flaxseeds

½ teaspoon ground cinnamon

1½ cups 1% cottage cheese

¼ cup buttermilk

6 tablespoons honey

3 tablespoons whole grain flour

½ teaspoon grated orange zest

1½ teaspoons grated lemon zest

Juice of 1 lemon

1 tablespoon vanilla extract

4 eggs, separated

1 pint raspberries

½ cup raspberry all-fruit jam

1. Preheat the oven to 350°F. Butter the bottom and sides of an 8" springform pan. In a medium bowl, combine the oat bran, flaxseeds, and cinnamon and sprinkle the mixture into the pan, tilting the pan to lightly coat the sides. Press the crumbs into the bottom of the pan.

2. In a food processor, combine the cottage cheese, buttermilk, honey, flour, orange zest, lemon zest, lemon juice, and vanilla and puree until smooth. Add the egg yolks and pulse to combine. Transfer to a large bowl.

3. In another large bowl, with an electric mixer on high speed, beat the egg whites until stiff peaks form. Gently fold the egg whites and raspberries into the cottage cheese mixture.

4. Pour the batter into the pan. Drop the fruit spread by tablespoons onto the top of the batter. With a knife, swirl the spread into the batter. Bake for 40 minutes, or until puffed and set. Turn off the oven and open the door for 1 minute to reduce the heat. Close the door and let the cheesecake remain in the oven for 1 hour. Refrigerate for 4 hours or overnight. Remove the pan sides before serving.

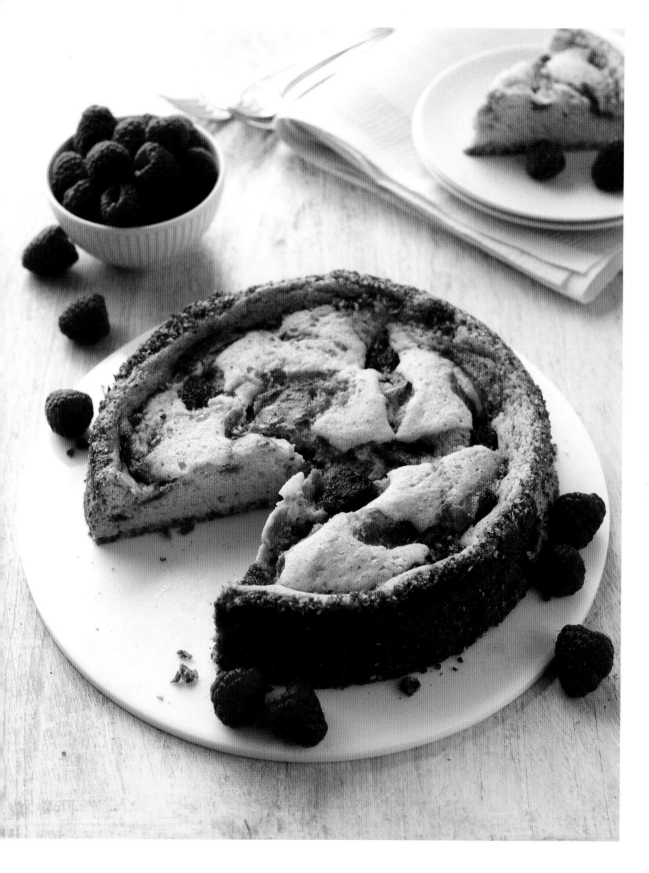

Makeover Magic

BEFORE		AFTER
420	CALORIES	229
16 g	FAT	14 g
4 g	SAT FAT	2 g
64 g	CARBS	22 g
1 g	FIBER	3 g
6 g	PROTEIN	5 g
300 mg	SODIUM	115 mg

Curb carbs: In order to cut the overall total grams of carbs per serving in this recipe, we substitute flaxseeds for some of the flour and use maple syrup as the main sweetener.

Fill up on fiber: Whole wheat pastry flour provides most of the fiber in this cake recipe.

Favor fats: Walnuts and flaxseeds add healthy fats. Instead of relying on butter, we use applesauce and whole eggs to give a moist tenderness to this cake.

MAPLE-WALNUT CAKE

PREP TIME: **30 MINUTES** ■ TOTAL TIME: **2 HOURS**

Makes 16 servings

½ cup canola oil

¾ cup maple syrup

½ cup unsweetened applesauce

4 omega-3–enriched eggs

1 teaspoon vanilla extract

1½ cups whole wheat pastry flour

¾ cup chopped walnuts

¼ cup ground golden flaxseeds

½ teaspoon baking soda

¼ teaspoon salt

⅔ cup reduced-fat sour cream

1. Preheat the oven to 300°F. Coat a 9" × 5" loaf pan with cooking spray.

2. In a large bowl, with an electric mixer on medium speed, beat the oil, syrup, and applesauce until light in color. Add the eggs one at a time, beating well after each addition. Beat in the vanilla.

3. In a medium bowl, whisk together the flour, walnuts, flaxseeds, baking soda, and salt. Alternately add the flour mixture and the sour cream to the maple mixture, beginning and ending with the flour mixture.

4. Pour the batter into the pan. Bake for 1 hour and 30 minutes, or until lightly browned and a wooden pick inserted in the center comes out clean.

5. Cool in the pan on a rack for 10 minutes. Run a spatula around the edges and invert the cake onto a rack. Turn upright and let cool completely on the rack.

COCONUT-LIME PUDDING CAKE

PREP TIME: **15 MINUTES** ■ TOTAL TIME: **50 MINUTES**

Makes 4 servings

3 limes

1 cup 1% milk

2 tablespoons canola oil

2 omega-3–enriched eggs, separated

⅛ teaspoon salt

⅓ cup whole grain pastry flour

½ cup unsweetened shredded coconut

1 egg white

¼ cup sugar

1. Preheat the oven to 350°F. Coat an 8" × 8" glass baking dish with cooking spray.

2. From the limes, grate 1½ teaspoons of zest and squeeze ⅓ cup of juice. In a large bowl, whisk together the milk, lime juice, oil, egg yolks, lime zest, and salt. Whisk in the flour and coconut until smooth.

3. In a separate large bowl, with an electric mixer on high speed, beat the 3 egg whites until soft peaks form. Gradually add the sugar while beating until stiff, glossy peaks form. Fold into the lime mixture. The batter will be lumpy and thin. Pour into the baking dish.

4. Place the baking dish in a large roasting pan. Fill with boiling water until it reaches halfway up the baking dish. Bake for 35 minutes, or until puffed and browned and the center of the cake is set. Cool on a rack for 15 minutes.

Makeover Magic

BEFORE		AFTER
580	CALORIES	203
41 g	FAT	12 g
27 g	SAT FAT	7 g
47 g	CARBS	19 g
1 g	FIBER	2 g
5 g	PROTEIN	4 g
270 mg	SODIUM	82 mg

Curb carbs: Enjoy the delicious flavors of a coconut cream pie—without all the carbs and calories.

Fill up on fiber: Coconut is a great source of fiber.

Favor fats: Be sure to use omega-3–enriched eggs and canola oil. They add diabetes-friendly fats.

BEFORE		AFTER
790	CALORIES	188
42 g	FAT	7 g
25 g	SAT FAT	4 g
104 g	CARBS	31 g
5 g	FIBER	2 g
10 g	PROTEIN	3 g
670 mg	SODIUM	104 mg

Curb carbs: Replacing sugar with maple syrup in the frosting is one quick way to curb carbs and make this cake diabetes-friendly.

Fill up on fiber: Whole grain pastry flour is a high-fiber alternative to white flour for this type of dessert.

Favor fats: Be sure to serve this dessert following a dinner high in healthy fats. Or experiment by replacing the butter in this recipe with 7 tablespoons of canola oil.

CHOCOLATE LAYER CAKE WITH MAPLE FROSTING

PREP TIME: **15 MINUTES** ■ TOTAL TIME: **1 HOUR 30 MINUTES**

Makes 16 servings

1½ cups whole grain pastry flour

½ cup unsweetened cocoa powder

1 tablespoon instant espresso powder

1 teaspoon baking soda

8 tablespoons butter, softened

1 cup sugar

1 egg

1 teaspoon vanilla extract

½ cup low-fat buttermilk

½ cup hot tap water

¾ cup maple syrup

3 egg whites

½ teaspoon cream of tartar

1. Preheat the oven to 350°F. Coat two 8" round cake pans with cooking spray.

2. In a medium bowl, mix the flour, cocoa powder, espresso powder, and baking soda. In a large bowl, place the butter and sugar. With an electric mixer on medium speed, beat for 3 minutes, or until creamy. Add the egg and vanilla. Beat on low speed until creamy.

3. With the mixer on low speed, beat in half of the flour mixture and all of the buttermilk. Beat in half of the remaining flour mixture and all of the water. Beat in the remaining flour mixture. Pour into the prepared pans.

4. Bake for 25 minutes, or until a wooden pick inserted in the center comes out clean. Cool in the pans on a rack for 10 minutes. Remove to the rack and cool completely.

5. In the top of a double boiler, combine the syrup, egg whites, and cream of tartar. Beat with an electric mixer on medium high until well blended. Place over rapidly boiling water. Beat for 7 minutes, or until stiff peaks form. Remove the top of the double boiler from the water and continue beating for 5 minutes, or until thickened and fluffy.

6. Place 1 cake layer on a serving plate. Spread 1 cup of the frosting over the cake. Top with the second cake layer. Spread the remaining frosting over the top and sides of the cake.

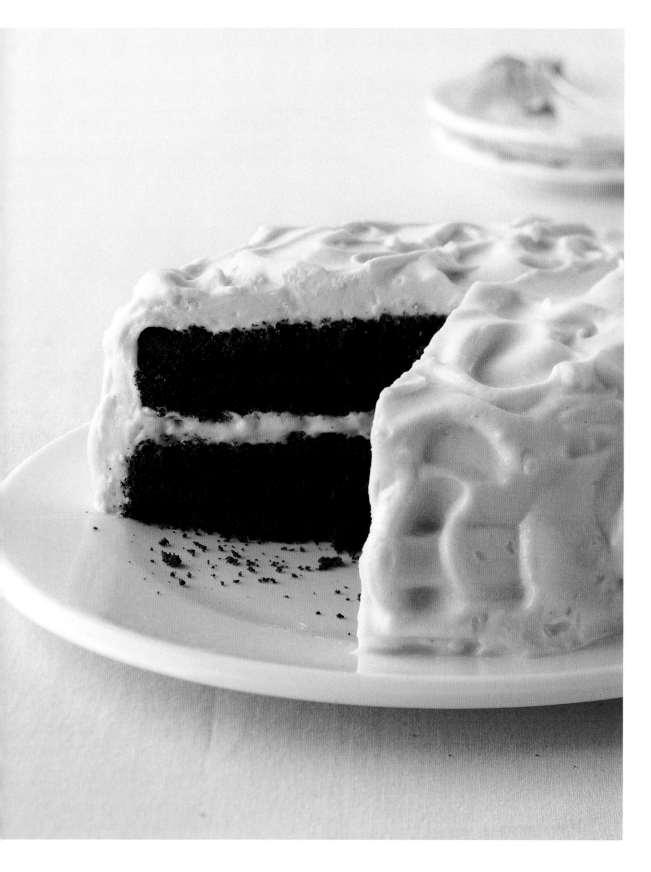

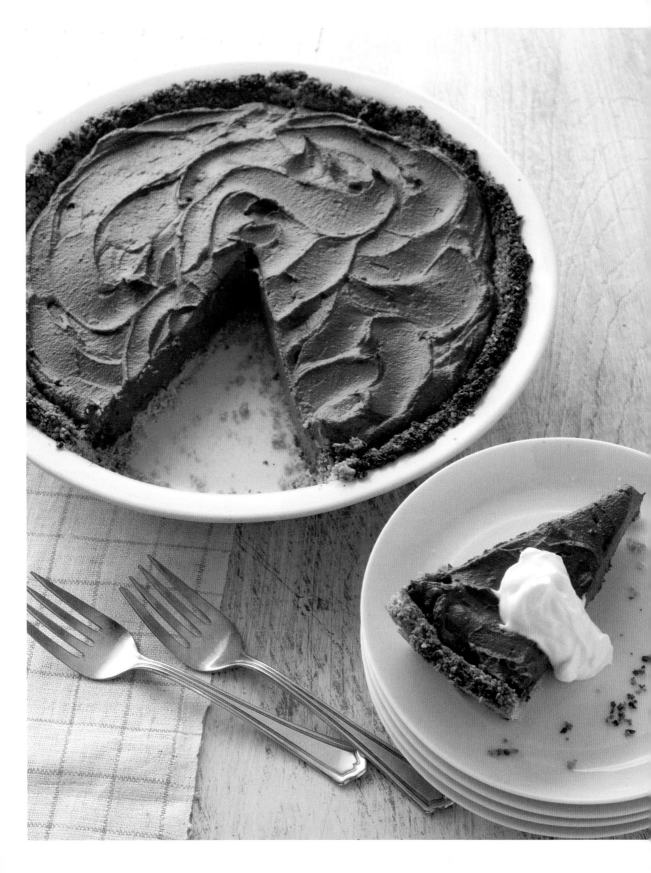

RICH CHOCOLATE CREAM PIE

PREP TIME: **20 MINUTES** ■ TOTAL TIME: **30 MINUTES + COOLING TIME**

Makes 12 servings

¾ cup almond meal or almond flour

¾ cup oat bran

¼ teaspoon baking powder

¼ teaspoon salt

2 tablespoons canola oil

1 tablespoon honey

2 packages (12 ounces each) silken tofu, drained

2 tablespoons unsweetened cocoa powder

1 tablespoon vanilla extract

8 ounces bittersweet (60–75%) chocolate, melted

1 cup plain 0% Greek yogurt

1. Preheat the oven to 350°F. In a large bowl, whisk together the almond meal or flour, oat bran, baking powder, and salt. Stir in the oil and honey until blended. Press into a 9" pie plate. Bake for 10 minutes, or until set and lightly browned. Remove to a rack and cool completely.

2. Meanwhile, in a food processor, place the tofu, cocoa, and vanilla and blend until smooth. Add the chocolate and blend for 1 minute. Scrape the sides with a rubber spatula and blend for 1 minute, or until incorporated. Pour into a large bowl.

3. Fold in the yogurt just until blended. Refrigerate.

4. When the pie shell is cooled, spread the chocolate mixture into the shell.

Makeover Magic

BEFORE		AFTER
305	CALORIES	206
19 g	FAT	12 g
10 g	SAT FAT	6 g
31 g	CARBS	21 g
1 g	FIBER	2 g
3 g	PROTEIN	6 g
90 mg	SODIUM	87 mg

Curb carbs: Relying on a small amount of honey and bittersweet chocolate for sweetness reduces the carbs in this recipe.

Fill up on fiber: Almond meal and oat bran add fiber to the crust.

Favor fats: Almonds and canola oil provide healthy fats.

THREE-BERRY PIE

PREP TIME: **45 MINUTES** ■ TOTAL TIME: **1 HOUR 30 MINUTES**

Makes 8 servings

CRUST

¾ cup whole grain pastry flour

¼ cup oat bran

¼ teaspoon salt

4 tablespoons chilled butter, cut into small pieces

3 tablespoons light sour cream

1½ tablespoons ice water, divided

¼ teaspoon almond extract

FILLING

2 cups fresh raspberries

1 cup fresh blackberries

1 cup fresh blueberries

3 tablespoons lemon juice

¼ cup honey

3 tablespoons cornstarch

3 tablespoons instant tapioca

CRUMB TOPPING

¼ cup whole grain pastry flour

1 tablespoon canola oil

2 teaspoons honey

SMARTSTART

In the Achieving and Repeating phases (see page 7), replace butter with canola oil. Add toasted oats to the crumb topping for an even more fiber-full recipe that will help your health.

1. **To make the crust:** In a food processor, pulse together the flour, oat bran, and salt until blended. Add the butter. Pulse until the mixture resembles coarse crumbs.

2. Add the sour cream, 1 tablespoon of the water, and the almond extract. Pulse just until the dough forms large clumps. (If the dough seems too dry, add a few more drops of remaining ice water.) Form into 1 ball and flatten into a disk. Cover and refrigerate for at least 15 minutes or up to 1 day.

3. Preheat the oven to 400°F. Coat a 9" pie plate with cooking spray. Line a baking sheet with foil.

4. On a well-floured surface, roll out each piece of dough into a 10" circle. Fit the dough into the pie plate, leaving the overhang.

5. **To make the filling:** In a large bowl, mix the raspberries, blackberries, blueberries, and lemon juice.

6. In a small bowl, mix the honey, cornstarch, and tapioca. Pour over the fruit, mix well, and let stand at room temperature for 15 minutes. Spoon into the pie plate.

7. **To make the topping:** Combine the flour, oil, and honey. Lightly sprinkle over the fruit filling.

8. Place the pie on the prepared baking sheet and bake for 40 minutes, or until the crust is golden brown and the juices bubble. Cool on a rack.

Makeover Magic

BEFORE		AFTER
650	CALORIES	169
24 g	FAT	6 g
15 g	SAT FAT	1 g
104 g	CARBS	29 g
7 g	FIBER	4 g
5 g	PROTEIN	3 g
270 mg	SODIUM	32 mg

Curb carbs: We cut back the amount of sweetener and let the natural flavor of the berries come through.

Fill up on fiber: Steel-cut oats are higher in fiber than regular or instant oats. Combine rolled oats and oat bran for even more fiber and texture.

Favor fats: Sliced almonds serve up a dish with MUFAs.

DOUBLE OAT–BLUEBERRY CRISP

PREP TIME: **15 MINUTES** ■ TOTAL TIME: **1 HOUR + STANDING TIME**

Makes 6 servings

2 tablespoons honey

1½ tablespoons arrowroot powder or cornstarch

3 cups fresh blueberries

⅛ teaspoon ground nutmeg

1½ teaspoons almond extract

½ cup old-fashioned steel-cut oats

¼ cup oat bran

4 tablespoons sliced almonds

1 tablespoon light brown sugar

2 tablespoons canola oil

Light whipped topping (optional)

1. Preheat the oven to 350°F. Coat an 8" × 8" baking pan with cooking spray.

2. In a large bowl, stir together the honey and arrowroot powder or cornstarch. Add the blueberries, nutmeg, and almond extract. Toss to coat the berries thoroughly. Transfer to the baking pan.

3. In the same bowl, combine the oats, oat bran, almonds, brown sugar, and oil. Toss to coat well. Sprinkle over the berry mixture.

4. Bake for 45 minutes, or until bubbling. Remove and let stand at room temperature for 5 minutes. Serve with a dollop of light whipped topping, if using.

SMARTSTART

Add lots of cinnamon to the crisp topping for glycemic balance!

PEAR-GINGER COBBLER

PREP TIME: **25 MINUTES** ▦ TOTAL TIME: **1 HOUR**

Makes 4 servings

4   cups sliced pears

2   tablespoons honey

1   large omega-3–enriched egg, well beaten

1   tablespoon quick-cooking tapioca

1   teaspoon grated fresh ginger

½   cup whole wheat pastry flour

½   cup oat bran

1   teaspoon baking soda

⅓   cup buttermilk

1   tablespoon butter, at room temperature

1. Preheat the oven to 425°F. Coat a 9" round baking dish with cooking spray.

2. In a medium bowl, combine the pears, honey, egg, tapioca, and ginger. Spread evenly over the bottom of the baking dish.

3. In another medium bowl, combine the flour, oat bran, baking soda, buttermilk, and butter to make a dough. On a well-floured surface, roll the dough to a ½" thickness. Prick the dough with a fork and place loosely over the pears. Bake for 25 minutes, until the filling is set and the topping is golden brown.

Makeover Magic

BEFORE		AFTER
300	CALORIES	196
9 g	FAT	3 g
5 g	SAT FAT	2 g
51 g	CARBS	39 g
5 g	FIBER	6 g
2 g	PROTEIN	6 g
90 mg	SODIUM	237 mg

Curb carbs: This dish uses honey instead of sugar for major carb reduction.

Fill up on fiber: Switching out some of the flour for oat bran increases the fiber. Pears are naturally a good source of fiber.

Favor fats: Be sure to use omega-3–enriched eggs. They are the secret source in this recipe.

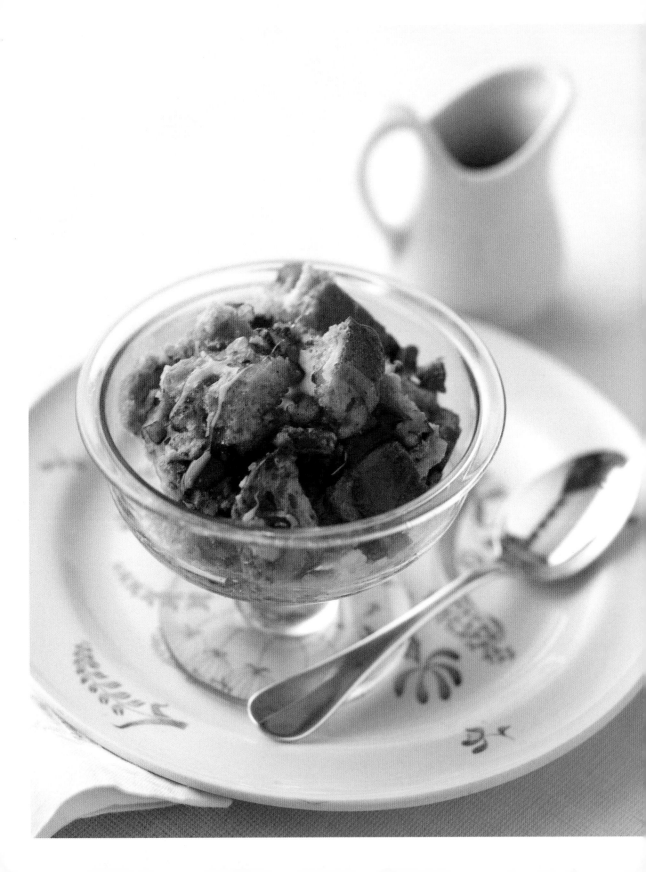

SOUTHERN PECAN BREAD PUDDING

PREP TIME: **15 MINUTES** ■ TOTAL TIME: **50 MINUTES**

Makes 9 servings

2 eggs, separated + 2 egg whites

Pinch of salt

1½ cups 1% milk

3 tablespoons + ¼ cup honey, divided

1 tablespoon vanilla extract

1 tablespoon canola oil

⅛ teaspoon ground nutmeg

3 cups cubed whole grain bread

¼ cup finely chopped pecans

1 tablespoon bourbon (optional)

Pinch of ground cinnamon

1. Preheat the oven to 350°F. Coat an 8" × 8" baking dish with cooking spray. Set aside.

2. In a large bowl, with an electric mixer on high speed, beat the 4 egg whites and salt until stiff, glossy peaks form.

3. In another bowl, beat the egg yolks with a fork. Add the milk, 3 tablespoons honey, vanilla, oil, and nutmeg. Beat to blend. Add the bread and pecans. Press with the back of a fork until the bread absorbs the liquid. Gently pour into the bowl with the beaten whites. Fold to incorporate. Transfer to the prepared pan.

4. Bake for 35 minutes, or until a knife inserted in the center comes out clean. If the top is browning too fast, cover lightly with a sheet of foil.

5. Meanwhile, in a microwaveable bowl, combine the remaining ¼ cup honey, bourbon (if using), and cinnamon. Microwave on high for 40 seconds, or until bubbling. Whisk until smooth. Spoon the warm pudding onto dessert plates. Drizzle with the honey mixture.

Makeover Magic

BEFORE		AFTER
976	CALORIES	156
64 g	FAT	5 g
30 g	SAT FAT	1 g
95 g	CARBS	22 g
3 g	FIBER	1 g
11 g	PROTEIN	5 g
558 mg	SODIUM	139 mg

Curb carbs: We reduced the amount of bread from a traditional recipe to keep carbs in range, yet still gooey and comforting.

Fill up on fiber: Whole grain bread and pecans add fiber.

Favor fats: Pecans add MUFAs to this classic southern dish.

BEFORE		AFTER
255	CALORIES	172
18 g	FAT	12 g
2 g	SAT FAT	2 g
22 g	CARBS	11 g
3 g	FIBER	3 g
6 g	PROTEIN	7 g
233 mg	SODIUM	25 mg

Curb carbs: Classic candied nuts are coated in sugar. Here we lightly sweetened the nut mixture with honey, cinnamon, and cardamom.

Fill up on fiber: Dried apples, as well as pecans and almonds, add fiber to this dish.

Favor fats: Nuts and pumpkin seeds are all great sources of desirable fats.

FRUIT AND NUT CLUSTERS

PREP TIME: **10 MINUTES** ■ TOTAL TIME: **1 HOUR**

Makes 8 servings

1 egg white

1 tablespoon honey

1 teaspoon ground cinnamon

1 teaspoon ground ginger

¼ teaspoon ground cardamom

½ cup pecans

½ cup almonds

½ cup raw pumpkin seeds (pepitas)

½ cup dried apples

1. Preheat the oven to 350°F. Line a baking sheet with parchment paper.

2. In a medium bowl, whisk the egg white, honey, cinnamon, ginger, and cardamom. Add the pecans, almonds, pumpkin seeds, and apples and toss to coat well. Spread the mixture onto the parchment paper. Bake for 20 minutes, or until browned.

3. Cool on a rack for 30 minutes, or until cooled. Break into bite-size pieces.

PISTACHIO KISSES

PREP TIME: **15 MINUTES** ■ TOTAL TIME: **1 HOUR 15 MINUTES +
STANDING TIME**

Makes 6 servings

2 egg whites, at room
temperature

¼ teaspoon cream of tartar

¼ cup maple sugar

½ cup unsalted roasted
pistachios, chopped

⅛ teaspoon ground
cardamom

1. Preheat the oven to 250°F. Line 2 large baking sheets with
parchment paper.

2. In a large bowl, beat the egg whites and cream of tartar with an
electric mixer on high speed until soft peaks form. Continue
beating while gradually adding the maple sugar, until very stiff
and glossy peaks form. Gently fold in the pistachios and
cardamom.

3. Drop by tablespoons onto the parchment paper. Bake for 1 hour.
Turn off the oven and leave in the oven for 1 hour without
opening the oven door.

4. Remove from the oven and store in an airtight container.

Makeover Magic

BEFORE		AFTER
130	CALORIES	120
6 g	FAT	5 g
2 g	SAT FAT	1 g
18 g	CARBS	11 g
0 g	FIBER	2 g
2 g	PROTEIN	5 g
55 mg	SODIUM	30 mg

Curb carbs: Using nuts
instead of flour in these cookies obliterates carbs while
leaving snackers satisfied.

Fill up on fiber: The pistachios provide half the belly-
filling fiber in this recipe.

Favor fats: Pistachios are also
a source of MUFAs.

Makeover Magic

BEFORE		AFTER
310	CALORIES	180
18 g	FAT	11 g
8 g	SAT FAT	4 g
32 g	CARBS	19 g
2 g	FIBER	2 g
4 g	PROTEIN	3 g
70 mg	SODIUM	26 mg

Curb carbs: This is one cool trick—instead of flour, use high-fiber black beans and watch half the carbs disappear!

Fill up on fiber: Black beans, pecans, and cocoa powder all add fiber to this dish.

Favor fats: Dark chocolate and pecans add MUFAs.

RICH BROWNIES

PREP TIME: **10 MINUTES** ■ TOTAL TIME: **50 MINUTES**

Makes 16 servings

1 can (14.5 ounces) no-salt-added black beans, rinsed and drained

3 eggs

½ cup honey

⅓ cup canola oil

¼ cup unsweetened cocoa powder

2 teaspoons ground cinnamon

6 ounces bittersweet (60–75%) chocolate, broken into pieces

½ cup chopped pecans

1. Preheat the oven to 350°F. Coat an 8" × 8" baking pan with cooking spray.

2. In a food processor or blender, combine the black beans, eggs, honey, oil, cocoa, and cinnamon. Pulse or blend until smooth. Add the chocolate and pulse until coarsely chopped.

3. Pour the batter into the pan. Sprinkle with the pecans. Bake for 45 minutes, or until a wooden pick inserted in the center comes out clean.

FIG BARS

PREP TIME: **15 MINUTES** ■ TOTAL TIME: **40 MINUTES**

Makes 16 servings

½ cup honey

⅓ cup plain 0% Greek yogurt

3 tablespoons canola oil

1 omega-3–enriched egg

1½ teaspoons vanilla extract

1½ cups chopped dried figs

¾ cup old-fashioned rolled oats

½ cup whole wheat pastry flour

⅓ cup ground golden flaxseeds

2 tablespoons chopped walnuts

½ teaspoon baking soda

1 tablespoon ground cinnamon

1. Preheat the oven to 350°F. Coat an 8" × 8" baking pan with cooking spray.

2. In a large bowl, whisk together the honey, yogurt, oil, egg, and vanilla until smooth. In another bowl, stir together the figs, oats, flour, flaxseeds, walnuts, baking soda, and cinnamon. Add to the first bowl. Stir to combine. Spread into the prepared pan.

3. Bake for 25 minutes, or until the top is browned and a wooden pick inserted in the center comes out with a few moist crumbs. Do not overbake. Remove to a rack to cool. Cut into 16 squares.

Makeover Magic

BEFORE		AFTER
279	CALORIES	149
11 g	FAT	5 g
11 g	SAT FAT	0.5 g
45 g	CARBS	25 g
3 g	FIBER	3 g
3 g	PROTEIN	3 g
157 mg	SODIUM	49 mg

Curb carbs: Honey is sweeter than sugar, so you can use less of it!

Fill up on fiber: Up the fiber with oats, walnuts, flaxseeds, and dried fruit. Just remember that dried fruit adds to your carb count quickly.

Favor fats: Walnuts and ground flaxseeds are a great source of ALA omega-3 fatty acids.

SMARTSTART

If you are at the Repeating or Time stages of START (see page 7), sprinkle each bar with 1 teaspoon of cinnamon for ideal blood sugar balance.

Makeover Magic

BEFORE		AFTER
300	CALORIES	125
14 g	FAT	4 g
8 g	SAT FAT	0.5 g
39 g	CARBS	20 g
0 g	FIBER	2 g
3 g	PROTEIN	3 g
230 mg	SODIUM	102 mg

Curb carbs: No need to add flour or too much sugar to these cookies. Honey and oats keep carbs curbed by removing flour and decreasing the overall sugar content.

Fill up on fiber: Oats, apple (with the skin on), and chia seeds all add fiber!

Favor fats: Olive oil and chia seeds provide MUFAs and omega-3 fatty acids to these sweet treats.

OATMEAL-APPLE COOKIES

PREP TIME: **10 MINUTES** ■ TOTAL TIME: **20 MINUTES**

Makes 4 servings

¾ cup old-fashioned rolled oats

1 apple, cored and shredded

2 egg whites

2 tablespoons honey

2 tablespoons white chia seeds

1 tablespoon 1% milk

1 tablespoon olive oil

1 teaspoon ground cinnamon

½ teaspoon baking powder

Pinch of salt

1. Preheat the oven to 350°F. Coat a baking sheet with cooking spray.

2. In a large bowl, combine the oats, apple, egg whites, honey, chia seeds, milk, oil, cinnamon, baking powder, and salt. Stir together until well blended.

3. Divide the dough into 8 equal pieces. Place on the baking sheet and flatten with the bottom of a glass.

4. Bake for 12 minutes, or until golden brown on the edges.

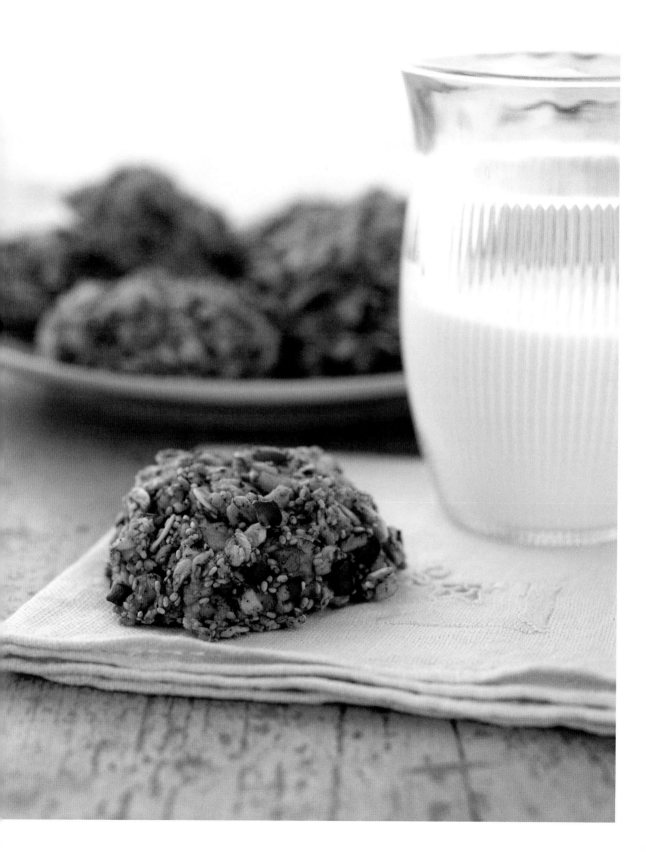

Makeover Magic

BEFORE		AFTER
180	CALORIES	100
5 g	FAT	4 g
1 g	SAT FAT	0.5 g
29 g	CARBS	13 g
1 g	FIBER	1 g
4 g	PROTEIN	2 g
160 mg	SODIUM	72 mg

Curb carbs: Our version of what is essentially a crispy rice treat uses honey instead of marshmallows and adds peanut butter for body and protein, while cutting carbs.

Fill up on fiber: Oat cereal adds just 1 gram of fiber, so this dessert would be great following a higher-fiber meal.

Favor fats: Nut butter is the favored fat providing MUFAs.

CRISPY OAT SQUARES

PREP TIME: **10 MINUTES** ■ TOTAL TIME: **10 MINUTES +
CHILLING TIME**

Makes 36 servings

3 cups oat "O" cereal

½ cup peanut or cashew butter

⅓ cup honey

1 tablespoon vanilla extract

1. Coat an 8" × 8" baking pan with cooking spray. Place the oat cereal in a large bowl.

2. In a medium saucepan over medium heat, stir the peanut or cashew butter, honey, and vanilla constantly for 3 minutes, or until melted. Remove from the heat and stir into the cereal.

3. Spread into the prepared pan. Cover and refrigerate for 1 hour. Cut into 36 squares.

Desserts

ALMOND RICE PUDDING

PREP TIME: **10 MINUTES** ■ TOTAL TIME: **1 HOUR 50 MINUTES +
CHILLING TIME**

Makes 8 servings

3 cups unsweetened
   soy milk

½ cup uncooked brown rice

2 tablespoons white chia
   seeds

2 tablespoons honey

1 teaspoon almond extract

⅛ teaspoon salt

⅛ teaspoon ground
   cinnamon

2 eggs

¼ cup sliced almonds,
   toasted

1. In a medium saucepan, stir the milk, rice, chia seeds, honey, almond extract, salt, and cinnamon. Bring to a boil over medium heat. Reduce the heat to low, cover, and simmer for 1½ hours, or until the rice is very tender. Remove from the heat and let cool for 5 minutes.

2. In a small bowl, lightly beat the eggs with a fork. Stir ½ cup of the hot rice mixture into the eggs. Gradually stir the egg mixture into the saucepan.

3. Place over medium-low heat and cook, stirring constantly, for 5 minutes, or until thickened. Remove from the heat and cool for 10 minutes. Pour into a serving bowl and cover the surface with plastic wrap. Refrigerate until cold. Sprinkle with almonds and serve.

Makeover Magic

BEFORE		AFTER
436	CALORIES	190
18 g	FAT	7 g
4 g	SAT FAT	1 g
59 g	CARBS	23 g
1 g	FIBER	2 g
12 g	PROTEIN	8 g
159 mg	SODIUM	119 mg

Curb carbs: Use unsweetened soy milk or even unsweetened almond milk to prevent this from being a blood sugar bomb.

Fill up on fiber: Brown rice and chia seeds provide a small amount of fiber.

Favor fats: Chia seeds can serve as fiber and fat. Sprinkling with sliced almonds adds the ultimate nutty flavor and favored fat.

Makeover Magic

BEFORE		AFTER
552	CALORIES	204
42 g	FAT	6 g
29 g	SAT FAT	4 g
41 g	CARBS	32 g
2 g	FIBER	5 g
6 g	PROTEIN	9 g
172 mg	SODIUM	52 mg

Curb carbs: Using Greek yogurt instead of sweetened whipped cream takes the carbs down in this sweet autumnal dish.

Fill up on fiber: Pumpkin is naturally high in fiber—each serving has 3 grams!

Favor fats: Chia seeds provide healthy fats in this dish.

CREAMY PUMPKIN MOUSSE

PREP TIME: **15 MINUTES** ■ TOTAL TIME: **1 HOUR 15 MINUTES**

Makes 4 servings

1 can (15 ounces) pumpkin

1 tablespoon chia seeds

2 tablespoons honey

1½ teaspoons pumpkin pie spice

1½ cups plain 0% Greek yogurt

2 ounces bittersweet (60–75%) chocolate, shaved

1. In a large bowl, combine the pumpkin, chia seeds, honey, and pumpkin pie spice. Gently fold in the yogurt until blended. Transfer to 4 individual serving bowls and top with the chocolate shavings.

2. Refrigerate for at least 1 hour before serving.

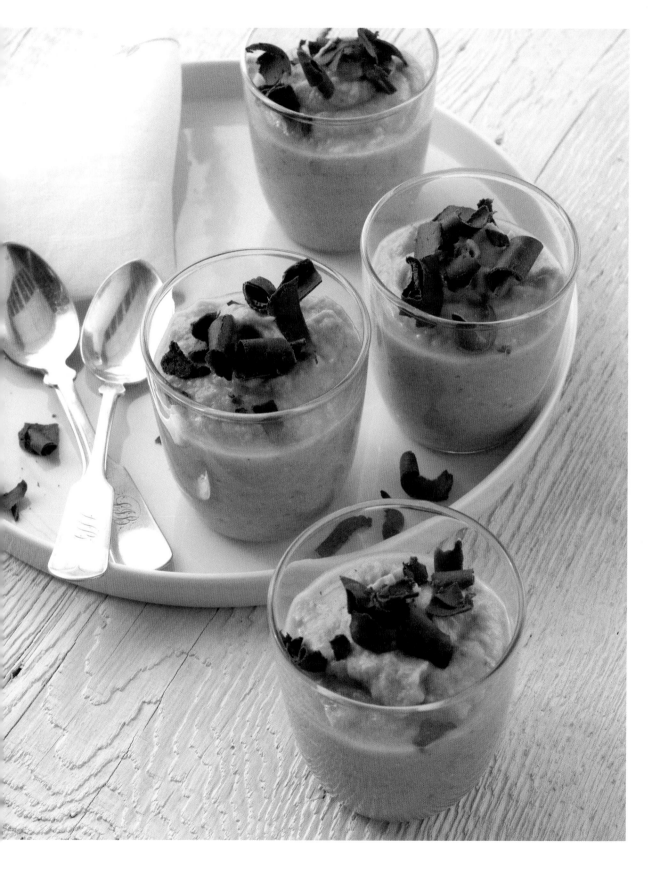

Makeover Magic

BEFORE		AFTER
694	CALORIES	216
41 g	FAT	10 g
23 g	SAT FAT	5 g
80 g	CARBS	29 g
3 g	FIBER	3 g
7 g	PROTEIN	7 g
170 mg	SODIUM	59 mg

Curb carbs: Streamlining the ingredients of a classic parfait helps cut calories. Layering nuts instead of cookies eliminates carbs—as does using bittersweet chocolate instead of milk.

Fill up on fiber: Even dessert can have fiber. Use sliced almonds for a combo of healthy fiber and fat.

Favor fats: Get rid of the unhealthy saturated fat in whipped cream by replacing it with a topping of slivered almonds, which are packed with MUFAs. Not only does bittersweet chocolate have less sugar than milk chocolate, but it is also a good source of antioxidants and MUFAs.

FROZEN MOCHA PARFAITS

PREP TIME: **5 MINUTES** ▪ TOTAL TIME: **5 MINUTES**

Makes 4 servings

1 teaspoon instant espresso powder

¼ cup bittersweet (60–75%) chocolate chips

2 cups low-fat chocolate frozen yogurt

4 tablespoons sliced almonds, toasted

1. In a small glass bowl, place the espresso powder and chips. Microwave on medium for 2 minutes, stirring every 30 seconds, or until smooth. Let cool for 5 minutes.

2. Place 1 small scoop (¼ cup) of the yogurt into 4 parfait glasses. Drizzle each with 1 teaspoon of the chocolate mixture and ½ tablespoon of the almonds. Repeat the layers. Serve immediately or freeze for up to 1 hour.

CHOCOLATE MALT

PREP TIME: **5 MINUTES** ■ TOTAL TIME: **5 MINUTES**

Makes 1 serving

2 tablespoons unsweetened cocoa powder

1 tablespoon unsweetened malted milk powder

¼ cup warm water

¾ cup 1% milk

2 teaspoons vanilla extract

⅓ cup crushed ice

1. In a blender, pulse the cocoa powder, malted milk powder, and water until well blended. Blend in the milk, vanilla, and ice for 1 minute, or until the mixture is thick and frothy.

2. Pour into a frosted glass and serve immediately.

Makeover Magic

BEFORE		AFTER
496	CALORIES	156
23 g	FAT	4 g
14 g	SAT FAT	3 g
64 g	CARBS	21 g
3 g	FIBER	4 g
10 g	PROTEIN	9 g
211 mg	SODIUM	119 mg

Curb carbs: Milk contains about 12 grams of carbs per cup. By using unsweetened cocoa and malted milk powder, you can keep the carbs curbed. You may need to halve this recipe if your snacks are limited to 15 grams of carbs.

Fill up on fiber: Surprised to see fiber in this drink? It comes from the cocoa powder, which adds almost 2 grams per tablespoon.

Favor fats: Add a tablespoon of chia seeds for a dose of omega-3 and omega-6 fatty acids.

Steps 4 and 5: Repeating and Time—
An Easy-to-Use 2-Week Meal Plan

You have reached the Repeating step. You are ready to consistently implement everything you have learned, whether it is journaling in your food log, observing your hunger/fullness cues, or curbing your carbs. To make this stage easy for you, we have created a delicious and comforting 2-week meal plan. So grab your sneakers and your canvas bags and head to the grocery store to get your ingredients for success.

Keep in mind that all meals curb carbohydrates to 45 grams. Men, feel free to add 15 grams of carbs to each of your three main meals per day to ensure that they are nutritionally adequate and you don't feel deprived. Each individual may add one to three snacks per day. This will depend on your internal regulation system, personal weight-loss goals, level of physical activity, and the quantity of food you were previously eating. Your meal plan is created with three meals and one snack. Add or reduce planned snack times depending on how feasible three meals and one snack are. Ask yourself, "Am I satiated? Can I wait 2 to 4 hours between snacks or meals?" Consider whether you are eating less than before. In most cases, you should be eating less than you were when you started reading this lifestyle cookbook. If you are choosing snacks, we recommend a midmorning snack, a midafternoon snack, and/or a nighttime snack each equal to 15 grams of carbs for women and 30 grams of carbs for men.

If you have already been diagnosed with diabetes and use a glucometer, you can take your meal plan a step further. Be proactive in achieving optimal blood sugar management by taking your blood sugar before eating and then 2 hours after your meal. This will help to ensure that the amounts and combinations of foods you are eating work for your body. In other words, check to be sure your blood sugar is generally less than 180 mg/dl 2 hours after meals, consistent with the recommendations of the American Diabetes Association. Remember that this number varies for each individual and is best determined with your personal diabetes care team when discussing diabetes self- management education.

And finally, if you love a particular recipe or food—especially one that is high in grams of carbohydrates per serving—learn to spread this food choice throughout the day to prevent a sugar roller coaster. So if you can't get enough of the Fruit and Nut Clusters (page 316), feel free to have one at breakfast and one at lunch, just not two at the same meal. This action plan will keep you happy and your body healthy.

HAPPY EATING AND SNACKING GUIDE

All portions are equal to 1 serving unless otherwise noted.

WEEK 1

SUNDAY

³⁄₄ cup 0% plain Greek yogurt

¹⁄₄ cup cooked wheat berries

1 small apple, cubed

2 tablespoons walnuts

¹⁄₈ cup mixed berries

Lunch
Chicken-Veggie Bowl: 4 ounces grilled
and shredded chicken strips and
2 cups cooked vegetables (¹⁄₂ cup yellow
onion, sliced; 1¹⁄₂ cups red, orange, and
yellow bell peppers, chopped; 1 clove
garlic, diced; and 2 teaspoons canola oil
sautéed over medium heat). Serve in
a bowl and, on the side, include a whole
wheat wrap spread with 1 tablespoon
olive hummus.

Chocolate-Almond Cake (page 301)

Dinner
Pasta with Summer Vegetables (page 257)

Baked Salmon: 4 ounces wild salmon
spread with 2 teaspoons Dijon mustard
and sprinkled with 2 teaspoons ground
flaxseeds. Bake at 375°F for 10 minutes,
or until the salmon is opaque.

Snack
15 grams of carbs:

> 2 tablespoons almonds and
> ¹⁄₂ large orange

30 grams of carbs:

> ¹⁄₄ cup almonds with 1 large orange

MONDAY

Breakfast
1 cup plain 0% Greek yogurt

1 cup mixed berries

1 tablespoon wheat germ

1 Fruit and Nut Cluster (page 316)

Lunch
Broccoli-Walnut Farfalle Toss (page 293)

1 Fruit and Nut Cluster (page 316)

Dinner
1¹⁄₂ servings *Herb-Roasted Chicken Breast
with Vegetables (page 206)*
Cheese and Vegetable Bake (page 280)

Snack
15 grams of carbs:

> 10 to 15 olives and five 1-ounce high-fiber
> crackers (the size of a Wheat Thin)

30 grams of carbs:

> ¹⁄₄ cup guacamole with 10 to 15
> (1.5 ounces) low-sodium baked tortilla
> chips and 1 cup carrot sticks for
> dipping

TUESDAY

Breakfast

Eggs Un-Benedict: 2 poached eggs,
 ¼ cup steamed spinach, and 2 toasted
 English muffins. Spread half the spinach
 over each side of a muffin and top with
 1 poached egg and the other muffin half.

1 clementine

Lunch

Turkey and Bean Quesadillas (page 224)

1 small apple

Dinner

Beef Ragù over Polenta (page 174)

Spinach Salad: 2 cups raw spinach dressed
 with 1 tablespoon slivered almonds,
 1 teaspoon Parmesan cheese, and
 1 tablespoon Lemon–Olive Oil Dressing
 (1 teaspoon lemon juice mixed with
 2 teaspoons olive oil and salt and ground
 black pepper to taste)

Snack

15 grams of carbs:

  6 ounces plain 0% plain Greek yogurt,
   sprinkled with 1 crushed small cookie

30 grams of carbs:

  6 ounces 0% fruit-flavored Greek
   yogurt, mixed with ½ cup berries
   and 1 tablespoon wheat germ

WEDNESDAY

Breakfast

1 cup higher-fiber, moderate-carbohydrate
 cereal (such as Kashi GOLEAN or Kashi
 GOLEAN Vanilla Graham Clusters)

¾ cup 0% blueberry Greek yogurt

Lunch

Asparagus Swiss Quiche (page 265)

Spiced Sweet Potato Chips (page 143)

Dinner

6 ounces grilled wild trout

1 cup Brussels sprouts roasted with
 1 teaspoon olive oil and 1 teaspoon garlic

1 cup steamed summer squash

Pear-Ginger Cobbler (page 313)

Snack

15 grams of carbs:

  2 tablespoons pecans and 1 small
   banana

30 grams of carbs:

  ¼ cup pecans and 1 banana

THURSDAY

Breakfast

Peanut Butter and Strawberry Sandwich:
2 slices multigrain toast spread with
1 tablespoon + 1 teaspoon natural
no-salt-added peanut butter and
¼ cup sliced strawberries

Lunch

*Corn, Black Bean, and Edamame Salad
(page 109)*

Turkey Wrap with Hummus: 4 ounces
turkey, 1 tablespoon hummus, and ⅓ cup
spinach wrapped in a whole wheat wrap

Dinner

Italian Sausage and Linguine (page 191)
(optional: pesto sauce for MUFAs)

Snack

15 grams of carbs:

1 higher-fiber, lower-carb, higher-protein
bar (~5 grams fiber, 15 grams carbs,
7 to 14 grams protein); e.g., Almond
Blueberry Zing bar or Gnu bar,
any variety

30 grams of carbs:

1 granola bar (6 grams fiber, 25 to
28 grams carbs, 10 to 14 grams protein
or healthy fats); e.g., Kind bar, LäraBar,
and/or Zing bar

FRIDAY

Breakfast

Lox Omelet: Combine 1 whole egg and
2 egg whites mixed with ¼ cup bell
peppers, 1 ounce lox, and ½ ounce feta
cheese. Cook in a skillet coated with
canola oil spray.

1 toasted pita (whole wheat, oat bran,
or spelt)

½ cup orange slices

Lunch

MUFA Salad: Toss together 3 cups mixed
greens, ½ cucumber, 8 olives, ⅛ avocado,
and 1 tablespoon sunflower seeds. Top
with 2 tablespoons olive oil balsamic
vinaigrette.

1 oat bran pita

Dinner

Mom's Meat Loaf (page 167)

*Roasted Vegetable Mac and Cheese
(page 258)*

Snack

15 grams of carbs:

Upside-Down Ambrosia: 4 ounces
low-sodium, low-fat cottage cheese
and 1 teaspoon shredded coconut
sprinkled over ¾ cup fresh pineapple

30 grams of carbs:

Upside-Down Ambrosia: 4 ounces
low-sodium, low-fat cottage cheese,
8 chopped nuts, and 1 teaspoon
shredded coconut sprinkled over
1¼ cups fresh pineapple

SATURDAY

Breakfast

Sunrise Oatmeal (page 85)

6 ounces 0% plain Greek yogurt

Lunch

Citrus–Grilled Shrimp Salad (page 106)

Coconut-Lime Pudding Cake (page 305)

Dinner

4 ounces filet mignon or top round sirloin, grilled

1 small baked sweet potato

1½ cups broccoli cooked in 1 teaspoon olive oil with 2 teaspoons garlic

Snack

15 grams of carbs:

2 tablespoons guacamole and ½ toasted whole wheat pita

30 grams of carbs:

¼ cup hummus and 20 to 25 (1.5 ounces) whole grain pretzels

WEEK 2

SUNDAY

Breakfast

Spiced Apple Pancakes (page 80)

½ cup 1% cottage cheese

Lunch

Grilled Cheese: 2 slices sodium-free whole wheat bread filled with 2 slices provolone cheese. Cook in a skillet coated with canola oil spray.

1 cup Amy's Organic Soups, Light in Sodium Low Fat Cream of Tomato

Dinner

Beef Stroganoff (page 160)

2 cups steamed spinach

1 Pistachio Kiss (page 317)

Snack

15 grams of carbs:

10 to 23 almonds and ½ large orange

30 grams of carbs:

15 to 25 almonds with 1 large orange

MONDAY

Breakfast

2 whole grain waffles (packaged, frozen: should equal 20 grams carbs, using magic carbs)

1 tablespoon natural peanut butter

2 teaspoons agave nectar or honey

1 teaspoon ground cinnamon

Lunch

Tuna Salad Wrap (page 122)

1/4 cup hummus

1/2 apple

1/2 cup baby carrots

Dinner

Asian Lettuce Cups (page 192)

2/3 cup cooked quick wild rice

Snack

15 grams of carbs:

   6 ounces 0% fruit-flavored Greek yogurt

30 grams of carbs:

   6 ounces 0% plain Greek yogurt with 1 small apple and 1/2 cup berries

TUESDAY

Breakfast

Tex-Mex Breakfast Pizza (page 75)

2 tablespoons chopped avocado

Lunch

Almond Butter Sandwich: 1 slice sprouted wheat bread spread with 1 tablespoon + 1 teaspoon natural salt-free almond butter, covered with 1/2 green apple, thinly sliced, and topped with 1 slice sprouted wheat bread

6 ounces 0% plain Greek yogurt

Dinner

2 ounces sprouted grain pasta

1/2 cup natural tomato sauce (made with olive oil, no sugar)

4 ounces browned ground turkey

1/4 cup diced raw carrot

8 olives, sliced, sprinkled over the pasta, sauce, meat, and carrot

1 1/2 cups steamed broccoli

Snack

15 grams of carbs:

   1/4 cup hummus, 1 cup raw cauliflower florets, and 1/2 apple, unpeeled and sliced

30 grams of carbs:

   1/4 cup hummus with 1 cup carrots and 3/4 whole wheat/spelt pita, toasted and cut into triangles

WEDNESDAY

Breakfast

1 Raspberry-Lemon Muffin (page 82)

6 ounces fruit-flavored 0% Greek yogurt

Lunch

Turkey Sandwich: 1 slice sprouted wheat
bread with 1 tablespoon olive tapenade,
topped with 4 ounces turkey breast and
1 slice bread

1 cup watermelon chunks

Dinner

5 ounces wild salmon, grilled or broiled

*Chilled Cilantro–Soba Noodle Salad
(page 112)*

1½ cups steamed mixed vegetables: Tuscan
kale, carrots, and broccoli

Snack

15 grams of carbs:

1 ounce hard cheese and 15 grapes

30 grams of carbs:

1½ ounces hard cheese, 15 grapes,
and 1 slice sprouted wheat toast

THURSDAY

Breakfast

1 cup bran flakes

¾ cup unsweetened almond milk

2 tablespoons slivered almonds

1 teaspoon chia seeds

1 teaspoon wheat germ

1 cup blueberries

Lunch

Tuna Sandwich: 4 ounces low-sodium
chunk light tuna in water mixed with
1 tablespoon canola oil mayonnaise
on a toasted Thomas' English muffin

1 cup baby carrots and/or cauliflower florets

¼ cup hummus

Dinner

4 ounces herbed pork tenderloin

8 grilled stalks asparagus

Barley Pilaf with Artichokes and Kale
(page 289)

Chocolate Malt (page 327)

Snack

15 grams of carbs:

Upside-Down Ambrosia: 4 ounces
low-sodium, low-fat cottage cheese
and 1 teaspoon shredded coconut
sprinkled over ¾ cup fresh pineapple

30 grams of carbs:

Upside-Down Ambrosia: 4 ounces
low-sodium, low-fat cottage cheese,
8 chopped nuts, and 1 teaspoon
shredded coconut sprinkled over
1¼ cups fresh pineapple

FRIDAY

Breakfast

Grilled Steak and Eggs (page 66)

2 pieces whole grain toast spread with
2 tablespoons mashed avocado

Lunch

Apple and Blue Cheese Salad (page 103)

Veggie Burger Wrap (page 263)

Dinner

5 ounces roasted chicken (no skin)

1 baked potato with 2 teaspoons olive oil
(instead of butter)

1 cup steamed broccoli

1 Pistachio Kiss (page 317)

Snack

15 grams of carbs:

6 ounces 0% plain Greek yogurt topped
with 1 crushed small cookie

30 grams of carbs:

6 ounces 0% fruit-flavored Greek
yogurt, mixed with ½ cup berries and
1 tablespoon wheat germ

SATURDAY

Breakfast

Salmon Breakfast Burrito (page 68)

1 cup mixed berries

2 tablespoons chopped walnuts

Lunch

1½ servings Vegetable Pizza (page 271)

Dinner

Vegetable Stir-Fry: 3 cups mixed vegetables,
½ cup shelled edamame, 1 cup cubed
firm tofu, and 2 tablespoons low-sodium
teriyaki sauce, served over ¾ cup whole
wheat couscous and sprinkled with
1 tablespoon toasted sesame seeds

Snack

15 grams of carbs:

Higher-fiber, lower-carb, higher-protein
bar (~5 grams fiber, 15 grams carbs,
7 to 14 grams protein); e.g., Almond
Blueberry Zing bar or Gnu bar, any
variety

30 grams of carbs:

1 granola bar (6 grams fiber, 25 to
28 grams carbs, 10 to 14 grams
protein or healthy fats); e.g., Kind bar,
LäraBar, and/or Zing bar

Calories, Carbs, and Fiber of Common Foods

Use this list to design your own meals, modify your favorite comfort food recipes, and build your own meal plans to follow the Diabetes Comfort Food Diet. The serving size of each food is included, as well as the total calories, carbohydrates, and fiber, so that you can take the "magic carbs" effect into account.

VEGETABLES

FOOD	SERVING	CALORIES	CARBS (G)	FIBER (G)
Artichokes:				
Whole	1 medium	60	13	7
Hearts, marinated	4	35	7	1
Asparagus	4 spears	25	3	1
Bamboo shoots	½ cup	12	2	1
Beans, green	½ cup	41	5	2
Beans, yellow wax	½ cup	22	5	2
Beets	½ cup	24	6	1
Bok choy	½ cup	5	1	0.5
Broccoli:				
Raw	½ cup	12	2	1
Cooked	½ cup	26	5	3
Broccoli rabe	½ cup	4	1	0.5
Brussels sprouts	½ cup	32	6	3
Cabbage:				
Chinese	½ cup	8	1	1
Green	½ cup	17	3	2
Red	½ cup	14	3	1
Savoy	½ cup	20	4	2
Carrots:				
Sliced	½ cup	43	6	2
Whole, 7½", raw	1	30	7	2

FOOD	SERVING	CALORIES	CARBS (G)	FIBER (G)
Cauliflower:				
Raw	½ cup	13	3	1
Steamed	½ cup	19	4	2
Celeriac	½ cup	5	1	21
Celery:				
Cooked	½ cup	14	3	1
Raw	1 rib	6	1	1
Chard	½ cup	14	3	2
Collards	½ cup	22	4	2
Corn:				
On the cob	1 ear	58	14	2
Cream style	½ cup	92	23	2
Kernels	½ cup	66	15	2
Cucumber	½ cup	7	1	0.5
Dandelion greens	½ cup	17	3	2
Eggplant	½ cup	14	3	1
Endive	½ cup	4	1	1
Fava beans	½ cup	94	17	5
Fennel:				
Cooked	½ cup	12	3	1
Raw	½ cup	13	3	1
Garlic cloves	1	3	1	0.5
Jerusalem artichoke	½ cup	57	13	1
Jicama, raw	½ cup	25	6	3
Kale	½ cup	18	4	1
Kohlrabi	½ cup	24	6	1
Lettuce:				
Boston/Bibb	½ cup	4	1	0.5
Iceberg	½ cup	4	1	0.5
Mixed greens	½ cup	5	1	0.5
Romaine	½ cup	4	1	0.5

(continued)

FOOD	SERVING	CALORIES	CARBS (G)	FIBER (G)
Mushrooms:				
Portobello	4 ounces	40	6	3
Shiitake, cooked	½ cup	40	10	2
Straw, canned	½ cup	29	4	2
Whole white, raw	½ cup	1	2	0.5
Mustard greens	½ cup	14	2	2
Okra	½ cup	23	5	2
Onions, raw	½ cup	32	8	1
Parsnips	½ cup	55	13	3
Peas, snow	½ cup	34	6	2
Peas	½ cup	55	10	3
Peppers:				
Green, uncooked	½ cup	15	4	1
Red, uncooked	½ cup	19	5	2
Potatoes:				
Baked	½ cup	78	15	2
Boiled	½ cup	83	16	1
Radicchio	½ cup	5	1	0.5
Radishes	10	9	2	1
Rutabaga	½ cup	33	7	2
Sauerkraut	½ cup	14	3	2
Scallions	½ cup	6	4	1
Shallots	½ cup	58	13	1
Sorrel, cooked	½ cup	0	2	1
Spinach:				
Frozen, steamed	½ cup	33	5	4
Raw	½ cup	3	0.5	0.5
Summer squash:				
Raw	½ cup	9	2	1
Cooked	½ cup	18	4	1
Zucchini:				
Raw	½ cup	9	2	1
Steamed	½ cup	19	4	1

FOOD	SERVING	CALORIES	CARBS (G)	FIBER (G)
Sweet potatoes:				
Baked, medium	½ potato	51	12	2
Boiled	½ cup	76	18	3
Tomatoes:				
Cherry	10	31	7	2
Plum	1	11	2	1
Small, fresh	1	16	4	1
Sun-dried, in oil	5 pieces	32	4	1
Turnip greens	½ cup	5	4	3
Turnips	½ cup	16	4	2
Water chestnuts	½ cup	40	10	2
Watercress	½ cup	2	0.5	0.5
Winter squash:				
Acorn, baked	½ cup	57	15	5
Butternut, baked	½ cup	41	11	3
Hubbard, boiled	½ cup	35	8	3
Pumpkin, boiled	½ cup	5	6	1
Pumpkin, canned	½ cup	58	10	4
Spaghetti, cooked	½ cup	21	5	1

FRUIT

FOOD	SERVING	CALORIES	CARBS (G)	FIBER (G)
Apple	½ medium	36	10	2
Applesauce:				
Sweetened	½ cup	97	25	2
Unsweetened	½ cup	52	14	2
Apricots:				
Canned in juice	3 halves	52	13	2
Dried	6 halves	50	13	2
Fresh	3 whole	50	12	2
Avocado:				
Hass	½ cup	192	10	8
Florida	½ cup	138	9	6

(continued)

FOOD	SERVING	CALORIES	CARBS (G)	FIBER (G)
Bananas	1 small	90	23	3
Blackberries:				
Fresh	½ cup	31	7	4
Frozen, sweetened	½ cup	93	25	2
Frozen, unsweetened	½ cup	48	12	4
Blueberries:				
Fresh	½ cup	41	11	2
Frozen, sweetened	½ cup	93	25	2
Frozen, unsweetened	½ cup	40	9	2
Boysenberries:				
Fresh	½ cup	31	7	4
Frozen, unsweetened	½ cup	33	8	4
Cherries:				
Sour, canned in water	½ cup	44	11	1
Sour, fresh	½ cup	26	6	1
Sweet, canned in water	½ cup	57	15	2
Sweet, fresh	½ cup	42	10	1
Cranberries, fresh	½ cup	23	6	2
Dates:				
Dry, chopped	½ cup	240	62	6
Fresh	3	68	18	2
Figs:				
Canned, in water	½ cup	30	17	3
Fresh	1 small	30	8	1
Fruit cocktail:				
Canned in heavy syrup	½ cup	91	24	1
Canned in water	½ cup	38	10	1
Gooseberries	½ cup	33	8	3
Grapefruit	½ cup	37	10	2
Grapes:				
Green seedless	½ cup	57	14	1
Red seedless	½ cup	57	14	1
Guava	½ cup	56	12	5

FOOD	SERVING	CALORIES	CARBS (G)	FIBER (G)
Kiwi	1	46	11	3
Kumquats	4	54	12	5
Lemon juice	2 tablespoons	8	3	0.5
Loganberries	½ cup	37	9	4
Mango:				
Dried	1 piece	16	4	0.5
Fresh	½ cup	54	14	2
Melons:				
Cantaloupe, cubes	½ cup	31	7	1
Cantaloupe	¼ of melon	97	12	1
Crenshaw melon, cubes	½ cup	22	5	1
Honeydew, cubes	½ cup	30	8	1
Watermelon, cubes	½ cup	25	6	0.5
Nectarine	1 whole	60	14	2
Oranges:				
Sections	½ cup	42	11	2
Fresh, medium	1 whole	64	16	3
Papaya:				
Dried	1 piece	59	15	3
Fresh, small	½ of fruit	59	15	3
Passion fruit	¼ cup	57	14	6
Peaches:				
Canned in water	½ cup	29	8	2
Dried	2 halves	62	16	2
Fresh, small	1 whole	31	8	1
Pears:				
Canned in water	½ cup	35	10	2
Fresh, Bartlett	1 whole	98	25	4
Fresh, Bosc	1 whole	82	21	3
Persimmon	½ cup	59	16	3
Pineapples:				
Canned, in water	½ cup	39	10	1
Fresh, chunks	½ cup	38	10	1

(continued)

FOOD	SERVING	CALORIES	CARBS (G)	FIBER (G)
Plums:				
Fresh	1 whole	16	4	0.5
Canned, in water	½ cup	51	14	1
Pomegranate	¼ whole	26	7	0.5
Prunes:				
Fresh	4 whole	80	21	2
Canned in heavy syrup	½ cup	123	33	5
Raisins:				
Golden	1 tablespoon	31	8	0.5
Seedless	1 tablespoon	31	8	1
Raspberries:				
Fresh	½ cup	30	7	4
Frozen, sweetened	½ cup	129	33	6
Rhubarb	½ cup	13	3	1
Strawberries:				
Fresh	½ cup	24	6	1
Frozen, sweetened	½ cup	122	33	2
Frozen, unsweetened	½ cup	39	10	2
Tangerine	1 whole	37	9	1

BEANS (LEGUMES) AND TOFU

FOOD	SERVING	CALORIES	CARBS (G)	FIBER (G)
Black beans	½ cup	114	20	8
Black-eyed peas	½ cup	111	20	5
Chickpeas	½ cup	147	25	7
Great Northern beans	½ cup	130	20	6
Kidney beans	½ cup	110	20	8
Lentils	½ cup	110	19	8
Lima beans	½ cup	115	21	7
Navy beans	½ cup	127	24	10
Pink beans	½ cup	126	24	5
Pinto beans	½ cup	117	22	7
Soybeans, green	½ cup	127	10	4

FOOD	SERVING	CALORIES	CARBS (G)	FIBER (G)
Split peas	½ cup	116	21	8
Tofu:				
Firm	½ cup	183	5	3
Regular	½ cup	94	2	0.5
Silken, firm	½ cup	70	3	0.5
Silken, soft	½ cup	62	3	0.5

GRAINS

FOOD	SERVING	CALORIES	CARBS (G)	FIBER (G)
Barley, cooked	½ cup	97	22	3
Bran, oat	2 tablespoons	10	3	1
Bran, wheat	2 tablespoons	16	5	3
Bulgur, cooked	½ cup	76	17	4
Cornmeal	2 tablespoons	63	13	1
Kasha, cooked	½ cup	77	17	2
Millet, cooked	½ cup	104	21	1
Quinoa, dry	1¼ cups	159	29	3
Noodles and pasta (cooked):				
Couscous	½ cup	88	18	1
Egg noodles	½ cup	106	20	1
Japanese somen	½ cup	115	24	1
Plain pasta	½ cup	88	20	3
Rice noodles	½ cup	96	22	1
Thai rice	½ cup	105	25	1
Udon (brown rice)	½ cup	103	20	2
Whole wheat pasta	½ cup	100	27	3
Pasta from other grains (cooked):				
Corn pasta	½ cup	100	23	3
Quinoa pasta	½ cup	90	18	1
Rice pasta	½ cup	105	22	0.5
Semolina pasta	½ cup	300	61	3
Spelt pasta	½ cup	95	20	3

(continued)

FOOD	SERVING	CALORIES	CARBS (G)	FIBER (G)
Rice:				
Arborio, cooked	½ cup	121	27	1
Basmati, dry	¼ cup	160	36	0
Brown, cooked	½ cup	108	22	2
White, cooked	½ cup	121	27	0
Wild, cooked	½ cup	83	18	2

NUTS AND NUT BUTTERS

FOOD	SERVING	CALORIES	CARBS (G)	FIBER (G)
Almond butter	2 tablespoons	203	7	1
Almonds, slivered	2 tablespoons	102	3	2
Almonds, whole	24	166	6	3
Brazil nuts	7	186	3	2
Cashew butter	2 tablespoons	188	9	1
Cashews, whole	18	161	9	1
Chestnuts, roasted	6	138	30	3
Hazelnuts, whole	12	177	5	3
Macadamia butter	2 tablespoons	230	5	0
Macadamias, whole	12	203	4	2
Peanut butter	2 tablespoons	190	6	2
Peanuts, whole nuts	35	164	6	2
Pecans, whole	15	191	4	3
Pine nuts	2 tablespoons	96	2	1
Pistachio nuts, whole (no shells)	49	161	8	3
Pumpkin seeds, hulled	2 tablespoons	36	4	0.5
Sesame seeds	2 tablespoons	103	4	2
Soybeans, roasted	¼ cup	133	10	5
Sunflower seeds, hulled	3 tablespoons	165	7	3
Sunflower seed butter	2 tablespoons	200	7	4
Walnut halves	14	185	4	2

FATS AND OILS

FOOD	SERVING	CALORIES	CARBS (G)	FIBER (G)
Canola	1 tablespoon	124	0	0
Coconut	1 tablespoon	116	0	0
Corn	1 tablespoon	120	0	0
Olive	1 tablespoon	119	0	0
Peanut	1 tablespoon	119	0	0
Safflower	1 tablespoon	120	0	0
Sesame	1 tablespoon	120	0	0
Soybean	1 tablespoon	120	0	0

DAIRY PRODUCTS

FOOD	SERVING	CALORIES	CARBS (G)	FIBER (G)
Milk:				
Buttermilk, 1% fat	1 cup	110	13	0
Condensed	2 tablespoons	123	21	0
Evaporated, 2%	2 tablespoons	29	4	0
Evaporated, whole	2 tablespoons	42	3	0
Low-fat (1%)	1 cup	102	12	0
Nonfat (skim)	1 cup	83	12	0
Reduced fat (2%)	1 cup	122	11	0
Whole	1 cup	146	13	0
Cream:				
Half-and-half	1 tablespoon	20	1	0
Heavy cream	1 tablespoon	51	0.5	0
Nondairy creamer	1 tablespoon	20	2	0
Whipped heavy cream	2 tablespoons	52	0.5	0
Whipped light cream	1 tablespoon	29	1	0
Cheese:				
Blue, hunk	1 ounce	100	1	0
Blue, crumbled	½ cup	238	2	0
Brie	1 ounce	95	0.5	0
Cheddar, sliced	1 ounce	114	0.5	0

(continued)

FOOD	SERVING	CALORIES	CARBS (G)	FIBER (G)
Cheese *(cont.):*				
Cheddar, shredded	½ cup	288	1	0
Colby, sliced	1 ounce	110	1	0
Colby, shredded	½ cup	223	1	0
Cottage cheese, 1% milkfat	1 cup	163	6	0
Cream cheese	1 tablespoon	50	1	0
Feta, crumbled	½ cup	198	3	0
Fontina, sliced	1 ounce	109	0.5	0
Fontina, shredded	½ cup	210	1	0
Gouda, sliced	1 ounce	101	1	0
Monterey, sliced	1 ounce	104	0.5	0
Mozzarella, sliced	1 ounce	85	1	0
Mozzarella, shredded	½ cup	168	1	0
Muenster, sliced	1 ounce	103	0.5	0
Parmesan, hard	1 ounce	111	1	0
Provolone, sliced	1 ounce	98	1	0
Ricotta, part-skim	½ cup	170	6	0
Sour cream, reduced fat	1 tablespoon	22	1	0
Swiss, sliced	1 ounce	106	2	0
Swiss, shredded	½ cup	205	3	0

FISH (COOKED UNLESS NOTED)

FOOD	SERVING	CALORIES	CARBS (G)	FIBER (G)
Bass, sea	6 ounces	252	0	0
Bass, striped	6 ounces	211	0	0
Bluefish	6 ounces	270	0	0
Catfish	6 ounces	313	0	0
Cod	6 ounces	208	0	0
Flounder	6 ounces	225	0	0
Haddock	6 ounces	208	0	0
Haddock, smoked	6 ounces	197	0	0
Halibut	6 ounces	238	0	0
Herring in sour cream	1¼ cups	120	8	0
Mackerel	6 ounces	377	0	0
Mahi-mahi	6 ounces	193	0	0
Perch	6 ounces	199	0	0
Salmon	6 ounces	291	0	0
Salmon, canned	6 ounces	245	0	0
Salmon, smoked	6 ounces	199	0	0
Sardines, canned in mustard	6 ounces	316	1	0
Sardines, canned in oil	6 ounces	354	0	0
Scrod	6 ounces	218	0	0
Shad	6 ounces	429	0	0
Swordfish	6 ounces	301	1	0
Trout	6 ounces	319	0	0
Tuna	6 ounces	259	0	0
Whitefish, canned in oil	6 ounces	316	0	0
Whitefish, canned in water	6 ounces	194	0	0

SHELLFISH

FOOD	SERVING	CALORIES	CARBS (G)	FIBER (G)
Clams	6 ounces	157	6	0
Crab	6 ounces	174	0	0
Crawfish	6 ounces	122	0	0
Lobster	6 ounces	167	2	0
Mussels	6 ounces	293	13	0
Oysters	6 ounces	104	6	0
Scallops	6 ounces	228	5	0
Shrimp	6 ounces	241	2	0
Squid	6 ounces	36	6	0
Surimi	6 ounces	174	17	0

BEEF

FOOD	SERVING	CALORIES	CARBS (G)	FIBER(G)
Brisket	6 ounces	563	0	0
Calf liver	6 ounces	240	5	0
Chuck	6 ounces	498	0	0
Eye round	6 ounces	410	0	0
Ground chuck	6 ounces	562	0	0
Ground round	6 ounces	454	0	0
Jerky stick	5 ounces	39	1	0
Prime rib	6 ounces	667	0	0
Rib-eye roast	6 ounces	667	0	0
Roast	6 ounces	576	0	0
Short ribs	6 ounces	660	0	0
Sirloin steak	6 ounces	344	0	0
Skirt steak	6 ounces	276	0	0
Tenderloin	6 ounces	258	0	0
Top loin	6 ounces	332	0	0
Top sirloin	6 ounces	342	0	0
Veal cutlet	6 ounces	483	0	0

LAMB

FOOD	SERVING	CALORIES	CARBS (G)	FIBER(G)
Leg of lamb	6 ounces	325	0	0
Lamb chops	6 ounces	614	0	0

PROCESSED MEATS

FOOD	SERVING	CALORIES	CARBS (G)	FIBER (G)
Bacon	3 pieces	81	0.5	0
Beef bologna	3 slices	129	2	0
Beef hot dog	1 hot dog	194	3	0
Canadian bacon	3 pieces	129	1	0
Ham	6 ounces	174	2	0
Liverwurst	6 ounces	556	5	0
Pastrami	6 ounces	248	0	0
Pepperoni	5 pieces	128	1	0
Salami	3 slices	110	1	0
Sausage				
Breakfast sausage	1 link	90	0	0
Chorizo	2 ounces	258	1	0
Kielbasa	2 ounces	126	2	0
Pork and beef sausage	1 link	51	0.5	0
Pork sausage	1 piece	82	0.5	0
Turkey sausage	2 ounces	97	0.5	0

PORK

FOOD	SERVING	CALORIES	CARBS (G)	FIBER (G)
Center cut, bone-in	6 ounces	344	0	0
Loin chop, bone-in	6 ounces	549	0	0
Loin roast	6 ounces	422	0	0
Pancetta	1 ounce	200	0	0
Prosciutto	6 ounces	331	1	0
Sausage, Italian	2 ounces	192	2	0
Spare ribs	6 ounces	427	0	0
Tenderloin	6 ounces	279	0	0

(continued)

CHICKEN

FOOD	SERVING	CALORIES	CARBS (G)	FIBER (G)
Breast, skinless	6 ounces	243	0	0
Breast, with skin	6 ounces	335	0	0
Drumstick, skinless	6 ounces	348	0	0
Drumstick, with skin	6 ounces	367	0	0
Light and dark, meat only	6 ounces	379	0	0
Thigh, boneless, with skin	6 ounces	420	0	0

OTHER POULTRY

FOOD	SERVING	CALORIES	CARBS (G)	FIBER (G)
Duck breast, no skin	6 ounces	238	0	0
Turkey breast, no skin	6 ounces	230	0	0
Turkey jerky	0.5 ounce	50	1	0

SWEETENERS

FOOD	SERVING	CALORIES	CARBS (G)	FIBER (G)
Natural sweeteners:				
Agave nectar	1 teaspoon	20	4	0
Brown rice syrup	1 teaspoon	20	5	0
Evaporated cane juice	1 teaspoon	15	4	0
Honey	1 teaspoon	21	6	0
Maple syrup	1 teaspoon	22	5	0
Molasses	1 teaspoon	16	4	0
Sugar, brown	1 teaspoon	17	5	0
Sugar, raw (turbinado)	1 teaspoon	16	4	0
Sugar, white	1 teaspoon	16	4	0
Noncaloric sweeteners:				
Equal	1 packet	0	0	0
Splenda	1 packet	4	1	0
Stevia	1 packet	4	1	0
Sugar Twin	1 packet	0	0.5	0
Sweet'N Low	1 packet	0	<1	0

BEVERAGES

FOOD	SERVING	CALORIES	CARBS (G)	FIBER (G)
Beer:				
Beer, light	12 ounces	99	0–5	0
Beer, regular	12 ounces	154	13	0
Wine/liquor:				
Hard liquor (all)	1 fluid ounce	82	0	0
Red	5 fluid ounces	88	3	0
Sherry, dry	3½ fluid ounces	72	1	0
Sherry, sweet	3½ fluid ounces	158	12	0
White	5 fluid ounces	85	3	0
Wine cooler	5 fluid ounces	49	6	0
Tea:				
Brewed (black, green, white)	8 fluid ounces	2	1	0
Herbal, brewed	8 fluid ounces	2	1	0
Soda:				
Cola	12 fluid ounces	153	36	0
Diet soda	12 fluid ounces	0	0	0
Ginger ale	12 fluid ounces	124	32	0
Grape	12 fluid ounces	124	32	0
Lemon-lime	12 fluid ounces	147	38	0
Root beer	12 fluid ounces	152	39	0
Seltzer/club soda	12 fluid ounces	0	0	0
Fruit juice:				
Apple	4 fluid ounces	58	15	0.5
Apricot	4 fluid ounces	70	18	1
Cranberry juice cocktail	4 fluid ounces	72	18	0.5
Grape	4 fluid ounces	77	19	0.5
Grapefruit, sweetened	4 fluid ounces	58	14	0.5
Grapefruit, unsweetened	4 fluid ounces	47	11	0.5
Guava	4 fluid ounces	74	19	1
Lemon	2 tablespoons	6	2	0.5
Lime	2 tablespoons	6	2	0.5

(continued)

FOOD	SERVING	CALORIES	CARBS (G)	FIBER (G)
Fruit juice *(cont.)*:				
Mango	4 fluid ounces	73	19	1
Orange	4 fluid ounces	56	13	0.5
Passion fruit	4 fluid ounces	63	17	0.5
Peach	4 fluid ounces	67	17	1
Pear	4 fluid ounces	66	16	0.5
Pineapple	4 fluid ounces	66	16	0.5
Prune	4 fluid ounces	91	22	1
Vegetable juice:				
Carrot	4 fluid ounces	47	11	1
Tomato	4 fluid ounces	21	5	1
Vegetable juice cocktail	4 fluid ounces	23	6	1

ENDNOTES

CHAPTER 1

[1]Merriam-Webster.com, s.v. "diet" (accessed January 21, 2013).

[2]National Diabetes Information Clearinghouse (NDIC). Insulin resistance and prediabetes. http://diabetes.niddk .nih.gov/dm/pubs/insulinresistance/index.aspx#what (accessed January 21, 2013).

[3]Ibid.

[4]National Diabetes Information Clearinghouse. http:/diabetes.niddk.nih.gov/dm/pubs/preventionprogram (updated November 6, 2012).

[5]American Diabetes Association. Nutrition recommendations and interventions for diabetes. *Diabetes Care* 31: S61–S78. doi:10.2337/dc08-S061.

[6]See note 4.

[7]L. Haas et al. National standards for diabetes self-management education and support. *Diabetes Educator* 38: 619–25.

[8]G. W. Greene et al. Dietary applications of the stages of change model. *Journal of the American Dietetic Association* 99: 673–78.

[9]Diabetes Prevention Program's Lifestyle Change Program, Appendix A: Session 4 or 2: Be a fat detective, page 6. http://www.bsc.gwu.edu/dpp/lifestyle/dpp_dcor.html.

[10]M. J. Franz et al. The evidence of medical nutrition therapy for type 1 and type 2 diabetes in adults. *Journal of the American Dietetic Association* 110: 1857–83.

[11]Ibid.

[12]S. W. Ng and M. Slinging. Use of caloric and noncaloric sweeteners in US consumer packaged foods, 2005–2009. *Journal of the Academy of Nutrition and Dietetics* 112: 1832.

[13]American Diabetes Association. Nutrition recommendations and interventions for diabetes. *Diabetes Care* 31 (2008): S61–S78. doi:10.2337/dc08-S061.

[14]Position Statement of the American Diabetes Association. Standards of medical care in diabetes–2012. *Diabetes Care* 35: S24.

[15]S. R. Colberg et al. The American College of Sports Medicine and the American Diabetes Association: Joint position statement. *Diabetes Care* 33: 2692–96.

[16]S. Colberg. Increasing insulin sensitivity. *Diabetes Self-Management.* December 3, 2008. http://www .diabetesselfmanagement.com/articles/insulin/increasing_insulin_sensitivity (accessed December 21, 2012).

[17]G. E. Duncan et al. Exercise training, without weight loss, increases insulin sensitivity and postheparin plasma lipase activity in previously sedentary adults. *Diabetes Care* 26 (2003): 557–62. doi:10.2337/diacare.26.3.557.

CHAPTER 2

[1]G. E. Duncan et al. Exercise training, without weight loss, increases insulin sensitivity and postheparin plasma lipase activity in previously sedentary adults. *Diabetes Care* 26 (2003): 557–62. doi: 10.2337/diacare.26.3.557.

[2]J. Montonen, P. Knekt, R. Järvinen et al. Whole-grain and fiber intake and the incidence of type 2 diabetes. *American Journal of Clinical Nutrition* 77(3) (March 2003): 622–29.

[3]J. W. Anderson et al. Oat-bran cereal lowers serum total and LDL cholesterol in hypercholesterolemic men. *American Journal of Clinical Nutrition* 52 (1992): 495–99.

[4]J. Brand-Miller et al. *The New Glucose Revolution: The Authoritative Guide to the Glycemic Index—The Dietary Solution for Lifelong Health.* New York, NY: Marlowe & Company, 2007.

[5]American Diabetes Association and the American Dietetic Association. Exchange lists for meal planning. Alexandria, VA: American Diabetes Association, 1995

[6]A. Magistrelli and J. Chezem. Effect of ground cinnamon on postprandial blood glucose concentration in normal-weight and obese adults. *Journal of the Academy of Nutrition and Dietetics* 11 (November 2012): 1806–9.

[7]National Pesticide Information Center. Pesticides and pregnancy. October 8, 2012. Available at http://npic.orst .edu/health/preg.html (accessed January 21, 2013).

[8]C. Rico. Is agave nectar safe for people with diabetes? American Diabetes Association. undefined. Available at http://www.diabetes.org/living-with-diabetes/treatment-and-care/ask-the-expert/ask-the-dietitian/archives /is-agave-nectar-safe-for.html (accessed December 28, 2012).

[9]K. J. Melanson et al. Effects of high-fructose corn syrup and sucrose consumption on circulating glucose, insulin, leptin, and ghrelin and on appetite in normal-weight women. *Nutrition* 23 (2007): 103–12.

[10]M. J. Franz et al. The evidence of medical nutrition therapy for type 1 and type 2 diabetes in adults. *Journal of the American Dietetic Association* 110 (2010): 1857–83.

[11]S. P. Fowler et al. Fueling the obesity epidemic? Artificially sweetened beverage use and long-term weight gain. *Obesity* (Silver Spring, MD) 16 (2008): 1894–1900.

[12]Q. Yang. Gain weight by "going diet?" Artificial sweeteners and the neurobiology of sugar cravings: Neuroscience 2010. *Yale Journal of Biology and Medicine* 83 (2010): 101–108.

[13]Position Statement of the American Diabetes Association. Standards of medical care in diabetes—2012. *Diabetes Care* 35 (2012), Supplement 1, S24.

[14]R. Larson. *The American Dietetic Association's Complete Food and Nutrition Guide.* New York, NY: American Dietetic Association, 1998: 160–68.

[15]K. A. Meyer et al. Carbohydrates, dietary fiber, and incident type 2 diabetes in older women. *American Journal of Clinical Nutrition* 71 (2000): 921–30.

[16]C. B. Breneman and L. Tucker. Dietary fibre consumption and insulin resistance—The role of body fat and physical activity. *British Journal of Nutrition* (December 7, 2012): 1–9.

[17]Position Statement of the American Diabetes Association. Supplement 1, S11–S63. doi:10.2337/dc12-s011.

[18]M. Chandalia, A. Garg, D. Lutjohann et al. Beneficial effects of high dietary fiber intake in patients with type 2 diabetes mellitus. *New England Journal of Medicine* 342(19) (May 11, 2000): 1392–98.

[19]T. G. Kiehm, J. W. Anderson, and K.Ward. Beneficial effects of a high carbohydrate, high fiber diet on hyperglycemic diabetic men. *American Journal of Clinical Nutrition* 29(8) (August 1976): 895–99.

[20]Anne M. May et al. Combined impact of lifestyle factors on prospective change in body weight and waist circumference in participants of the EPIC-PANACEA study. MID: 2085032.

[21] L. Bozzetto et al. Liver fat is reduced by an isoenergetic MUFA diet in a controlled randomized study in type 2 diabetes patients. *Diabetes Care* 35 (2012): 1429–35.

[22] ———. The association of hs-CRP with fasting and postprandial plasma lipids in patients with type 2 diabetes is disrupted by dietary monounsaturated fatty acids. *Acta Diabetologica* (August 11, 2011). [Epub ahead of print]. Department of Clinical and Experimental Medicine, Federico II University, Via S Pansini 5, 80131, Naples, Italy.

[23] D. P. Brostow et al. Omega-3 fatty acids and incident type 2 diabetes: The Singapore Chinese health study. *American Journal of Clinical Nutrition* 94 (2011): 520–26.

[24] L. Djousse et al. Plasma omega-3 fatty acids and incident diabetes in older adults, *American Journal of Clinical Nutrition* 94 (2011): 527–33.

[25] United States Environmental Protection Agency. What should I know about eating fish that might contain mercury or other pollutants? Where can I find information about eating fish caught in a particular body of water? November 22, 2012. http://publicaccess.supportportal.com/link/portal/23002/23012/Article/24361/What-should-I-know-about-eating-fish-that-might-contain-mercury-or-other-pollutants-Where-can-I-find-information-about-eating-fish-caught-in-a-particular-body-of-water (accessed January 21, 2013).

[26] F. B. Hu et al. Dietary fat intake and the risk of coronary heart disease in women. *New England Journal of Medicine* 337 (1997): 1491–99.

[27] National Institutes of Health. Third report of the national cholesterol education program expert panel on detection, evaluation, and treatment of high blood cholesterol in adults (adult treatment panel III). Bethesda, MD: National Institutes of Health, 2001. NIH Publication 01–3670.

[28] S. Margens. *The Wellness Encyclopedia of Food and Nutrition.* New York, NY: Health Letter Association, 1992: 271–82.

[29] Ibid.

[30] R. Sinha et al. Dietary intake of heterocyclic amines, meat-derived mutagenic activity, and risk of colorectal adenomas. *Cancer Epidemiology, Biomarkers & Prevention* 10 (2001): 559–62.

[31] Ibid.

[32] K. Van Ittersum and B. Wansink. Plate size and color suggestibility: The Delboeuf illusion's bias on serving and eating behavior. *Journal of Consumer Research* 39(2): 215–28. doi:10.1086/662615.

INDEX

Underscored page references indicate sidebars. **Boldface** references indicate photographs.

B

Bacon, turkey
    Bacon and Apple Grilled
        Cheeses, 121
    Bacon-Wrapped Chicken, 212
    Stuffed Potato Skins, **144**, 145
Baked Chicken with Mustard
    Sauce, 205
Baked Pasta and Vegetables, 261
Baked Risotto, 292
Baked Salmon, <u>329</u>
Baked Spaghetti with Turkey Meat
    Sauce, 227
Baked Ziti with Turkey, 228, **229**
Baking foods, 38
Bananas
    Chocolate-Banana-Stuffed
        French Toast, **78**, 79
    Sundae Breakfast Smoothie, 88
Barbecue sauce
    Barbecue Shrimp Wraps, 124
    Slow-Cooker Pork Barbecue, 180
Barbecuing foods, 38
Barley, 22
    Barley Pilaf with Artichokes and
        Kale, 289
    Beef Barley Soup, 95
    Mushroom-Barley Stuffing, 288
    Salmon-Barley Bake, **242**, 243
Bars
    Crispy Oat Squares, 322
    Fig Bars, 319
    Rich Brownies, 318
Basil
    Fettuccine with Basil-Walnut
        Sauce, 296
Beans
    African Stew, 267
    Bean Enchiladas, 269
    Black Bean Burgers, 270
    calories, carbs, and fiber in,
        <u>342–43</u>
    for carb curbing, 22
    as carbohydrates, 19
    Chicken with Pinto Beans Skil-
        let, 214

Corn, Black Bean, and Edamame
    Salad, 109
Cornmeal Catfish with Black-
    Eyed Peas, 238
Couscous and Chickpea Salad,
    110, 111
Fiesta Turkey Soup, 92, **93**
Fire-Roasted Chili, 268
Grand Slam Nachos, 147
Kicked-Up Tomato Soup, 100
Layered Chicken and Bean
    Enchiladas, 213
Mexican Dip, 149
Minestrone, 94
Rich Brownies, 318
Scallops with Beans and Aru-
    gula, 251
Steak Burrito Bowl, 164, **165**
Tex-Mex Pasta and Beans, 297
Turkey and Bean Quesadillas,
    224, **225**
Wild Mushroom and White
    Bean Risotto, **254**, 255
Beef
    Beef Barley Soup, 95
    Beef Goulash, 173
    Beef Ragù over Polenta, 174,
        175
    Beef Stroganoff, 160–61
    calories, carbs, and fiber in,
        <u>348</u>
    Chinese Beef and Vegetables,
        162–63
    Cobb Salad–Style Buffalo Dogs,
        176
    Country-Fried Steak, 154–55
    Go-To Spaghetti and Meatballs,
        172
    grass-fed, <u>169</u>
    Grilled Steak and Eggs, 66, **67**
    Mom's Meat Loaf, 167
    Philly Cheese Steaks, 114, **115**
    Roast Beef Rolls, 125
    Salisbury Steak, 168
    Shepherd's Pie, 166
    Sizzlin' Beef Fajitas, 159
    Steak Burrito Bowl, 164, **165**

Steak with Mushroom Sauce
    and Roasted Artichokes,
    156–57
Traditional Slow-Cooker Pot
    Roast, 158
Un-Stuffed Peppers, 169
Zesty Italian Cheeseburgers,
    170, 171
Beef Barley Soup, 95
Beef Goulash, 173
Beef Ragù over Polenta, 174, **175**
Beef Stroganoff, 160–61
Beer, 27, <u>27</u>, 28, 52
    calories, carbs, and fiber in, <u>351</u>
Behavioral eating, 39, 51
Behavior changes, for weight loss, 12
Belgian Waffles, 81
Beverages
    alcoholic, 27–28, <u>27</u>, 52, <u>351</u>
    calories, carbs, and fiber in,
        <u>351–52</u>
    Chocolate Cake Smoothie, 89
    Chocolate Malt, 327
    glasses for decreasing intake of, 38
    seltzer, 27, 53, 56
    sugar-sweetened, limiting, 11
    Sundae Breakfast Smoothie, 88
    water, 27, 38, 53, 56
Bison
    Ground Bison with Spaghetti
        Squash, 177
Black beans
    Bean Enchiladas, 269
    Black Bean Burgers, 270
    Corn, Black Bean, and Edamame
        Salad, 109
    Fiesta Turkey Soup, 92, **93**
    Grand Slam Nachos, 147
    Kicked-Up Tomato Soup, 100
    Layered Chicken and Bean
        Enchiladas, 213
    Mexican Dip, 149
    Rich Brownies, 318
    Steak Burrito Bowl, 164, **165**
    Tex-Mex Pasta and Beans, 297
    Turkey and Bean Quesadillas,
        224, **225**

CONVERSION CHART

These equivalents have been slightly rounded to make measuring easier.

VOLUME MEASUREMENTS			WEIGHT MEASUREMENTS		LENGTH MEASUREMENTS	
U.S.	IMPERIAL	METRIC	U.S.	METRIC	U.S.	METRIC
¼ tsp	–	1 ml	1 oz	30 g	¼"	0.6 cm
½ tsp	–	2 ml	2 oz	60 g	½"	1.25 cm
1 tsp	–	5 ml	4 oz (¼ lb)	115 g	1"	2.5 cm
1 Tbsp	–	15 ml	5 oz (⅓ lb)	145 g	2"	5 cm
2 Tbsp (1 oz)	1 fl oz	30 ml	6 oz	170 g	4"	11 cm
¼ cup (2 oz)	2 fl oz	60 ml	7 oz	200 g	6"	15 cm
⅓ cup (3 oz)	3 fl oz	80 ml	8 oz (½ lb)	230 g	8"	20 cm
½ cup (4 oz)	4 fl oz	120 ml	10 oz	285 g	10"	25 cm
⅔ cup (5 oz)	5 fl oz	160 ml	12 oz (¾ lb)	340 g	12" (1')	30 cm
¾ cup (6 oz)	6 fl oz	180 ml	14 oz	400 g		
1 cup (8 oz)	8 fl oz	240 ml	16 oz (1 lb)	455 g	2.2 lb 1kg	
			2.2 lb	1 kg		

PAN SIZES		TEMPERATURES		
U.S.	METRIC	FAHRENHEIT	CENTIGRADE	GAS
8" cake pan	20 × 4 cm sandwich or cake tin	140°	60°	–
9" cake pan	23 × 3.5 cm sandwich or cake tin	160°	70°	–
11" × 7" baking pan	28 × 18 cm baking tin	180°	80°	–
13" × 9" baking pan	32.5 × 23 cm baking tin	225°	105°	¼
15" × 10" baking pan	38 × 25.5 cm baking tin	250°	120°	½
	(Swiss roll tin)	275°	135°	1
1½ qt baking dish	1.5 liter baking dish	300°	150°	2
2 qt baking dish	2 liter baking dish	325°	160°	3
2 qt rectangular baking dish	30 × 19 cm baking dish	350°	180°	4
9" pie plate	22 × 4 or 23 × 4 cm pie plate	375°	190°	5
7" or 8" springform pan	18 or 20 cm springform or	400°	200°	6
	loose-bottom cake tin	425°	220°	7
9" × 5" loaf pan	23 × 13 cm or 2 lb narrow	450°	230°	8
	loaf tin or pâté tin	475°	245°	9
		500°	260°	–